EAT TO WIN
for the
21st CENTURY

EAT TO WIN
for the
21ˢᵗ CENTURY

THE SPORTS NUTRITION BIBLE
FOR A NEW GENERATION

ROBERT HAAS, MS

 NEW AMERICAN LIBRARY

New American Library
Published by New American Library, a division of
Penguin Group (USA) Inc., 375 Hudson Street,
New York, New York 10014, USA
Penguin Group (Canada), 10 Alcorn Avenue, Toronto,
Ontario M4V 3B2, Canada (a division of Pearson Penguin Canada Inc.)
Penguin Books Ltd., 80 Strand, London WC2R 0RL, England
Penguin Ireland, 25 St. Stephen's Green, Dublin 2,
Ireland (a division of Penguin Books Ltd.)
Penguin Books (Australia), 250 Camberwell Road, Camberwell, Victoria 3124,
Australia (a division of Pearson Australia Group Pty. Ltd.)
Penguin Books India Pvt. Ltd., 11 Community Centre, Panchsheel Park,
New Delhi - 110 017, India
Penguin Group (NZ), cnr Airborne and Rosedale Roads, Albany,
Auckland 1310, New Zealand (a division of Pearson New Zealand Ltd.)
Penguin Books (South Africa) (Pty.) Ltd., 24 Sturdee Avenue,
Rosebank, Johannesburg 2196, South Africa

Penguin Books Ltd., Registered Offices:
80 Strand, London WC2R 0RL, England

First published by New American Library,
a division of Penguin Group (USA) Inc.

First Printing, January 2005
10 9 8 7 6 5 4 3 2 1

NEW AMERICAN LIBRARY and logo are trademarks of Penguin Group (USA) Inc.

LIBRARY OF CONGRESS CATALOGING-IN-PUBLICATION DATA:

Haas, Robert, 1948–
    Eat to win for the 21st Century : the sports nutrition bible for a new generation / Robert Haas.
        p.   cm.
    Includes bibliographical references.
    ISBN 0-451-21402-1 (trade pbk.)
    1. Athletes—Nutrition. I. Title.
    TX361.A8H2997 2005
    613.2'024'796—dc22   2004021111

Set in Ehrhardt
Designed by Helene Berinsky

Printed in the United States of America

PUBLISHER'S NOTE
Every effort as been made to ensure that the information contained in this book is complete and accurate. However, neither the publisher nor the author is engaged in rendering professional advice or services to the individual reader. The ideas, procedures, and suggestions contained in this book are not intended as a substitute for consulting with your physician. All matters regarding your health require medical supervision. Neither the author nor the publisher shall be liable or responsible for any loss or damage allegedly arising from any information or suggestion in this book. The opinions expressed in this book represent the personal views of the author and not of the publisher.

CONTENTS

Section I

Eat to Win for the 21st Century

THE MEDITERRASIAN DIET MIRACLE

I t was twenty years ago today.

Eat to Win was the number one best-selling diet book in the world. The Eat to Win Diet helped people around the world achieve their perfect body weight, enjoy phenomenal stamina and energy, lower their blood pressure and blood cholesterol into the ideal range, and reverse type 2 diabetes and heart disease.

More than a few professional athletes set world records and became legends in their own time once they embraced the Eat to Win Diet. World-champion athletes such as Jackie Joyner-Kersee, Martina Navratilova, Ivan Lendl, and scores of pros in the NBA, NFL, PGA, LPGA, ATP, NHL, WTA, NASCAR, AL, and NL used the Eat to Win Diet to excel at their respective sports. Active celebrities including Cher, Carly Simon, Daryl Hall and John Oates, Glenn Frey, George Foreman, Woody Harrelson, Marlo Thomas, Don Johnson, and Mike Nichols became avid Eat-to-Winners.

Immediately after the publication of *Eat to Win*, untold numbers of people around the world grew enviably thin, healthy, and fit. Saturated fats, cholesterol, and most vegetable oils were considered the enemies of good health and peak performance. Baked potatoes were in. Carbs were king.

A SHORT HISTORY OF EAT TO WIN

In 1980, I used the term *peak performance* for the first time to describe the high-energy- and stamina-producing effects of the Eat to Win Diet. During this Dark Age of nutrition, most professional athletes followed the questionable advice of coaches, trainers, and locker-room lore, which included swallowing protein supplements and salt tablets. Training-table fare reflected the prevailing steak-and-eggs mentality of the time; pasta and potatoes were proscribed. Coaches and trainers withheld water during training to build discipline.

The Eat to Win Diet, which I originally began developing in 1970 to solve my own health problems, led to a historic sports nutrition revolution by establishing the essential role carbohydrates play in helping athletes go faster, higher, and farther.

Shortly after its publication in 1984, the Eat to Win Diet become the gold standard of peak-performance eating for weekend and world-class athletes alike. More world-champion athletes have relied on the Eat to Win Diet to set new world records than any other eating plan. The reason? It works.

The Eat to Win Diet is not based on armchair theories and speculation, as are most fad diets. I conducted clinical trials of the diet in my own health center staffed with physicians, nurses, and lab technicians. I've traveled the world many times over working with top professional athletes to field-test the diet in real-life competition. The Eat to Win Diet has also been successfully tested in a formal scientific study conducted by impartial physicians and registered dietitians.

Thousands of studies published in peer-reviewed medical and nutritional journals support the safety and efficacy of the nutritional principles of the Eat to Win Diet. All major sports and health organizations agree that these dietary principles are safe, effective, and healthy. As you will discover, these organizations do *not* say this about most currently popular diets.

After the publication of *Eat to Win*, I received thousands of letters (there was no e-mail in those days) from active people and professional athletes in all sports who recounted their success stories on my diet. The national and international press reported many of the success stories of professional athletes who had embraced the Eat to Win Diet.

WHO EATS TO WIN TODAY?

That's easy—thousands of professional and amateur athletes around the world.

The reason is quite simple: No other diet provides better endurance, stamina, or mental focus. No other diet keeps professional athletes at their leanest and fittest. Even athletes who have never heard of the Eat to Win Diet have learned that if they don't follow its nutritional principles, they will quickly lose to athletes who do.

Lance Armstrong knows a lot about eating to win. After winning the Tour de France six times, a feat that was heretofore thought impossible, and beating cancer to boot, Lance stands as living proof that the right diet can make mincemeat of the competition.

Lance isn't secretive about how he eats. He gladly shares his training table with the rest of the world. (Okay, he might keep just a few of his special dietary supplements close to the vest.) Lance fuels his body with the same type of diet and peak-performance foods that you will enjoy on your new Eat to Win Diet.

To stay at his healthiest and fittest, Lance obtains about 70 percent of his calories from carbohydrates—you know, the foods that diet doctors tell you will make you fat, unfit, and unhealthy. Don't tell that to the crème de la crème of endurance cycle racers who dominated professional cycling and conquered his biggest foe of all—cancer.

Does Lance eat a high-fat diet? Not on your life! Lance gets just 15 to 20 percent of his calories from fats and oils. This is the Eat to Win diet prescription for success. Lance knows that a high-fat diet would lead him straight to the back of the pack. Here's what Lance has learned, in his own words:

The body can store fat very well, and even extremely lean riders have plenty of fat to use for fuel. In contrast, there is a limit to the amount of carbohydrate you can store in muscles and in the liver. The importance of carbohydrate cannot be overstated. Not only is it the primary fuel source for endurance performance, it is the only fuel the brain and central nervous system can use.

Armchair diet-book authors who have never worked with world-champion athletes or trained even half as hard as Lance Armstrong does clearly don't possess the nutritional training and practical experience to know what he has learned through years of competition. Lance Armstrong's incomparable *six* Tour de France championships have earned him a place in history next to other such nutrition-savvy athletes as Martina Navratilova and Ivan Lendl.

When Lance retires from endurance cycle racing, he could have a bright future as a sports nutritionist and diet-book author.

THE "SNACKWELL'S SNAFU": HOW DIETERS LOST THEIR WAY

The message of *Eat to Win* is that a diet consisting of natural whole foods rich in complex carbohydrates and low in fats would boost energy, endurance, and longevity. On the Eat to Win Diet, people reach their ideal weight as a side effect of the diet. Many who followed the diet weren't trying to lose weight; it happened naturally as a consequence of eating the proper mix of high-complex carbohydrate foods, animal and vegetable proteins, and biologically friendly fats. Published studies show that an Eat to Win–type diet leads people directly to successful very-long-term weight loss.

Collectively, the lay public misinterpreted the message of *Eat to Win* to mean that they could eat any carbohydrate-rich food or food product in any quantity desired provided it contained little or no fat. The fallacy of this belief is that calories don't matter. People took this to mean they could gorge themselves on prefab, no- and low-fat food products that flooded the marketplace during the Eat to Win era, just as today's low-carb dieters wolf down any food product labeled as having low "net carbs."

This gross misinterpretation of the Eat to Win Diet eventually led to a backlash against all carbs that I call the "SnackWell's Snafu" (named after a popular line of nonfat baked goods). I recall asking a friend of mine who was in the midst of consuming an entire bag of Nabisco SnackWell's brand cookies in a single sitting what possessed him to do so. He glanced at the bag's nutrition panel and said, in all seriousness, "Because there's nothing in 'em."

Simply replacing fat in the diet with carbohydrate does not automatically lead to lasting slenderness. For example, nearly 60 percent of the people of South Africa are overweight even though they consume, on average, a diet with less than 22 percent of calories from fat. This indicates that a national obesity epidemic can occur even with fat intakes that are generally considered to be low.

Regrettably, the focus on eating a low-fat diet alone distracts from the real causes of obesity: high total energy intake and low physical activity levels. The Eat to Win Diet emphasizes replacing saturated and trans fats with monounsaturated oils and enjoying a reduced-calorie diet that balances energy intake from both carbohydrates and fats with regular physical activity.

During the next decade, dieters consumed more non- and low-fat food products loaded with sugar and began to eat *more* fat. At the same time, food manufacturers, fast-food chains, and restaurants started supersizing their products and menu items. Americans now ate more sugar and fat than ever before, increased their daily caloric intake, on average, by 300 to 500 calories a day, and became less active.

Opportunistic diet-book authors blamed carbohydrates for the ensuing American obesity epidemic even though Americans were eating more fat calories and total calories as well. This led to a collective knee-jerk reaction against almost all carb-rich foods and helped authors promote the polar opposite diet: the high-protein/high-fat, carb-limited diet. This type of diet is artificially high in protein and fat and artificially low in carbohydrate-rich foods.

Curiously, most proponents of this diet are physicians who

unashamedly appropriated the diet from each other or from the original high-fat, low-carb diet devised by the 19th-century British surgeon Dr. William Harvey. Like Dr. Harvey, these 20th-century diet doctors made carbohydrates the scapegoat and dietary fat and protein the holy grail of weight loss and good health.

A new crop of diet "experts" told a nation of confused dieters that carbohydrates were the reason they got fat. Frustrated dieters made easy marks for these mealtime messiahs who promised to lead them into the land of full-fat milk and low-net-carb honey. These carb-bashing diet gurus appeared on cue and brought with them a new diet mantra for the masses: Pass the Alfredo; hold the fettuccini!

MILLIONS OF AMERICANS MAKE A TERRIBLE MISTAKE

You can't blame people for wanting to try a high-fat diet. Who wouldn't be seduced by the promise that one can lose weight while enjoying the same rich, fatty, and calorically dense foods that made them fat in the first place?

Diets that severely limit carbs and promote rich, fatty foods may work in the short run because they create the appetite-suppressing symptoms of illness: dehydration, nausea, diarrhea, constipation, joint pain, headache, lethargy, and halitosis. Just like when they're ill, dieters lose their appetites and consume fewer calories. The excessive protein in these diets forces the body to increase its metabolic rate, thereby creating extra ammonia and burning extra calories to convert the protein into sugar. Eventually, the body rebels and dieters realize there is only one cure for their self-inflicted malady: carbohydrates.

Some people can enjoy short-term success on high-fat, low-carb diets simply by eliminating much of the 150 pounds of sugar they eat, on average, each year. Eating fewer sugar calories is better for everyone, but these diets also limit many phytonutrient-rich[1] grains, vegetables,

---

1. Phytonutrients, found only in complex-carbohydrate foods, including whole grains, fruits, and vegetables, are like industrial-strength vitamins. They help protect against heart disease, cancer, and other serious health problems. The MediterrAsian-style Eat to Win Diet contains a much higher proportion of phytonutrients than a high-fat, low-carb diet.

and fruits. There's nothing magical about these diets other than the fact they severely limit calories from sugar *and* an entire group of healthy foods.

DIET DOCTORS: THE LEADING SOURCE OF QUESTIONABLE DIET ADVICE

As the 21ˢᵗ century commences, people are being seduced by quick-weight-loss diets that offer scientifically meritless advice: "Eat high-fat for a healthy heart" "Eat like a Neanderthal," "Eat foods based on your blood type," "Add fat to meals to lose weight." A century from now, historians will look back upon this era of diet disasters and will likely find it quite amusing, just as we do today when we watch a movie about the Old West depicting a snake-oil salesman peddling nostrums to a group of gullible townsfolk.

David L. Katz, MD, MPH, from the Yale Preventive Medicine Research Center in New Haven, Connecticut, maintains that such low-carbohydrate diets as the Atkins and the South Beach diets are based on a premise that is "so utterly wrong as to be insane." Many highly respected health researchers, physicians, and health organizations take issue with the questionable rationale for such diets.

The current crop of high-fat, low-carb diet books is really a case of old wine in new bottles. With minor variations, all of these books serve up the same tired message that recalls the dietary dogma of the 1950s, when the centerpiece of restaurant diet plates was a ground-beef patty—hold the bun.

Their theory is clear: Eating carbs will make you fat; eating fat will make you thin. Try telling that to native Okinawans who've enjoyed five thousand years of superb longevity and health without following a ketogenic[2] or other type of high-fat, low-carb diet. Nearly seventy percent of

---

2. Ketogenic diets force the body into a deranged metabolic state known as ketosis. Ketosis causes the body to burn stored fat and convert dietary protein into carbohydrate for energy to make up for the deficit in carbohydrate intake. The body responds by attempting to rid itself of the toxic waste products of protein metabolism (urea and ammonia) and those of incomplete fat metabolism (keto acids). Ketosis has been linked with serious health problems and death.

the daily calories in the traditional Japanese diet comes from white rice and other carb-rich foods. Okinawans who continue to eat their traditional high-carb diet remain among the thinnest and longest-lived people on the planet. When they change their diet to one that more closely resembles popular American low-carb diets, they suffer from higher rates of heart disease and other health problems.

Diet doctors who promote ketogenic and other types of high-fat, low-carb diets promise that people can still enjoy the "good life" by eating large amounts of meat, cheese, butter, mayonnaise, vegetable oil, and cream without putting their health at risk. They also hold out the unfulfilled promise of lasting fat loss.

This type of diet has enjoyed recurring popularity every decade or so for the last half century. After more than fifty years, there are still no credible, long-term scientific studies that show dieters can stick with this type of diet in the long run or that the diet leads people to long-term fat loss. In fact, published studies have revealed that in addition to the diet's ability to raise blood cholesterol scores and cause a host of other health problems, it confers no weight-loss advantage over lower-fat diets in the long run. These studies have also established that dieters can't stick with these eating plans for long.

I am convinced that most dieters will fail on a diet that drastically limits consumption of delicious and nutritious complex-carbohydrate-rich foods because such a diet ignores the fact that people find it extraordinarily difficult to endure "carb-privation" indefinitely. It is possible for the rare, highly disciplined person to stay on this type of a diet, but given the unpleasant side effects, unfavorable changes in cardiovascular risk factors, and the dire warnings issued by leading health experts and medical organizations, what dieter would choose to do so?

Sadly, the vast majority of low-carb dieters don't realize that carbohydrate cravings will eventually derail their diets. Even more liberal variations of this type of diet tend to limit carbs to such an extent that dieters eventually begin to add back the carbs they miss the most.

Referring to ketogenic and low-carb diets, George Blackburn, MD, director of nutrition at Harvard Medical School, observes: "Dieters just can't go without one of the food groups and be satisfied with the limited variety of foods on this diet."

At some point, many low-carb dieters realize they can't live without the carbs they love and announce:

"I'm on a *modified* version of the _____ Diet" (fill in the name of your favorite carb-restricted fad diet).

Here's what the dieter is actually saying: "My brain and body crave carbs."

I usually tell the person to put their own name on the diet, because at that point, it's another diet altogether.

THE DIET'S THE SAME; ONLY THE NAME HAS CHANGED

For the millions of Americans who have fallen head-over-steak-knife for ketogenic and low-carb diets, the Eat to Win Diet represents nutritional heresy and stands for everything that proponents of ketogenic diets proclaim make people fat.

The Atkins and South Beach diets are currently the two most popular low-carb diets in the United States. They both use the same questionable diet strategy—severe carbohydrate restriction and then low-carb maintenance diets. Stewart Trager, MD, medical director of Atkins Nutritionals, says that the South Beach Diet is a copycat diet and admits that the Atkins and South Beach diets offer the same level of healthy carbs and healthy fats. As proof, he points to a food-by-food, calorie-by-calorie diet analysis of published Atkins and South Beach diet menus:

> Independent analysis of the menus in both books reveals that there is no statistically significant variation between levels of healthy fats and healthy carbs between the Atkins and South Beach programs.

If this is true, it isn't welcome news for Dr. Arthur Agatston, creator of the South Beach Diet, nor is it good news for the millions of South Beach dieters who believe that they are following a healthier version of the Atkins Diet.

Scientists at Tufts University School of Nutrition Science, in the May 2004 *Health & Nutrition Letter*, call the South Beach Diet "a fad wrapped within a gimmick."

Tufts scientists criticize the book's author, Agatston, for cashing in on the low-carb craze and believe that his diet book, *The South Beach Diet*, is "replete with faulty science, glaring nutrition inaccuracies, contradictions, and claims of scientific evidence minus the actual evidence."

Dr. Agatston, who admits to taking a statin drug (a prescription medication taken by people with elevated blood lipid scores) and blood-cholesterol-lowering fish-oil supplements, prescribes a high-fat, carb-restricted diet for his readers and labels critics' health warnings about ketosis as "overstated."

PHYSICIANS FIGHT BACK AGAINST
FAT-PUSHING DIET DOCTORS

In 2002, the Physicians Committee for Responsible Medicine (PCRM) established a Web site (www.AtkinsDietAlert.org) that alerts dieters to scientific studies and news regarding ketogenic and other high-fat diets and provides them with a registry for reporting health problems on these diets. According to the site, of 188 registrants who logged on to the site shortly after the registry's start-up, 22 percent complained of kidney problems (11 percent kidney stones, 9 percent reduced kidney function, 2 percent infections), while 20 percent reported such heart-related problems as heart attack, heart-rhythm abnormalities, or elevated cholesterol levels. Eleven percent of registrants reported gallbladder problems. Registrants also reported episodes of gout, a painful form of arthritis.

The *Southern Medical Journal* reported the death of a sixteen-year-old girl following the Atkins Diet, and two studies that compared the Atkins Diet to a low-fat diet revealed that two people following the Atkins Diet died and 30 percent saw a worsening of their blood-cholesterol scores. One Florida man has filed suit, with the help of the PCRM, against the Atkins Diet organization because he claims he developed serious coronary artery blockage and had to undergo surgery to treat it.

Dr. Atkins, who himself appeared "grossly overweight," according

SCIENTISTS AND FOOD GROUPS WARN AGAINST
THE ATKINS, SOUTH BEACH, AND ZONE DIETS

The following organizations have banded together to warn dieters about the risks of following the South Beach, Atkins, Zone, and other popular high-fat, low-carb diets. A recent press release by the Partnership for Essential Nutrition, led by former U.S. Surgeon General C. Everett Koop's Shape Up America!, states that such diets can "stress the kidneys and increase the risk of liver disorders, gout, coronary heart disease, diabetes, stroke and several types of cancer."

The following organizations are part of the coalition or have contributed time, money, and resources to help it achieve its public health goals:

- Alliance for Aging Research
- American Association of Diabetes Educators
- American Institute for Cancer Research
- American Obesity Association
- Centers for Disease Control and Prevention affiliate organization
- Gerber Food Products
- National Women's Health Resource Center
- Pennington Biomedical Research Center in Baton Rouge, LA
- Society for Women's Health Research
- University of California—Davis Department of Nutrition
- Yale-Griffin Prevention Research Center in Derby, CT

to John A. McDonald, MD, a physician who knew him for years, was diagnosed with coronary artery disease, high blood pressure, and cardiomyopathy (loss of functioning heart muscle), and suffered at least one cardiac arrest. Information published on the Atkins Diet Web site and the medical examiner's postmortem report suggest Dr. Atkins had an angioplasty.

Dr. Atkins never disclosed to his readers that he had high blood pressure, coronary artery disease, and surgery to repair it. He may also have hidden this information from his personal physician, who shortly

REPORTED ADVERSE EFFECTS OF HIGH-FAT, LOW-CARB DIETS

As compiled by the Physicians Committee for Responsible Medicine (PCRM), as of December 15, 2003, 429 individuals reported, via the PCRM online registry, experiencing problems with high-fat/high-protein, low-carb diets.

COMMON PROBLEMS REPORTED BY REGISTRANTS
44 percent reported constipation
40 percent reported loss of energy
40 percent reported bad breath
29 percent reported difficulty concentrating
19 percent reported kidney problems: kidney stones (10 percent), severe kidney infections (1 percent), or reduced kidney function (8 percent)
33 percent reported heart-related problems, including 13 individuals reporting heart attack, stent placement, or bypass surgery, 26 reporting arrhythmias, 42 reporting other cardiac problems, and 58 reporting elevated serum cholesterol levels
9 percent reported gallbladder problems or removal
5 percent reported gout
4 percent reported diabetes
4 percent reported colorectal (1 percent) or other cancers (3 percent)
3 percent reported osteoporosis

OTHER PROBLEMS REPORTED BY SEVEN OR MORE INDIVIDUALS
31 reported severe gastrointestinal problems including irritable bowel syndrome, diverticulitis, ulcers, heartburn, vomiting, severe abdominal pain, or cramps
19 reported severe mood swings, apathy, general malaise, or depression
18 reported peripheral neuropathy, pain, cramps, tingling, or numbness in their limbs
16 reported chronic or severe diarrhea
15 reported experiencing hypoglycemia or feeling fatigued, shaky, and weak
15 reported vertigo, dizziness, fainting, or light-headedness
15 reported severe or repeated headaches
10 reported menstrual irregularities or severe menstrual problems

8 reported chest pain
8 reported high blood pressure
7 reported nausea
7 reported increasing weight or failure to lose weight

before Dr. Atkins's death publicly stated that Dr. Atkins had healthy coronary arteries.

Dr. Atkins staunchly maintained to his death that a low-carb diet is safe enough to recommend to millions of dieters and to those, like him, who have documented cardiovascular disease.

It is ironic that two cardiologists have handed the nation a prescription for eating an array of fatty, cholesterol-rich foods as mainstays of their "heart-healthy" diets. Both cardiologists argue that this diet strategy is safe and effective, despite the passionate protestations of many leading health organizations and medical researchers.

Dr. Atkins prescribes ketosis to his readers. Although Dr. Agatston does not specifically prescribe ketosis, many South Beach dieters report they find themselves experiencing the symptoms of ketosis on the first phase of his diet, which drastically curtails carbohydrate intake. Published reports link ketosis to serious health problems, including the deaths of children and adults who suffered a cardiac arrhythmia (an abnormal heartbeat that often leads to sudden death) while following a ketogenic diet.

Dr. Agatston greatly admires William Castelli, MD, and calls him "a brilliant researcher and charismatic teacher." Yet Dr. Castelli, a longtime director of the ongoing Framingham Heart Study, which began in 1948, is convinced that the foods Dr. Agatston recommends in bulk quantities on the South Beach Diet are the very ones responsible for killing millions of Americans each year—animal protein foods and fats.

"If Americans adopted a vegetarian diet, the whole thing would disappear," Castelli says of the coronary heart disease epidemic. According to Dr. Castelli, we have been "brainwashed to eat meat," and it's killing us.

Studies published in peer-reviewed medical journals show that a high-animal-protein, low-carb diet can dramatically increase LDL cholesterol levels (commonly called "bad" cholesterol) in the blood of susceptible people and that it can precipitate attacks of angina pectoris—pain in the heart muscle due to oxygen insufficiency.

Even exceptionally healthy professional athletes and exercise enthusiasts could put themselves at risk of dehydration and heatstroke while following a ketogenic diet. Fortunately, many dieters find ketosis so unpleasant that they cannot follow this type of diet for more than a few days or a few weeks.

Some physicians have warned that dieters will have trouble becoming pregnant on a ketogenic diet and, if already pregnant, could harm the fetus and themselves. Even Dr. Atkins advises women to avoid his ketogenic diet when pregnant. Since such diets may cause painful inflammation of the joints, lethargy, mineral losses from the skeleton, thinning hair, headaches, kidney stones, and dizzy spells, what mother would want to subject herself to these unpleasant side effects as she begins to breast-feed her newborn child?

Since millions of Americans apparently believe that a high-fat, carb-restricted diet can lead them to permanent fat loss, fitness, and better health, I have devoted Chapter 2 to exposing the scientifically meritless theories and incorrect nutritional beliefs of diet-book authors. Afterward, you will likely know more about safe and sound dieting than the diet-book authors who devised these diets.

HIGH-FAT, ANIMAL-PROTEIN-RICH DIETS LINKED TO IMMUNE DISEASES

A 2004 study by Yale researchers found that consuming foods high in animal protein, eggs, and dairy could lead to an increased risk of developing non-Hodgkin's lymphoma (NHL), a cancer that attacks the lymphatic system—part of the body's immune system.

In sharp contrast, the study revealed that diets high in dietary fiber—tomatoes, broccoli, and other vegetables—were associated with a reduced risk of NHL.

"An association between dietary intake and NHL is biologically plausible because diets high in protein and fat may lead to altered immunity, resulting in increased risk of NHL," said principal investigator Tongzhang Zheng, associate professor of epidemiology and environmental health at Yale School of Medicine.

"So far, risk of NHL associated with animal protein and fat intakes has only been investigated in American women, in three studies," said Zheng. "If the association could also be demonstrated in American men, it would provide important information towards understanding the cause of NHL."

The incidence of non-Hodgkin's lymphoma has increased dramatically over the last couple of decades. Once relatively rare, it is now the fifth most common cancer in the United States. The reason for these dramatic increases is unknown.

HIGH-FAT DIETS CRIPPLE ATHLETIC PERFORMANCE

If you're a professional athlete and want to get on the fast track to a short career, jump on the high-fat, low-carb diet bandwagon. The glycogen depletion that occurs on carb-restricted diets will help you quickly reach your goal. Even ordinary exercise enthusiasts can suffer a decline in endurance and athletic performance on such diets. Here's why:

Glycogen (carbohydrate fuel stored in the liver and muscles) is like money in the bank to professional athletes. Lance Armstrong knows it and now you do as well.

Okay, so you're not Lance Armstrong. Will you benefit from glycogen?

Glycogen allows *all* active people to compete at peak performance levels and outlast the competition. It doesn't matter if you cycle, swim, racewalk, play golf, or hike with your children.

Ketogenic and other high-fat, carb-limited diets can deplete the body of its glycogen reserves. This forces the body to convert some of the excessive amounts of protein in these diets to sugar. This is quite inefficient and wasteful because the body must use a great deal of energy to detoxify the protein (which creates the harmful by-products,

ammonia and urea, that dehydrate the body). Then the body must convert the remnant protein molecules to glucose. It is this wasted energy
that allows dieters in ketosis to lose a few extra pounds. As studies show,
they tend to gain it all back, but not until developing a taste and possibly an addiction for rich, fatty foods.

According to the National Weight Registry, which has tracked long-
term successful dieters since 1996, 99 percent of the people who enjoy
lasting fat loss (more than 70 pounds lost and kept off for over six years)
don't use ketogenic or high-protein, low-carb diets. They use *high-carb*
diets.

High-protein, low-carb diets force the body to use fats and proteins
for fuel because they're low in carbs. The rapid burning of protein and
fat for fuel helps raise the ammonia level of the blood during exercise.
Research conducted in Poland showed that people exercising on the
Atkins Diet suffered reduced endurance and exercise capacity and an
increase of the stress hormone, norepinephrine, in the blood.

It would be sheer folly to follow a ketogenic diet if you wanted to
compete in the New York Marathon, the Tour de France, or the Hawaii
Ironman Triathlon. It would be equally self-defeating for an amateur
golfer or soccer or tennis enthusiast. Weekend and world-class athletes
all require more complex carbs for peak physical performance than a
ketogenic diet allows.

Following a ketogenic or another carb-limited diet makes it all but
impossible to recover quickly from strenuous exercise. Any athlete in
hard training usually learns, if only by trial and error, that a high-carb
diet makes recovery after training much easier and faster.

During the last twenty years, world-champion athletes in all sports
have tested the Eat to Win Diet under the most grueling conditions
possible—real-life competition with their careers on the line. To this
day, the Eat to Win Diet remains the de facto dietary gold standard for
professional athletes and active people. The Eat to Win Diet for the 21st
century incorporates all of the important research findings of the last
twenty years. Now, more than ever, it provides professional athletes
with a blueprint for career success and longevity. It gives all active people and sports enthusiasts a chance to eat like the champions eat. The

21ˢᵗ-century Eat to Win Diet is healthier than ever due to its Mediterr-Asian nutrient-rich profile. Nutritional science has never devised a better way to eat for maximum energy, endurance, stamina, performance, and health.

If you're a weekend warrior or a world-class athlete, don't just eat to eat—eat to *win*.

WANT TO LOSE BODY FAT PERMANENTLY? CONTROL CALORIES, NOT CARBS

The Eat to Win Diet, combined with regular walking or other activity, forces your body to surrender its fat. At the same time, the food chemistry of the Eat to Win Diet lowers your LDL cholesterol and blood pressure, and normalizes your blood sugar level. Calorie for calorie, it supplies more disease-fighting phytonutrients and fiber than any popular high-protein, low-carb diet.

You don't have to deprive yourself of enjoying carbs in order to be lean and healthy. The Eat to Win Diet uses *Automatic Calorie Control* to help you achieve lifelong slenderness and fitness. Automatically controlling calories, not carbs, ultimately determines how thin you will become and how long you will maintain your weight loss.

Your total daily caloric intake will also determine to a large extent *how long you will live.* As you will discover in the next two chapters of this book, it is your total calorie intake and not your intake of carbs that controls your weight-loss destiny, your risk of disease, and how long you will live. All of the positive weight-loss results of high-fat, low-carb diets you read about in the media result from consuming fewer calories and not from eating fewer carbs.

The Eat to Win Diet for the 21ˢᵗ century contains the healthiest nutritional elements of the traditional diets followed by natives of Crete and Okinawa (until their diets changed in the 1960s due to modernization). This MediterrAsian diet design allows much less fat than is today consumed by people who eat modern Mediterranean and Japanese diets. Sadly, these once-healthy diets have become "Americanized" and now more closely resemble popular high-protein diets. On one level, the Eat to Win Diet takes you back to a healthier, slimmer era when you could enjoy pasta without guilt or weight gain. On another, it takes you to the cutting edge of 21st-century nutritional science.

An eating plan that does not advocate regular exercise does dieters a disservice. You can become quite lean on the Eat to Win Diet without ever exercising, but you stand a much better chance of remaining lean for life by walking or enjoying other physical activity *at least* five hours each week. All walking beyond what you would normally do counts, irrespective of whether you do it at a mall, in your neighborhood, on a treadmill in your home or at a gym. Aerobic exercise promotes cardiovascular fitness and helps lower your blood cholesterol score, blood sugar levels, and triglyceride levels (blood fats). It promotes a healthy skeleton and lifelong weight control, and it helps avert diabetes and many types of cancer. Chapter 10 contains exercise information and a simple walking plan for beginners.

AUTOMATIC CALORIE CONTROL

The Eat to Win Diet uses the principle of Automatic Calorie Control.

You don't have to learn how to do it because it's already built into your brain!

Automatic Calorie Control is no gimmick. It is based on well-established scientific principles that have been clinically tested in people and established as scientifically valid and reliable. Nutritionists have known for years that it works like a dream. Automatic Calorie Control causes dieters to reduce their calorie intake without feelings of hunger or lack of satiety. Dieters remain blissfully unaware that they are on the road to lasting fat loss.

The calorie density of the foods you will enjoy on the Eat to Win Diet is relatively low, but the nutrition and satiety of these foods is very high—much higher than is possible on a ketogenic or other type of high-fat diet. This means that on the Eat to Win Diet, you will consume fewer calories than you normally would, yet feel wonderfully satisfied and full. Your body will respond as if you eat like a king or queen, but your belly, thighs, and butt will look like you eat like a champion.

The Eat to Win Diet has helped people achieve their professional dreams and their weight-loss goals for twenty years. That's because the Eat to Win Diet is the world's most scientific and advanced performance-based eating system. Now it is yours as well.

CALORIC DENSITY: THE SECRET OF LASTING FAT LOSS

Diet-book authors who promote popular high-fat, low-carb diets do so in an attempt to keep dieters' blood sugar and blood insulin levels within normal limits. They believe that eating foods that rank high on the glycemic index (GI) elevate blood levels of both, which leads dieters to hunger and obesity. The GI rates individual foods on their ability to raise blood sugar levels relative to white bread or glucose.

These authors attempt to lower sugar and insulin levels in the blood of their readers by encouraging the consumption of calorically dense foods with low GI ratings. This is precisely the opposite of what they should recommend to their readers.

The safe and effective way to achieve healthy sugar and insulin levels in the blood and to enjoy lasting fat loss is to consume phytonutrient-rich foods with low caloric densities, irrespective of their GI ratings.

The typical portions of such phytonutrient-rich foods you'll enjoy on the Eat to Win Diet contain more bulk and far fewer calories than the fat-heavy and protein-dense foods you'll gorge on by following a popular low-carb fad diet. Lower-calorie, phytonutrient-rich foods are the cure for high blood levels of insulin and sugar. They also provide a lasting cure for obesity.

If the caloric density of a diet is sufficiently low, it doesn't matter what the GI rating of a food may be or what the glycemic load of a meal is (the product of the amount of carbohydrate in a food and its GI rating). Dieters will lose weight and lower blood cholesterol scores, blood pressure, and blood sugar without denying themselves lifesaving, phytonutrient-rich carbohydrate foods.

Lasting fat loss and peak health have always been about the *calories* and not the carbs.

The GI rating of foods has relevance only for dieters who consume more calories during snacks and meals than their body can adequately handle.

Diet-book authors who promote low-carb diets encourage their readers not to restrain themselves while eating. This is when eating foods with a low GI becomes important. But it also limits the dieter's intake of disease-fighting phytonutrients, so it's self-defeating.

The easiest way to overwhelm the body's ability to digest, absorb, and assimilate calories is to consume foods with a high-calorie density—the kinds of foods promoted on high-fat, low-carb diets. Fats possess little satiety value, especially when compared to the phytonutrient-rich, low-calorie foods emphasized on the Eat to Win Diet.

Dieters who eat according to Eat to Win dietary principles will be able to consume foods with high GI ratings such as carrots, potatoes, and watermelon with adding fat to their bodies and without risking obesity or jeopardizing health. The same cannot be said about dieters following ketogenic diets or other fad diets that promote consumption of calorie-dense foods.

SUBWAY PROVES AN EAT TO WIN–TYPE DIET CAUSES LONG-TERM FAT LOSS

Subway, the national fast-food sandwich chain that currently licenses the term "Atkins-friendly" for use with some of its high-fat, low-carb sandwiches, inadvertently helped prove that a carb-rich Eat to Win–type diet leads to long-term extraordinary fat loss.

Subway also unintentionally helped to discredit the fundamental theory behind low-carb diets—that eating carbs and foods that rank high on the glycemic index leads to obesity.

How did the fast-food franchise unwittingly accomplish all of this?

Subway shot itself in the foot-long sub by featuring a not-so-average-weight Joe named Jared Fogel in a national TV advertising campaign. Jared lost an eighth of a ton of excess body weight simply by eating a *high-carb, low-fat* diet exclusively at Subway. Each day for a little over two years, Jared enjoyed two sandwiches made with high-carb bread, tomato, lettuce, processed turkey meat, low-fat dressing, two diet sodas, and two bags of high-carb/low-fat snack chips.

Jared's well-publicized weight loss while using a high-carb, low-fat diet singlehandedly made mincemeat of the pseudoscientific theories that carb-bashing doctors use to sell their books.

Jared Fogel didn't need to read a diet book named after a doctor or city, nor did he have to purchase specially prepared diet foods or join an expensive weight-loss center. He just sat his fat fanny down at a local Subway and followed, by chance, the weight-loss principles of the Eat to Win Diet. The result: Jared lost 245 pounds eating a high-carb diet. More impressively, Jared has kept almost all the weight off *for over five years* (he eats a more varied diet now).

Jared Fogel never took a single bite of an Atkins-friendly Subway sandwich during his two years as a steady Subway customer. Subway hadn't yet licensed the right to use the Atkins-friendly trademark, nor had it created a line of Atkins-friendly menu items. Had Jared done so, we might never have heard of him: Subway's Atkins-friendly high-fat wraps contain more than 100 extra calories over the low-fat subs Jared used to lose 245 pounds.

Jared Fogel's Subway diet taught America an important lesson about how to eat to lose: A low-fat, carb-rich diet that's naturally low in calories leads directly to extraordinary long-term weight loss. Jared's nutrient profile on the Subway diet approaches that of the even healthier Eat to Win weight-loss diet.

Thank you, Subway, for helping to establish that the glycemic index rating of a food is meaningless for extraordinary and long-term fat loss.

Thank you, Jared, for confirming that an Eat to Win–type diet works over the long run, even while dining out.

EAT TO WIN KEEPS YOU GOING AND GOING AND GOING

In the original *Eat to Win*, I went out on a limb and predicted that Martina Navratilova would be winning at Wimbledon long after the time that most tennis professionals retire from the sport. Sports pundits laughed at me for claiming that the Eat to Win Diet could help de-age the body and extend professional athletic careers.

In 2004, twenty-two years after my bold prediction, the forty-seven-year-old tennis legend won her first-round match at the celebrated tennis tournament. Martina was one of the first athletes to show how using a team of professionals—"Team Navratilova," as I called it—in the areas of coaching, training, computer match analysis,[3] and sports nutrition could turn a good player with a genetically endowed potential into a great champion. Martina was able to compete in a Grand Slam tennis tournament at an age when most players wouldn't consider stepping on center court because she has followed a healthy diet for most of her adult life.

Another athlete I currently counsel, Gregor Fucka, is considered by many of his fans to be the Michael Jordan of the Euroleague (European professional basketball league)—the equivalent of our NBA. (Before you raise an eyebrow, I should tell you that Gregor hails from Croatia, where his surname is pronounced *Foot-shka* and is quite common and socially acceptable.)

I have worked with Gregor for the last five years and he has since won the Euroleague MVP award and won the 2000 Italian National Championship with team Fortitudo (Bologna), the 2003 Euroleague Championships with FC Barcelona, and the 2003 and 2004 Spanish National Championships with team FC Barcelona. Gregor is now thirty-three years old and shows no signs of slowing down at an age when most players begin contemplating retirement. If he played in the NBA, he would rival the league's finest players.

Both Martina and Gregor are genetically gifted athletes, but neither rose to the top of their profession and stayed there for many consecutive years until they embraced the Eat to Win Diet. You may not possess the genetic endowments of these world champions, but the Eat to Win Diet can help you become the best you can be—at any age.

3. I believe that the computer analyses of Martina's matches against Chris Evert contributed to some extent to Martina's domination of her most well known rival. As Martina noted, "The computer is a good scout." Arthur Ashe wrote a favorable article in *World Tennis* magazine about my use of computers to analyze tennis matches and predicted that one day, such analyses would become ordinary practice in professional tennis. I believe that Martina was the first professional tennis player to use computers to analyze matches of her opponents (recall that this was 1981!).

WHAT THIS BOOK WILL DO FOR YOU

Since the Eat to Win Diet does not eliminate whole groups of foods, you get to enjoy most of your favorite foods in scientifically safe and effective amounts. Do you love lobster, adore apples, crave chocolate, covet coffee, pine for pasta, long for lasagna, savor sake, or whine for wine? You'll get to enjoy all those foods and beverages and much more while becoming lean and fit.

Perhaps you aspire to win Wimbledon or Olympic gold. The Eat to Win Diet has already made such dreams come true for professional athletes; it could do the same for you or even your children.

When you read most diet books, you're not really reading the author's own words, because almost every diet-book author uses a ghostwriter or a professional "book doctor." Fortunately, my graduate training in nutrition and food science, my years of clinical nutrition experience, and my work with the world's foremost professional athletes allow me to articulate my knowledge. The result: You will read my words, thoughts, and analyses of diet and health issues and not some hired gun's interpretation of what I *should* say or what I *meant* to say. Surprisingly, I remain the only number one best-selling diet-book author in history who has earned a graduate degree in nutrition. Does all this make a difference? I think it does.

I wrote this book because I want you to enjoy the thrills of peak performance, achieving better health, and reaching your weight-loss goals. None of these come easy, and all take dedication and discipline. But I believe that once you are armed with correct information about diet and nutrition, you will be more likely to make rational and informed mealtime choices, even when they are at odds with your desire to wolf down a double scoop of your favorite premium ice cream.

Toward this end, I have devoted extra effort to making you aware of the dangers associated with following many of today's most popular diets and to clearing up common diet myths and misconceptions that could prevent you from reaching your fitness, health, and weight-loss goals. I want to help you to avoid common diet scams that will make you fatter, not thinner. And of course, I want to help active people and professional athletes reach new heights of performance and help them excel at their chosen sport.

Once you embrace the Eat to Win Diet, you'll begin to lose your excess body fat as a side effect of eating this way. From the first day of your new diet, you'll start to "de-age" your blood. This is not hype: Your blood chemistry will begin to resemble the healthier one you enjoyed as a child. Your risk of heart disease, type 2 diabetes, high blood pressure, and many types of diet-related cancers will decline dramatically. Your endurance, energy, and stamina will dramatically improve. You'll get to enjoy pasta, rice, and potatoes again. You'll stay younger longer. Your breath won't smell of ketones.

The Eat to Win Diet gives you the power to become enviably thin, if that is one of your goals. For a woman, this could mean wearing size-four dresses instead of trying to squeeze into a size eight; for a man, this might mean wearing slim-cut jeans with a thirty-inch waist instead of filling out a "relaxed fit" pair with a thirty-eight-inch waist.

I want to show you how to optimize your diet to suit your favorite sport with my sports-specific diets. If you're lucky enough to have the genetics of an Ivan Lendl, Martina Navratilova, or Jackie Joyner-Kersee, you could very well dominate your sport and set a world record of two. You'll discover why there is no other diet in all of muscledom that can compete with the Eat to Win Diet.

That's why I can promise that when you embrace the Eat to Win Diet, you will not only be following a lifelong eating plan that is supported by published robust scientific data—you will be following a diet that has been field-tested by world-champion athletes for the last twenty-years. More athletes have set world records and dominated their sports while eating to win than on any other diet.

The Eat to Win Diet makes it easy to enjoy eating in and outside of the home. If and when you need to deviate from the diet, I'll show you how to do so without jeopardizing your long-term goals. That's because the Eat to Win Diet keeps you in nutritional balance at all times. Do you enjoy salmon, ham, turkey, and steak? Do you miss pasta and potatoes? What about beer, wine, and coffee? Perhaps you embrace a vegetarian philosophy. All are welcome on the Eat to Win Diet. What about choco-late? Within limits, it's perfectly okay.

Now *that's* a diet most people can live with—for a long, long time.

Q & A

Q. What's the big deal about calories? I thought carbs were all I had to count to be thin and fit.

A. Diet doctors–turned–diet-book authors who promote ketogenic and other high-fat diets recommend counting carbs, not calories, to be-come thin and fit. Most of them encourage their readers not to limit food consumption on these diets. While many people who follow this questionable advice do lose weight in the short run, only a very small percentage of dieters will be able to keep that weight off in the long run. That's not speculation; published studies have established this beyond any reasonable doubt.

The only way to ensure permanent fat loss *and* optimal health is to eat healthy foods rich in bulk, fiber, and satiety and low in caloric density. This eliminates the need for counting calories or carbs.

As a general rule, the amount of calories you consume, regard-less of where they come from, determine how slender you will look, how long you will live, and how healthy you will be. Scientists who study calorie-moderated diets in any number of species—from worms to spiders to dogs to monkeys—all agree that consuming fewer calories translates to longer, healthier lives.

Scientists have every reason to believe that humans respond the same way. A growing body of published evidence supports this theory. Even short-term experiments in caloric restriction reveal that when humans consume 25 percent fewer calories than they ordinarily would eat, all of their biologic signs, including amount of body fat, fasting blood sugar score, blood cholesterol score, and blood pressure, improve dramatically. Their blood chemistry resembles that of a much younger person. The infamous Biosphere Experiment proved that caloric re-striction improves these "biomarkers" of health and longevity.

Q. How many calories should I eat each day?

A. Genetics, physical activity (intensity and duration are important in determining caloric needs), gender, and type of diet all play a role in an individual's need for daily calories. I have counseled sedentary women who could not lose body fat on as few as 1,400 calories a day. I have also counseled extremely active people who required more than 6,000 calories each day in order to maintain their weight. Ivan Lendl, the tennis champion who dominated men's professional tennis for five consecutive years while on the original Eat to Win Diet, is a good example of someone who needed to eat an enormous amount of calories each day just to maintain his weight during strenuous training and competition.

I believe that no diet should provide fewer than 1,000 calories per day on average, because the body responds to fewer calories than that by going into a "starvation" mode. This slows down the body's metabolic rate and, consequently, you will burn fewer calories each day.

Most sedentary people will consume between 1,000 and 1,400 calories each day on the Eat to Win Diet. Very active people will be able to enjoy a few hundred more calories each day and still achieve their health and fitness goals. Professional athletes will, of course, be able to consume many more calories, depending upon the duration, frequency, and intensity of their training and competition.

Q. Are the ratios of protein-to-fat-to-carbohydrate important? One popular diet emphasizes a 40/30/30 ratio of fat-to-protein-to-carbohydrate. Are these healthy ratios?

A. Most leading health organizations, including the American College of Sports Nutrition, have discredited the "40/40/30" ratio hypothesis. On the Eat to Win Diet, you'll consume 20 to 25 percent protein (the majority from low-fat, low- to no-cholesterol foods), 20 to 25 percent fat (mostly from monounsaturated- and omega-3-fat-rich foods), and 50 to 60 percent complex carbohydrates (from natural whole foods). Once you reach your ideal weight, these ratios will change to about 15 percent protein, 20 percent fat, and 65 percent carbohydrate. The only thing "magical" about these ratios is that they are healthy because they embody the phytonutrient-rich MediterrAsian foods on the diet and provide an exceptionally healthy and highly palatable eating strategy for athletes and couch potatoes alike.

Elite endurance athletes will typically consume a great percentage of their daily calories as complex carbohydrates—up to 70 percent— while consuming about 15 percent of their calories as protein. While this creates the impression that elite athletes will consume less protein than a couch potato, in truth, elite athletes eat much more protein each day than sedentary people due to the large amount of daily calories they require. It's only because their complex-carb intake is so high that their protein ratio appears relatively low compared to the protein ratio consumed by an inactive individual.

Q. Is it healthy to consume fewer calories even when weight loss is not an issue?

A. The level of calorie reduction on the Eat to Win Diet (about 25 percent fewer calories than a typical American weight-maintenance diet), slows the rate at which your body ages and helps delay the onset of diet-related degenerative disease. In addition, the phytonutrient-rich foods on the Eat to Win Diet (especially those rich in polyphenols) mimic the antiaging effects of calorie restriction by stimulating a class of cellular enzymes known as sirtuins. Sirtuins promote DNA stability by stimulating DNA repair of older cells, thereby rejuvenating them. Even if you don't need to shed any weight, the level of calorie reduction on the Eat to Win Diet will keep you healthier and allow you to live longer than if you ate a healthy diet but did not reduce your caloric intake.

Q. The author of a popular low-carb diet book claims that eating fat, not carbs, leads to improved athletic performance. Is this true?

A. The theory that eating more fat improves athletic performance over eating carbs enjoys scant evidence in the published biomedical literature. In general, the body tends to burn fats and carbs for energy in roughly the ratio found in the diet. During exercise, that ratio begins to shift, based on exercise intensity. When exercise intensity reaches 63 to 65 percent of maximum effort, the body shifts to burning more fat than carbs, but intense exercise always burns more fat for fuel than does light exercise, even though the ratio of fat-to-carbohydrate burning remains higher during light exercise.

Some diet-book authors and athletes mistakenly believe that athletes need to eat more fat to boost athletic performance because fat contains over twice the energy value (calories) of carbs. They demonstrate their ignorance of two well-established principles of intermediary metabolism:

1. The fat we burn for fuel does not come directly from the foods we eat but rather from stored fatty acids in adipose tissue. These fatty acids originally came from the fat, carbohydrate, and protein in our foods. So it doesn't matter how much fat is in the diet itself—it won't be used directly for energy during exercise.
2. No one runs out of fat during a 26.2-mile marathon or grueling triathlon, but many athletes run short on carbohydrates. This condition, known as "hitting the wall," makes it difficult to continue the event. Conditioned athletes store only about 1,000 or so calories of readily usable carbohydrate but store 150,000 or more calories as fat.

Here's another way to see the lack of merit of such claims by diet-book authors: During a marathon, runners often drink a fat-free electrolyte-glucose sports beverage. The reason is simple: The carbs in the sports drink can be used directly and immediately for energy. If there were any fat in the drink, it would first have to be broken down into its component fatty acids, repackaged as triglycerides (three fatty acids combined in one molecule), transported to adipose tissue in carriers called chylomicrons, and then stored in fat cells. Only then could the fatty acids be released into the bloodstream and used by the body for energy. A marathon runner would already be at home enjoying dinner by the time that fat would become available for energy. So you can see that eating fat has nothing to do with improving sports endurance, stamina, or performance.

Published research has shown that on an Eat to Win–type diet, it takes only one day to restore glycogen to optimal levels after strenuous physical activity. It takes five to seven days on a low-carb diet. That's a zone no athlete wants to enter.

Q. Why should I follow the Eat to Win Diet rather than one devised by a diet-book author with a medical degree?
A. Unless the diet-book author/physician also earned a graduate degree in nutrition or has devoted many years to study in the field, I wouldn't recommend blindly trusting the dietary musings of such a physician. As physicians readily admit, they receive their training in medicine and not in nutrition.

Physicians, like other diet-book authors, write books and magazine articles on diet and nutrition that dispense highly questionable information. One popular diet doctor claims that our blood type determines which diet is best for us. Another claims that eating large quantities of foods loaded with saturated fats and cholesterol *reduces* the risk of cardiovascular disease.

One cardiologist/diet-book author admits to taking a statin drug (these drugs are designed to keep elevated blood cholesterol levels in check). Why would a cardiologist who presumably eats a "heart-healthy" diet take a prescription cholesterol-lowering drug with potentially harmful side effects? Does this mean that all people who embrace his diet should gobble statins as well?

My experience with cardiologists has shown that they don't always make the most informed decisions when it comes to diet. For example, many years ago I approached Dr. Phillip Sammet, the head of the Department of Cardiology at Mount Sinai Hospital in Miami Beach, Florida, to help determine if the Eat to Win Diet could reverse coronary artery blockage. This was a decade before another physician, Dr. Dean Ornish, established that this could indeed be accomplished with diet and lifestyle change instead of surgery and

drugs. Dr. Sammet invited me to present my proposal to his Department of Cardiology.

After my formal presentation, Dr. Sammet decided against testing my diet in a handful of patients with angiographically documented coronary artery blockage. I was, of course, surprised by his
decision. His biggest concern was that the local press would catch
wind of this trial and report it to the public. God forbid if it was lifesaving news that could help his patients! The publicity-shy Dr. Sammet could have been the first cardiologist in history to establish that
heart disease was reversible through dietary intervention—a full ten
years before Dr. Ornish achieved worldwide fame for doing so.

**Q. Are you implying that cardiologists and other physicians
lack the nutritional knowledge to advise people how to eat?**
A. Not at all. There are a number of brilliant cardiologists and physicians who have devoted their careers to the study of nutrition and
who make significant contributions to the field. Regrettably, such
clinicians and researchers usually don't write best-selling diet
books. You have to read biomedical journals to learn of their work.

Most physicians in private practice probably have not had sufficient graduate training or clinical experience in nutritional science
to qualify as credible diet-book authors. Book publishers tend to
give book contracts to medical doctors because they believe the ca-
chet of "MD" after their name will automatically establish credibility and help sell books. The publishers are evidently correct.
Judging from book sales of popular diet books authored by physicians, the general public apparently believes that physicians are as
qualified to practice nutrition as they are to practice medicine. As
you will discover in the following chapters of this book, this as-
sumption is questionable.

**Q. Has the Eat to Win Diet ever been tested in a formal medical
study?**
A. Yes. Medical researchers associated with the Chicago Heart Association, Northwestern University, and the University of Chicago

Medical School learned of my research and diet and evaluated its fundamental principles. Dr. Robert W. Wissler, a world-renowned atherosclerosis researcher at the Specialized Center for the Research of Atherosclerosis, Department of Pathology, University of Chicago, invited me to make a formal presentation to the physicians, researchers, and hospital dietetic staff at Northwestern University. Among them were some of the world's leading health experts, including Dr. Wissler himself and Dr. Jeremiah Stamler of Northwestern University.

My presentation met with such success that researchers agreed to conduct a small pilot study drawn from a very large government-sponsored study at the time called MR FIT (an acronym for Multiple Risk Factor Intervention Trial). The results of the test of my diet in participants who were already enrolled in the MR FIT study were excellent.

The pilot study's principal investigator, Dr. David Berkson, president of the Chicago Heart Association, noted that my diet achieved good short-term results in lowering a number of measurable risk factors for heart disease (e.g., blood cholesterol scores, blood pressure, body weight). Dr. Berkson reported that my diet also produced a surprising and unintended result: By chance, there were a number of alcohol-dependent participants who were in the pilot study group testing my diet. In every case, these study participants were able to abstain from drinking while enrolled in the pilot study.

Q. Do newspapers and magazines print accurate information about popular diets?

A. I wish I could answer yes to this question because it takes the wind out of my sails when I read some of the dreadful press coverage about diet and nutrition. Even some of the most respected publications are not immune to misreporting and lack of fact checking. Here's one notable example:

In 2002, our national collective fear of eating too much fat seemed to evaporate after the publication of an article on the Atkins

Diet in the prestigious *New York Times Magazine*. The article, written by science writer Gary Taubes, "What If It's All Been a Big Fat Lie?" quoted a group of world-renowned researchers and health experts from such prestigious institutions as Harvard and Stanford universities as supporting the Atkins dietary approach. Until this point, the vast majority of reputable diet experts had warned of the health risks of following the Atkins Diet and copycat high-fat diets. The *Times* article depicted a sudden and radical reversal of the long-standing and nearly universal scientific consensus regarding the Atkins Diet.

The *Times* article and the ensuing media hype it generated probably did as much to sell the high-fat ketogenic diet to a fat-fearing public as all previous publicity combined. Much of the media fell into lockstep behind the parade of health authorities quoted in the *Times* article. The nation took note and started to eat fatty, rich foods while drastically limiting their intake of potatoes, carrots, legumes, many forbidden fruits, and other high-complex-carb foods.

The *New York Times Magazine* article set off a huge media frenzy by creating the impression that the fat-heavy Atkins Diet had earned the blessing of some of the world's leading health experts; it caused no less of a stir throughout the scientific and medical communities—particularly among those who were quoted by Taubes in his article.

Skeptical journalists who checked the veracity of Taubes's reportage discovered that Taubes had practiced what appeared to be a manipulative and deceptive form of bait-and-switch journalism: The scientists he quoted had acknowledged that certain fats can be part of a healthy diet—specifically, unsaturated fats from plant and fish oils—and they told him that people would be better off if they ate fewer refined carbohydrates, but *none* of the scientists recommended that people follow a diet like the one promoted by Dr. Atkins. To the contrary, they recommended that Americans embrace a Mediterranean-type diet, low in saturated animal fats and rich in vegetables, whole grains, beans, and fruits, and omega-3 and omega-9 fats from fish oils and nuts and seeds, respectively. No researcher or health expert interviewed by Mr. Taubes recommended that people should follow Dr. Atkins's advice to consume generous amounts of red meat and butter, both laden with saturated fat. In fact, they recommend that these foods should be eaten sparingly.

Professor Walter Willett, MD, PhD, from the Harvard School of Public Health, quoted liberally in the *Times* article, told Taubes during the interview that eating large amounts of steak and butter is unhealthy and that the primary problem with the Atkins Diet is that it is extremely high in animal fats, which raises the risk of heart disease, colon cancer, and prostate cancer. Professor Willett maintains that he told this to Taubes several times but that Taubes had omitted this crucial warning in his article.

In the Center for Science in the Public Interest's November 2002 "Nutrition Action Health Letter," John Farquhar, professor emeritus of medicine at Stanford University's Center for Research in Disease Prevention, called the *New York Times Magazine* article "a disaster" and complained that he was "greatly offended at how Gary Taubes tricked us all into coming across as supporters of the Atkins Diet." Stanford University obesity researcher Gerald Reaven, a leading health and obesity expert quoted by Taubes in the article, said he was "horrified" by the piece.

Q. Are there other ways the media enables distortions of the truth about diets?

A. I'm always amused when the news media report that a celebrity uses a particular diet to stay slender. What the media doesn't reveal is that more often than not, that celebrity is addicted to nicotine. When people use cigarettes to stay thin, it doesn't matter what diet they follow because nicotine lowers the body's set point for storing fat by 10 to 20 pounds. Smokers will store less body fat and burn more stored fat than nonsmokers, all else being equal. Smoking lowers insulin levels and stimulates the release of stored fat to be burned as energy. Interestingly, a similar metabolic scenario occurs during ketosis. Once dieters cease using tobacco or ketosis to take

off the pounds, their set points for fat increase to former levels and
their body fat is restored at a faster rate than it was lost.

Women in particular apparently find the prospect of being 10 to
20 pounds lighter without dieting enough of an enticement to use a
product that could lead them directly to cancer, cardiovascular disease, emphysema, and many other serious health problems. Female
smokers outnumber male smokers, and for the first time in history,
lung cancer rates in women have surpassed those in men. As someone who has nutritionally counseled people battling lung cancer, I
can assure you that being 10 to 20 pounds overweight is far more
preferable.

The next time you admire the slender figure of a celebrity, check
to see if that celebrity uses tobacco to stay thin. In most cases, that's
their real weight-loss "diet."

Q. So is there a bias in the press in favor of the ketogenic diet?
A. I'm not a conspiracy theorist, but the treatment it has received in
the press sometimes makes me question whether I should become
one! Here's just one of many examples:

When the United States Department of Agriculture (USDA)
published an important diet study in 2002, few U.S. newspapers reported it, although it received wide coverage in European countries.
Your taxpayer dollars financed this important study, yet you never
heard or read about it.

The press is often reluctant to waste valuable space on studies
that show that eating diets high in complex carbs and low in saturated fats is the healthiest way to eat. These types of headlines don't
play well across all time zones; the press likes controversy, sensa-
tionalism, and mass appeal. There's nothing sexy about whole
grains, fruits, and vegetables, save for the fact that the people who
eat them generally enjoy healthier sexual function than those who
avoid them.

The press knows that many Americans want to read and hear
about diets that say it's okay to eat lots of meat and cheese and eggs.
There are many studies published to show that lower-fat, high-

complex-carb-rich diets are healthier, but we don't hear or read about them very often. Every time a new high-fat diet study is published, however, we're going to read or hear about it.

The USDA study and other stories you never hear or read about reveal that dieters who follow ketogenic or other high-fat, low-carb diets can't stick with them in the long run. The data reveal that these eating plans almost guarantee that dieters will eventually jettison them. Only 1 percent of successful long-term dieters tracked by the National Weight Control Registry at the University of Colorado follow a high-fat/low-carb diet! The registry, which began in 1996, now contains data on over six thousand adult Americans who have lost at least 30 pounds and kept it off for a year. The registry has also collected data to show that almost every one of its registrants who has lost about 70 pounds and kept it off for six years did so on a reduced-fat, high-carb diet. To join the registry, call 1-800-606-NWCR.

Q. **Diet-book authors claim that eating such cholesterol-rich foods as eggs, mayonnaise, butter, cream, and cheese won't affect my blood cholesterol score. Is this true?**
A. A number of published studies that showed that adding cholesterol-rich foods to the diet doesn't raise blood cholesterol scores very much have thrown many diet-book authors off the right track simply because they have no training in nutrition and are therefore unequipped to evaluate the flawed published studies purporting to show that consuming such foods does not adversely affect blood cholesterol scores.

Many physicians remain unaware that once blood cholesterol scores rise above 150 (and LDL cholesterol scores rise above 70 or 80), the risk of coronary artery disease significantly increases. Research shows that individuals and populations that consume cholesterol-rich diets do not enjoy blood cholesterol scores, on average, anywhere near 150.

For example, studies that test whether egg yolks raise blood cholesterol scores usually involved people with blood cholesterol scores of 190 to 240. People who have such scores already ingest so much

dietary cholesterol that they have trouble absorbing more cholesterol from their diet, so feeding them additional cholesterol in eggs
won't cause a significant rise in their cholesterol scores.

What many diet-book authors don't tell you is that when you add
the same cholesterol-rich foods to the diets of healthy people with
cholesterol scores of 150 and below, you see a dramatic and dangerous increase in their blood cholesterol score.

According to Dr. William Castelli, longtime lead investigator of
the famous Framingham Heart Study, a cholesterol score of 150 is a
score that confers immunity from premature heart attack:

> We've never had a heart attack in Framingham in 35 years in
> anyone who had a cholesterol level under 150. Three-quarters
> of the people who live on the face of this Earth never have a heart
> attack. They live in Asia, Africa, and South America, and their
> cholesterols are all around 150.

Cholesterol- and fat-pushing diet doctors are either unaware of
the published data (highly unlikely in the case of the Framingham
Heart Study) or perhaps choose to ignore the data because it destroys their basic premise that a high-fat, high-cholesterol diet isn't
dangerous.

Another confounding variable is that it's not just dietary cholesterol alone, but the combination of cholesterol and saturated fat in
the diet that causes blood cholesterol scores to increase. In fact, saturated fats (and trans fats) play significant roles in raising blood
cholesterol scores. Some studies show a rise of 30 to 100 points in
blood cholesterol scores in people who begin a ketogenic or other
high-fat/high-cholesterol diet. Mixing large amounts of dietary
cholesterol and saturated fats creates a recipe for atherosclerosis.
There are a number of additional dietary factors that will raise your
blood cholesterol score, including sugar and excess calories from all
food sources, but dietary cholesterol and saturated fats account for
the high blood cholesterol scores that eventually lead to heart disease. High-cholesterol diets generally contain large amounts of

arachidonic acid, a compound that raises the body's production of cholesterol.

Q. I've read that a Mediterranean diet is a healthy diet. What, exactly, is a Mediterranean diet?

A. A comparison of the various diets consumed by inhabitants of Mediterranean countries, including southern Italy, Spain, Greece and Crete, and Maghreb (coastal northwestern Africa), reveals that the Mediterranean diet is not a single homogeneous diet. Foods rich in various phytonutrients, cereals and grains, fats and oils, and alcohol consumption vary greatly among residents of these areas.

People in Mediterranean countries consume more total fat than many northern European countries, but most of the fat is in the form of monounsaturated fatty acids from olive oil and omega-3 fatty acids from fish, vegetables, and certain meats like lamb. For example, natives of Crete consume 40 percent of their total calories as fat, mostly from olive oil. They also consume alpha-linolenic acid by eating herbs, walnuts, seeds, snails, purslane, and lamb.

In 1993, the Lyon Diet Heart Study demonstrated that a diet resembling the Cretan diet provided superior protection from the recurrence of heart attacks compared to the American Heart Association's well-known "prudent diet." The Lyon Diet Heart Study provided the first clinical proof that a Mediterranean-type diet exerted a protective effect on cardiovascular disease.

The modern Mediterranean diet does not promote body-fat loss, but it does contain an exceptionally high amount of disease-fighting phytonutrients. Such phytonutrients from garlic, onions, cocoa, wine, tea, olive oil, colorful vegetables, and whole grains confers health advantages even to obese people who consume a Mediterranean diet. All of these foods contain nutrients that can lower the risk of coronary artery disease and many types of cancer.

Q. Aren't high-fat foods more satisfying than carb-rich foods?

A. One of the greatest distortions of the truth promoted by carb-bashing diet doctors is that protein does not stimulate the production of insulin as much as carbs do. Most of these authors believe that in- sulin spikes in the blood promote hunger and, therefore, obesity. These diet docs apparently remain unaware that for the last half century, diabetes researchers have used protein to check the body's ability to produce insulin by administering arginine, an essential amino acid found in all foods that contain protein. In truth, con- suming beef raises insulin output more than eating whole-grain pasta. Cheese, another highly touted food on a high-fat diet, raises insulin levels more than pasta made from refined flour; fish in- creases insulin output more than oatmeal.

With respect to satiety, the baked potato—taboo on a high-fat diet—produces twice the level of satiety as beef or cheese. (I'll tell you more about the satiety index of foods in Chapter 2.)

2

"Net Carbs" and Other Diet Myths and Misconceptions

As a nation, we've been down this road before. During the low-fat frenzy of the 1980s and early 1990s, food manufacturers and restaurateurs acceded to the public demand for eating lower-fat foods by concocting nonfat and low-fat products and menu items. People devoured food products labeled "nonfat" and "low-fat," but instead of stopping at one serving, they believed they were entitled to consume three or four (the SnackWell's Snafu). The fear of fat had blinded them to the calories in these foods—the same calories that helped fuel the U.S. obesity epidemic of the 21st century.

Today's dieters are about to repeat the mistakes of the past, only this time the SnackWell's Snafu has a new name—*net carbs.*

IT'S DÉJÀ VU ALL OVER AGAIN

Contemporary carbophobes can now enjoy 21st-century prefab low-net-carb foods with the same relish that 20th-century low-fat dieters savored sugary nonfat foods. Food manufacturers are again capitalizing on dieters' fears with new lines of low–"net carb" products. Such low-net-carb products will be the undoing of the low-carb diet, reminiscent of how the SnackWell's Snafu derailed the low-fat diet of the 1980s.

Eager to capitalize on a fear of all things "carb," food companies and restaurant chains have created products and menu items that create the appearance of being "low-carb" foods. The trouble is, there is no scientific consensus of what constitutes a low-carb food or menu item. The FDA is currently struggling to come up with a standard of identity so that dieters won't continue to be confused or misled. In the meantime, food manufacturers and restaurant chains are using the terms "low carb" and "net carb" with impunity, often to the detriment of trusting dieters. The term "net carbs" at best is little more than a marketing tool. At worst, it is a food scam that deceives dieters into believing that certain carbs don't contain calories (they do) and that a product's total calories don't count (they most certainly do).

Nutrients that food manufacturers and diet-book authors don't count as "net carbs" include fiber, glycerin (also called glycerol, a common food additive), and other sugar alcohols with names like sorbitol and mannitol. Diet-book authors and food manufacturers tell their readers that these carbs don't matter.

The problem is, they do.

As one example, James E. Hoadley of the FDA's Office of Food Labeling points out, "There is no rational basis to consider glycerin (or glycerol) as anything but a carbohydrate."

A number of companies that make diet candy bars exclude the glycerin (glycerol) in their bars from the carb count. One-half of the thirty nutrition bars recently tested by an independent laboratory (ConsumerLab.com) exceeded their claimed levels of carbohydrates, often by large amounts. According to a statement released by the laboratory:

One product, which described itself as a low carbohydrate diet bar, claimed only 2 grams of carbohydrates, but was found to actually contain 22 grams. A clue as to why this discrepancy existed was a statement written in small type on the product's label indicating that it contained glycerin but that the manufacturer was not counting glycerin as a carbohydrate.

Many types of fiber are partially digestible and do in fact yield some metabolizable calories. Glycerin can be repackaged by the body to help form new carbs and can serve as part of the triglyceride "backbone" molecule—the storage form of body fat. Sugar alcohols are simply carbs masquerading under another name and contain measurable calories like other carbs.

Just as the SnackWell's Snafu made the low-fat diet unpopular, net carbs will eventually contribute to the demise of the low-carb diet. Many dieters will wolf down excessive calories from low-net-carb-labeled food products because they will mistakenly believe that such foods can be consumed with impunity. Dieters will consider these as "fantasy" foods, just as low-fat dieters did with products labeled as "low-fat" and "no-fat."

Many products designed for the low-carb diet demographic provide no weight-loss advantage whatsoever over the food products they are intended to replace. For example, an Atkins-brand chocolate candy bar contains 150 calories and 12 grams of fat. A regular chocolate candy bar typically provides 150 calories and 10 grams of fat.

Soon, millions of Americans will be compounding their first mistake—embracing a high-fat, low-carb diet—with a second one by consuming processed foods laced with unnatural amounts of sugar alcohols added to food products in order make them taste sweet and to lower their net-carb count. This could create a new set of health issues for dieters who have already placed themselves at risk for serious health problems by virtue of having embraced these diets.

"Net carbs mislead people into believing they are consuming fewer carbohydrates when those carbs should be counted," notes Gail Frank, a spokesperson for the American Dietetic Association. "A carbohydrate is a carbohydrate, whether or not it raises blood sugar."

FIGURE 2.1

CALORIE COUNTS OF COMMONLY USED POLYOLS NOT COUNTED AS "NET CARBS" IN LOW-CARB FOOD PRODUCTS

"Net carb"	Calories per gram
Erythritol	0.2
Glycerol	4.0
Hydrogenated starch hydrolysates	3.0
Isomalt	2.0
Lactitol	2.0
Maltitol	2.1
Mannitol	1.6
Sorbitol	2.6
Xylitol	2.4

Data courtesy of the Calorie Control Council.

THE "EATING FATS CURBS APPETITE" MYTH

Dr. Arthur Agatston believes this myth and perpetuates it by making the following statement in *The South Beach Diet* as if it were an established nutritional dictum:

> When we eat fats, we become satiated. As a result, we know when to stop eating.

Scientific studies have, in fact, shown just the opposite. Dr. Agatston's statement is not supported by scientific evidence and has been discredited many times over.

Recall the study conducted at the University of Pennsylvania I told you about in Chapter 1. The women in the study did not compensate for the additional fat calories served to them by eating less at dinner. They ate, on average, almost 60 percent more calories when served the largest portion of the highest-calorie (highest-fat) entrée than when served the smallest portion of the lowest-calorie (lowest-fat) entrée. *The amount of fat in the meals had no effect on satiety or fullness.*

Studies such as this one (you can find others in the reference bibliography at the end of this book) clearly show that people invariably overconsume fats and oils in their diets because these nutrients are not nearly as satiating as foods rich in complex carbohydrates. Most well-informed nutritional scientists and registered dietitians know from their academic training, published studies, and personal clinical experience that fats simply don't possess great satiety value.

Anyone who has eaten French fries and baked potatoes implicitly knows that compared to a baked potato, with its low calorie count and negligible fat content, one could easily consume many more calories from calorically dense French fries before feeling full. Despite Dr. Agatston's pronouncement, adding fat to the nonfat potato does not increase its satiety value.

It takes thousands of calories from several hundred ears of corn to yield just one cup of corn oil. You would probably feel full after eating two ears of corn but you could easily consume hundreds more calories from the corn oil used in meals and recipes and not feel full. Millions of people prove this every evening: Upon finishing a salad swimming in corn oil–based dressing, they go on to eat a full dinner (with more fat) plus dessert (still more fat). Only then do they feel full. Corn oil and other fats don't tell us when to stop eating.

Published studies reveal that on a per-calorie basis, fat has the lowest satiety value of any macronutrient. Dietary fat plays a number of roles in the body, but telling your appetite when to shut down, as Dr. Agatston contends it does, is *not* one of them. Fat doesn't fill you up—it fills you out. Alcoholic beverages provide the same poor satiety value as fat, which is why the Eat to Win weight-loss plan limits alcohol consumption to seven drinks each week.

Ironically, the only food group that Dr. Agatston restricts—the complex carbohydrate food group—possesses the highest satiety value of all food groups.

If Dr. Agatston knew about the satiety index (the satiety index measures how full and satisfied dieters feel hours after consuming a single serving of a food), he would probably not advise his readers that if they enjoy a baked potato for lunch, by late afternoon they would become ravenous. What single food do you think ranks at the very top of the satiety index? You guessed it—the baked potato.

MORE IS LESS: AN OLD TRICK FOR A NEW GENERATION OF DIETERS

During the low-fat frenzy of the 1980s, food manufacturers devised a clever trick to make dieters believe that their products were low in fat. The scam works like this:

A frozen "diet" dinner that contains 300 calories in which 30 percent of the calories comes from fat would ordinarily deter a low-fat dieter from purchasing it. So food manufacturers came up with a wonderfully deceptive scheme to trick consumers into believing the frozen dinner was, technically speaking, a true low-fat diet product: They simply added a sugar-laden dessert to the same frozen dinner entrée. Since the nonfat dessert added 100 additional carbohydrate calories to the frozen entrée, it lowered the percent of the total calories as fat, transforming it into an acceptable product in the eyes of unsuspecting low-fat dieters. Only now, dieters ate even more calories and sugar than they would have if they had purchased the original frozen "high-fat" diet dinner.

Today, food manufacturers simply adjust the amount of sugar alcohols, other sweeteners, and fiber in their products to create an "acceptable" net-carb count. In truth, this raises both the carb count and the calories in the food, much in the same way that food manufacturers in the eighties lowered the percentage of fat in their products by adding pure sugar to them.

QUESTIONABLE USE OF THE GLYCEMIC INDEX

Carb-bashing diet doctors convinced the nation that such high-carbohydrate foods as potatoes, oatmeal, carrots, and pasta were the reason everyone got fat. To prove their point, they employed their favorite piece of propaganda—the glycemic index.

Many sports nutritionists, coaches, trainers, and registered dietitians joined the carb bashers in hailing the glycemic index (GI) as a valuable tool that could help people pick the "healthiest" carbohydrate foods. I would like to cast doubt on the wisdom of all of these health and fitness experts in recommending the GI as a tool to lose weight. I am going to show you why it is a poor guide for helping people select foods to help them curb hunger. Then I'll show you the real index you should use to decide which foods to eat—the satiety index.

The GI is a table of data that contains the numerical ranking of an individual food's ability to raise blood glucose levels relative to a reference carbohydrate—usually glucose or white bread. Diabetics use the GI to help them make food choices and construct diets. The theory is that diabetics can better determine how to adjust their glucose-lowering medications by knowing which foods will raise blood sugar faster than others. Such thinking can be misleading, however, as you will see in a moment.

Low-carb diet promoters use the GI as a scare tactic to convince you that a high-complex-carbohydrate diet is unhealthy and inappropriate for weight loss. The GI measures the blood-glucose-raising effects of a single food. It doesn't work as well for food combinations, individual foods with added toppings or sauces, and whole meals. But even when used as intended, the GI can lead dieters to make some unhealthy food choices. Here's why:

Watermelon has a high GI rating—much higher than that of a chocolate candy bar. Watermelon is rapidly broken down in the digestive tract and absorbed quickly, but because it's low in calories and contains negligible amounts of fat, watermelon will not add fat to your body. A thick slice of watermelon contains only about 60 calories, so it doesn't matter if the calories are absorbed rapidly. There are simply too few to matter.

What about potatoes? Those rank high on the GI too. Will eating potatoes make you fat?

A medium russet potato contains about 110 calories. As with

watermelon, the body quickly absorbs the calories in a potato, but because it's a low-calorie food and contains almost no fat, it won't add fat to your body. But it will satisfy your appetite and make you feel full.

Recent research has shown that among all foods tested, the ordinary baking potato ranks highest on a more useful index for dieters than the GI—*one that carb-bashing diet-book authors don't tell you about.* It's called the satiety index. This index measures the ability of a single food to satisfy appetite and hunger. Potatoes rank highest, followed by other such "fattening" foods as oatmeal and pasta.

Pasta? Isn't that a refined carbohydrate?

Pasta is generally made from refined wheat flour and water, although many types of whole-grain and vegetable pasta abound in supermarkets and natural-food stores. Homemade pasta recipes usually call for egg yolks and therefore I do not recommend them. However, ordinary white pasta, as sold in most supermarkets and as served in many Italian restaurants, is a food you can enjoy (as long as you don't top it off with a high-fat sauce) without worrying about weight gain. Pasta (choose whole grain when available) is so filling that most people simply won't be able to eat enough of it to make them fat. And like potatoes, pasta contains not a hint of cholesterol and is very low in fat.

Ice cream, which enjoys a relatively low GI ranking—much lower, in fact, than rice—increases insulin levels in the body more than rice does—a food that low-carb diet doctors limit. This is because *dietary fat amplifies the insulin response to carbohydrate*—both of which are in plentiful supply in ice cream. Eating ice cream causes much more insulin output than does eating white rice despite ice cream's much lower GI score. Dietary protein also promotes greater insulin release. In fact, beef and full-fat dairy products cause a bigger insulin release than pasta.

These facts, of course, discredit the whole GI theory of obesity, which in turn, discredits the anticarbohydrate theories of diet-book authors who promote them.

The truth behind the GI myth is quite simple: *Total calories per snack or meal determine whether or not the foods you eat will add fat to your body.*

Only dieters who cross a certain "calorie threshold" at each meal or at each snack need to consult this questionable index. On a high-fat, low-carb diet, dieters routinely cross that threshold due to the caloric density of the foods on such diets and due to the diet doctors' exhortations not to limit the amount of food they eat. People following the Eat to Win Diet will rarely, if ever, exceed the calorie threshold for healthy eating.

If the GI does become relevant to what you are eating, it means *you're already eating too many calories for optimal health, longevity, and lasting fat loss.* Eating too many calories will shorten your life span and age you prematurely regardless of what you eat.

If you follow the prescription of diet-book authors not to limit your intake of foods, as Dr. Arthur Agatston recommends to South Beach dieters, the GI of foods will be a bit more relevant to your diet—but only marginally so. Dr. Agatston's prescription forces you to limit or abandon many nutritious foods that will get you thin and keep you thin and healthy.

Infants are born with a natural instinct for moderating food intake. Babies tend to eat when they are hungry and tend to stop when they are full. If they swallow too much at one feeding, they regurgitate the excess. When those infants become adults, they stuff their stomachs full of fatty foods and learn to take antacids to prevent nausea and regurgitation—and then stuff their stomachs again at the next meal.

Some diet-book authors who promote high-fat, low-carb diets permit eating liberal amounts of bacon and other high-fat foods. These diets keep you from staying in touch with your satiety instincts because fat has little satiety value. If you follow such a diet, keep those antacids and the GI handy!

THE SATIETY INDEX

Dr. Susanne Holt at the University of Sydney conducted studies that reveal the superiority of complex-carbohydrate foods over high-protein and high-fat foods in quelling hunger. Holt's research dispels the myth that such foods as potatoes, oatmeal, rice, and fruit make you hungry because the calories in these foods are digested and released into the blood faster than high-protein foods.

Using white bread as a control food (which she arbitrarily assigned a

value of 100), Holt asked study participants to score thirty-eight different foods on how effectively each food created feelings of fullness or satiety. Each participant fasted the night before and then ate a 240-calorie
portion of a specific food along with a glass of water. During the next two
hours, participants filled out a questionnaire to determine the degree of
hunger or satiety they felt. After two hours of no food, they were allowed
to eat freely from a wide variety of foods until they felt satisfied. Foods
scoring higher than 100 were considered more satisfying than white
bread, and those scoring under 100 were considered less satisfying.

As a group, fruits ranked at the top, with a satiety index 1.7 times
that of white bread, but the highest-ranking food was the very one the
carb-bashing diet doctors want you to avoid like the plague: the potato.
Other foods that scored high in satiety were oatmeal, pasta, apples, and
oranges. The irony is that these foods surpassed the ability of nearly all
of the high-protein, high-fat foods that low-carb-diet-book authors
recommend to quell hunger.

Dr. Arthur Agatston and other carb-bashing diet-book authors
claim that eating potatoes and certain fruits and vegetables will make
you hungry, fat, and unhealthy. This is food faddism at its worst. Unlike
the high-fat foods promoted by Dr. Agatston, which score low on the
satiety index, natural complex-carbohydrate foods contain disease-
fighting phytonutrients, fiber, and a much greater ability to effectively
suppress hunger.

Now you can understand why none of the carb-bashing diet-book
authors tell you about the satiety index. It destroys their fundamental
premise that carbohydrate-rich foods make you feel hungry and lead to
obesity. It discredits their use of the GI to prove their questionable theories of obesity. As Dr. Holt observed:

> Fatty foods are not satisfying, even though people expected them to
> be. We think the reason is that the body sees fat as a fuel, which
> should be used only in emergencies—it stores it in the cells instead
> of breaking it down for immediate use. Because it doesn't recognize
> the fat (in food) as energy for immediate use, the body does not tell
> the brain to cut hunger signals, so we go on wanting more.

Foods scoring highest on the satiety index contain fewer calories per gram than the steak, prime rib, cheese, and other rich foods promoted by low-carb-diet promoters. They have a negligible fat content and contain no cholesterol.

Holt conducted another study comparing the satisfying power of different breakfasts. She observed:

The two high-carb breakfasts tended to improve alertness to a greater extent than the two high-fat breakfasts. Also, because the subjects were not completely satisfied by the two high-fat meals, they tended to be grumpy and a bit more aggressive/disappointed.

FIGURE 2.2

THE SATIETY INDEX

All foods are compared to white bread, ranked as 100. **Boldface** type denotes low-calorie foods that provide greatest satiety.

Snacks & Confectionery	Carbohydrate-Rich foods	Protein-Rich foods	Breakfast Cereals	Fruits
Cake 65	Brown pasta 188	Baked beans 168	All-Bran 151	**Apples 197**
Cookies 120	Brown rice 132	Beef 176	Honey Smacks 132	Bananas 118
Crackers 127	French fries 116	Cheese 146	Mueslix 100	Grapes 162
Croissant 47	**Pasta 188**	Eggs 150	**Oatmeal 209**	**Oranges 202**
Doughnuts 68	**Potatoes 323**	Lentils 133	Special K 116	
Jelly beans 118	White bread 100			
Mars candy bar 70	White pasta 119			
Peanuts 84	White rice 138			
Popcorn 154	Whole-grain bread 157			
	Yogurt 88			

Carbohydrates curb your hunger:

Potatoes rank highest in satiety, nearly seven times higher than the least-satisfying food, croissants. Whole-grain bread is 57 percent more filling than white bread. High-fat foods normally classified as carbohydrates, such as cakes, cookies, and doughnuts, are among the least filling. Fish is more satisfying, per calorie, than lean beef or chicken.

THE "EGGS DON'T RAISE YOUR BLOOD CHOLESTEROL SCORE" MYTH

The American Egg Board, Dr. Atkins, and Dr. Agatston would like you to believe that eating whole eggs every day does not raise dangerous LDL cholesterol levels in your blood. I would like to take this opportunity to cast doubt on this position.

The American Egg Board has sponsored a number of studies that show adding eggs to an ordinary American diet doesn't significantly raise dieters' blood cholesterol scores, nor does it change the various particle sizes of LDL cholesterol that promote atherosclerosis, the same disease diagnosed in Dr. Atkins a few years before his death. Atherosclerosis progressively narrows arteries in the heart and elsewhere in the body.

In a study typical of most industry-funded egg research, scientists randomly assigned twenty-seven premenopausal women and twenty-five men to either an egg diet (containing 640mg of additional dietary cholesterol) or a placebo diet for thirty days. This flawed study design, similar to many previous studies that examined the impact of egg cholesterol on blood cholesterol scores, found that people who already eat cholesterol-rich diets would typically show a small but statistically insignificant rise in blood cholesterol scores when they add eggs to their diets.

The reason is deceptively simple: Your body's ability to absorb dietary cholesterol is already near its maximum if you consume a cholesterol-rich diet (e.g., the ordinary American diet, the Atkins Diet, the South Beach Diet, the Zone Diet). On these diets, adding more cholesterol to the diet will not appreciably raise the blood cholesterol score of a majority of dieters who already have blood cholesterol scores in excess of 150. For this reason, many of the study participants' "normal" blood cholesterol scores didn't rise considerably in response to eating excess egg-yolk cholesterol and cholesterol from all other animal foods. Most cardiologists consider a "healthy" cholesterol score to be 170 to 190. Regrettably, they are mistaken. This is still far too high to prevent heart attacks and strokes.

ONE EGG STUDY THE AMERICAN EGG BOARD DIDN'T FUND

A fourteen-year Japanese study, led by Dr. Yasuyuki Nakamura at Shiga University of Medical Science, which tracked the diets and health of 9,300 men and women, found that those who consumed one or more eggs a day were more likely to die prematurely than women who ate one or two eggs a week. Researchers measured study participants' blood pressure, cholesterol levels, and other health indicators at the start of the study, and deaths were tracked over the next fourteen years.

"Limiting egg consumption may have some health benefits, at least in women in geographic areas where egg consumption makes a relatively large contribution to total dietary cholesterol intake," concluded the researchers in a paper published in the July 2004 edition of the *American Journal of Clinical Nutrition.*

Researchers found that women who ate an egg a day were 22 percent more likely to die of any cause during the course of the study, compared with those who ate only a couple of eggs per week—regardless of factors such as age, smoking habits, and body weight. Those who ate two or more eggs a day showed a still higher death risk, but only a small number of women fell into that category.

Recall what William Castelli, MD, a former director of the Framingham Heart Study, concluded after studying which people in Framingham got heart disease and which people didn't:

We've never had a heart attack in Framingham in 35 years in anyone who had a cholesterol level under 150. Three-quarters of the people who live on the face of this Earth never have a heart attack. They live in Asia, Africa, and South America, and their cholesterols are all around 150.

Dr. Castelli's research group found that the carotid arteries (the main arteries in the neck that carry blood from the heart to the brain) of women who follow a high-fat, carbohydrate-restricted diet have nearly double the plaque (fatty deposits) of those on a higher-carbohydrate, lower-fat diet.

Most people cannot eat an ordinary American diet or a high-fat, low-carb diet and achieve a blood cholesterol score of 150 or below. Only an extremely rare and genetically endowed individual can eat this much cholesterol and not suffer the consequence of atherosclerosis. The overwhelming odds are that it's not you.

THE "ONLY SATURATED FATS MATTER" MYTH

A number of dietary factors in addition to saturated fats raise blood cholesterol scores: Trans fats, cholesterol, sugars, and consuming excess calories are among the worst offenders.

As I mentioned, the artery-clogging process proceeds between meals, as cholesterol-enriched particles, called chylomicrons, VLDL,[1] IDL, and LDL cholesterol, deliver their cholesterol payloads to arteries. Chylomicrons and free fatty acids (fats that freely circulate in the blood) increase in the hours after a meal and typically decline within eight hours. Most studies examine blood cholesterol scores only in people who have fasted overnight for twelve hours. By that time, cholesterol-enriched chylomicron and free-fatty-acid levels are low, and the damage they've done to arteries cannot be measured by an ordinary blood cholesterol test.

This creates the misconception that people with blood cholesterol scores between 170 and 190 enjoy reduced risk of succumbing to cardiovascular disease, when in fact their between-meal blood cholesterol scores are much higher than measured after a fast.

The best way to ensure that your blood cholesterol score remains in the safe range between meals is to follow a low-calorie diet with no added trans fats, and one low in saturated fats (no more than 5 percent of total calories) and low in dietary cholesterol (no more than 50mg/day).

The authors of high-fat, low-carb diets think that it's okay to eat bacon and eggs for breakfast. I think it's slow suicide.

---

1. VLDL (very-low-density lipoprotein) is a triglyceride-rich carrier molecule; IDL cholesterol (intermediate-density cholesterol) is now considered part of LDL cholesterol (low-density cholesterol). All contribute to atherosclerosis—the process by which arteries become clogged with cholesterol-filled plaque.

THE "INCOMPLETE" PLANT PROTEIN MYTH

It's positively mind-boggling! The notion that plant proteins are inferior to animal proteins persists even into the 21st century—even among "credible" sources.

How is it possible that this long-discredited notion remains firmly entrenched in the collective mind of millions of dieters, athletes, trainers, and physicians?

One reason could be that we currently find this myth circulating in such pop-culture publications as *Newsweek* magazine and in such scholarly publications as those proffered by the American Heart Association (AHA).

In 2001, the Nutrition Committee of the AHA published a warning to dieters about of the dangers of such high-protein diets as the Atkins, South Beach, Sugar Busters, and Zone diets. In this otherwise commendable report, the AHA's Nutrition Committee's stated: "Although plant proteins form a large part of the human diet, most are deficient in one or more essential amino acids and are therefore regarded as *incomplete* proteins" (my italics).

The AHA's Nutrition Committee uses the scientifically discredited 1971 pop diet book *Diet for a Small Planet*, written by Frances Moore Lappe, as a *scientific reference* to support their untenable position. Even the book's author long ago apologized for her blunder, admitting that she erred in speculating that vegetable proteins were "incomplete" proteins and had to be combined with other "incomplete" vegetable proteins to form the "complete" proteins found in animal muscle.

It's one thing for a newsmagazine such as *Newsweek* to misstate the facts; the American Heart Association's promulgation of such pop-science pap borders on nutritional quackery.

Let's look at the established scientific facts we know about plant proteins and decide for ourselves if they are adequate to support peak physical performance and excellent health:

- One hundred percent of all beef, poultry, and milk consumed on this planet comes from steers, chickens, and cows that eat *only* plant proteins. These creatures didn't need to eat a single molecule of animal protein to manufacture the "complete" protein in their own muscle tissue, eggs, and milk.

- A gorilla, which possesses the strength of four or more adult men, achieves its remarkable power and musculature from eating only plant foods.

- Sixty percent of all people alive today thrive on a diet in which the sole source of protein comes from plant foods. Most of these people have successfully avoided the diet-related diseases that kill most Americans.

- Natives living in New Guinea eat a diet consisting mainly of yams with a few other vegetables. They remain strong and hearty and don't suffer from premature cardiovascular disease, diabetes, hypertension, or obesity.

- When starving children in Africa are nursed back to health, it is generally on a diet consisting exclusively of vegetable proteins from corn, rice, wheat, and beans. Even though children recovering from starvation require many times more protein to catch up in developmental growth to healthy children, a diet exclusively of plant proteins easily meets their expanded protein needs.

- Most people don't know that just 500 calories of spinach, which contains no cholesterol and a very small amount of fat, would provide 65 grams of *complete* protein sufficient to meet a recreational athlete's daily protein needs. (See Figure 2.3.)

- Many elite athletes have won the Hawaii Ironman Triathlon while following a diet composed exclusively of vegetable protein foods.

- Upon cessation of breast-feeding, infants will thrive on a vegetable-protein-only diet. We typically feed infants oatmeal (15 percent protein), rice (9 percent protein), and potatoes (8 percent protein) with no effects other than excellent health and growth.

FIGURE 2.3

THE ESSENTIAL AMINO ACID PROFILE IN 500 CALORIES OF SPINACH

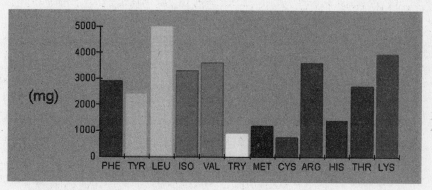

As little as 500 calories of boiled spinach supplies 65 grams of "complete" protein—more than enough to meet the protein needs most active adults. This chart lists the twelve most important amino acids (nine are essential for life, which means they must be obtained through food). The amino acid profile for spinach is nearly identical to that of beef. (See Figure 7.1, p. 150.)

THE "SHORT-TERM KETOSIS ISN'T HARMFUL" MYTH

All major health organizations have issued formal warnings about the long-term health risks linked to following a ketogenic diet (high in fat and cholesterol and relatively low in fiber and phytonutrient-rich carbohydrate foods). There's no need to belabor this point, but I would like to take a moment to dispel the myth that ketogenic diets are safe in the short run.

Dr. Arthur Agatston isn't concerned if South Beach dieters happen to stumble into ketosis because he believes "the specter of ketosis has been overstated."

Perhaps Dr. Agatston is unaware of the sad story of Rachel Huskey.

In a case widely covered by the British press but only marginally reported by the U.S. media, Rachel Huskey, a teenage girl who was worried about her weight, went on the Atkins Diet. Rachel, at five feet, nine inches and 238 pounds, was clinically obese.

For six weeks Rachel stuck to the Atkins plan, limiting her intake of carb-rich foods in favor of animal-protein foods. Despite her regular bouts of nausea (a common side effect of the Atkins and South Beach ketogenic diets), Rachel lost fifteen pounds—much of it water.

Without warning, Rachel collapsed while in school. Efforts to revive her failed. Today Rachel's family believes the Atkins Diet caused her death. Her mother, Lisa, warns: "I want people to know you can die doing something as stupid as this."

The coroner ruled that the cause of death was cardiac arrhythmia—due to an irregular heartbeat. Researchers from the University of Missouri, Rachel's home state, discovered her body had critically low levels of potassium and calcium, which could have caused the arrhythmia. They concluded that people in ketosis might be susceptible to this mineral imbalance because these diets have a strong a diuretic effect that accelerates the body's loss of minerals required for a healthy heartbeat. Health experts on both sides of the Atlantic have cautioned about the cardiac dangers of ketosis diets for the past thirty years.

3

Your Five Vital Values

A SIMPLE BLOOD TEST WILL TELL YOU WHICH LEVEL OF THE EAT TO WIN DIET IS RIGHT FOR YOU

All adults should have a simple and inexpensive blood test that can help determine if they are at risk for cardiovascular disease and diabetes. Every athlete I've ever counseled has learned how to eat to win based on his or her own blood chemistry. Although the Eat to Win Diet is based on nutritional principles that everyone follows, I make individual adjustments in the diets of champions that give them the competitive edge over their opponents. I can, to the extent possible in a book, do the same for you.

When I first presented this "revolutionary" idea for the original *Eat to Win* to my publisher/editor, Eleanor Rawson, over twenty years ago, I had some convincing to do. She rightly questioned whether people would be put off by having to visit their physician or a walk-in health-testing laboratory and paying for such a test. After all, she was the publisher who helped turn the Atkins Diet from a two-page article in *Vogue* magazine in 1970 into a full-fledged diet book. I've never forgiven her! (Just kidding, Eleanor.)

I pointed out that most people spend the equivalent of the price of such a test on a dinner for two at a medium-priced restaurant. Surely, one's health and longevity is worth the price of a dinner check! Eleanor Rawson saw the merit of my argument and agreed that it was a good idea.

Most diet-book authors don't tell their readers that this simple blood chemistry test is the only accurate way they can learn if a particular diet is making them healthier or sicker. Weight loss alone is no indicator of health.

A recent weight-loss study that examined the health effects of ketogenic and low-carb diets found that even as people lose weight on such diets their blood cholesterol scores often soar and their coronary arteries become blocked. In that same study, one low-carb dieter lapsed into a coma and two died.

Curiously, diet-book authors who are also physicians have no problem encouraging their readers to eat like gluttons but they don't insist on having them take this potentially lifesaving test. This test is one of the least expensive your doctor will ever perform for you. In my opinion, you can't afford *not* to take this test.

Your blood chemistry is unique and will help you individualize the Eat to Win Diet. There are three levels to the Eat to Win Diet, and one of them is right for you with your current blood values.

You can discover where to start your diet by having a simple and inexpensive laboratory test called a blood chemistry profile. You can get this test from a physician, public health center, walk-in testing center, or college or university health center. It will take less than ten minutes of your time, and a laboratory technician can rapidly evaluate the results.

You should refrain from eating or drinking after dinner the night before the test. This is not difficult to do if you schedule your test for early morning. Avoid eating or drinking anything except water after dinner. Have your blood test the next morning, and then eat breakfast. Only a fasting blood chemistry profile will yield accurate results.

After you receive that laboratory analysis of your blood (the blood chemistry profile) make sure that your physician has a copy if he or she did not order the original test.

Your unique blood chemistry profile can help determine your risk of diet-related diseases. This evaluation is the easiest and single most powerful screening test for many health conditions, including diabetes, liver and kidney disease, and elevated cholesterol levels. It will indicate if you are at risk for cardiovascular disease or other health conditions. Everyone, young and old, should have a blood chemistry profile done at least once every year.

YOUR FIVE VITAL VALUES

There are dozens of blood components that a blood chemistry profile will measure, but only five are essential to determine which level of the Eat to Win Diet is right for you. As your blood chemistry changes over time (which you will discover in subsequent tests), you will move from one level of the diet to the next until you reach the final and highest peak-performance level—level three. The three levels cover the entire range of normal human blood chemistry so that you will easily be able to find your appropriate starting level.

The five vital values to test for are:

- **Total cholesterol:** This value provides a general risk-factor indicator for the possibility of developing cardiovascular disease.

- **HDL cholesterol:** The level of HDL cholesterol is a strong indicator of risk of cardiovascular disease and can reveal whether an individual is getting enough aerobic exercise.

- **Triglycerides:** These blood fats can help determine if one is consuming too many calories and too much alcohol, sugar, and fat. Triglycerides are also predictive of heart disease and type 2 diabetes.

- **Glucose:** Fasting blood sugar levels can uncover latent diabetes, a tendency toward diabetes, metabolic imbalances, and a lack of exercise.

- **Uric acid:** High levels can indicate excessive protein and alcohol intakes and can indicate which people may be predisposed to kidney disease and gout (arthritis).

Health experts have discovered another blood value that may be worth testing. It's called a C-reactive protein test, and it can reveal the presence of inflammation in the body and is now being recognized as an important laboratory value in predicting heart disease and perhaps even cancer risk. Although it is still too early to recommend this test for everyone, you should discuss it with your physician to see if it's right for you.

The blood is a mirror of the body. The results of repeat blood chemistry just before, and four weeks after, you commence the Eat to Win Diet, will help confirm, in a clear and scientific manner, the health benefits of this eating plan.

HDL AND LDL CHOLESTEROL

You can raise your blood cholesterol score well above 150 simply by enjoying egg yolks, beef, fish, poultry, pork, full-fat dairy products, sugar, butter, lard, and trans fats (hydrogenated oils). Eating too many calories from any foods or being sedentary will also raise your blood cholesterol score.

Even though diet-book authors, registered dietitians, and medical writers refer to HDL cholesterol and LDL cholesterol as "good" and "bad" cholesterol, respectively, the HDL and LDL carriers each transport the same cholesterol molecule, which is neither good nor bad.[1]

The basic distinction between the two transporters of cholesterol, HDL and LDL, is that the cholesterol packaged in the HDL transporter is generally unavailable for deposition in arteries; in fact, the HDL transporter can whisk cholesterol away from arteries to prevent the buildup of plaque, a mix of cholesterol, protein, calcium, and other compounds that can form a tumorlike blockage in the wall of arteries.

The cholesterol packaged in the LDL transporter is generally available to arteries and other tissues. It's actually much more complicated

1. HDL stands for "high-density lipoprotein"; LDL stands for "low-density lipoprotein." Along with VLDL (very-low-density lipoprotein) and IDL (intermediate-density lipoprotein), these carrier molecules make up the important lipoprotein fractions in the blood that serve as transports for fat, cholesterol, and fat-soluble vitamins and phytonutrients.

than this because there are subfractions of HDL and LDL cholesterol (and other cholesterol carriers and subfractions), and there are varying particle sizes of LDL, some of which are more dangerous than others. For our purposes, it's sufficient to know that it's healthier to have a high HDL cholesterol score and a low LDL cholesterol score.

Weight loss, smoking cessation, and exercise will safely raise HDL levels, but the general level of HDL is usually predetermined by genetics. The only instance I can think of when you don't want to see your HDL cholesterol score increase is if you follow a ketogenic or high-fat, low-carb diet. A rise in your HDL cholesterol score on such a diet would most likely mean that your total cholesterol and LDL cholesterol scores have risen as well, which is not a good thing, despite any favorable changes you might see in your LDL-to-HDL ratio or total cholesterol.

Regrettably, studies designed to examine the significance of the ratios of such lipoprotein fractions have been poorly designed and have too many confounding variables that distort the true contribution of these fractions to an individual's overall cardiovascular risk profile. These studies have never compared the LDL-to-HDL ratios or total cholesterol of people following the Eat to Win Diet with those following ketogenic or high-protein/high-fat diets. If and when they do make such comparisons, they will discover that the *absolute level* of LDL cholesterol in the blood is the more important determinant of the risk for cardiovascular disease. They will also find that the Eat to Win Diet confers much greater protection against cardiovascular disease than these low-carb diets do.

The ability to predict the risk of heart disease, based on the ratio of HDL cholesterol to LDL cholesterol carried in the blood, has largely been misunderstood by the medical community for the last thirty years. In the original *Eat to Win*, I explained that HDL cholesterol loses much of its predictive significance once total blood cholesterol scores (which include HDL, LDL, and VLDL cholesterol) drop to 150 and below.

Some years ago, I counseled a man who was a member of the board of directors of a large and prestigious hospital in Miami Beach, Florida. He was worried about his elevated blood cholesterol score,

230. Many cardiologists at the time considered this to be a high-normal score. A "big-name" cardiologist on his hospital staff suggested that he take a cholesterol-lowering prescription drug to reduce his elevated cholesterol score. Diet modification was not mentioned.

The hospital board member decided to first consult with me about dietary change before taking a medication with unpleasant and dangerous side effects. After twelve weeks on the Eat to Win plan, his cholesterol score dropped 105 points to 125. His HDL cholesterol score dropped from 30 to 25. Cardiologists consider an HDL cholesterol score of 25 a cause for concern.

Ordinarily, such concern would be justified in an individual with this low of an HDL score who ate an ordinary American diet or in someone who followed a ketogenic or high-fat, low-carb diet. In truth, when one's blood cholesterol score drops below 150, the HDL cholesterol score loses a great deal of its ability to predict the risk of heart disease.

This is one reason why physicians need to establish new blood lipid guidelines in assessing the risk of heart disease in their patients. Another is that the typically healthy range of total blood cholesterol scores has always been too lenient. An LDL cholesterol score of 70 or below is ideal, yet for the last fifty years, most physicians believed scores well in excess of this number are healthy scores.

This hospital board member was greatly concerned until I showed him published research about a very fit and healthy group of Mexican Indians who had lipid profiles similar to his. Rates of heart disease among these natives are extraordinarily low. None of the cardiologists on staff at his hospital was aware of this research. Twenty years after I explained this in *Eat to Win*, many cardiologists still don't know that a low HDL cholesterol score is a safe score in a person with a total blood cholesterol score of 125 and especially in someone with an LDL cholesterol score of 80 or below (70 or below is even healthier). Exercise can help raise a low HDL cholesterol score without raising LDL cholesterol levels. In fact, regular exercise can lower LDL levels as well.

A person with an HDL cholesterol score of 25, a total blood cholesterol score of 125, and a triglyceride score of 80 enjoys far greater protection

*against cardiovascular disease than a person with an HDL cholesterol score
of 50, a total blood cholesterol score of 200, and a triglyceride score of 50.*

But these are just numbers that obscure the relevance of a high or
low HDL score. Whether a low HDL cholesterol score signals danger
really depends on what diet an individual follows and if there are any
other diseases present.

Most discussions of HDL cholesterol overlook additional and important roles this transporter plays in the body. For example, once
lutein and zeaxanthin—two phytonutrients found in green and yellow
plant foods that protect the eye lens and the retina from UV radiation
and oxygen—reach the liver, they are incorporated into HDL lipoproteins and transported through the blood.

It would be easy for a dieter who follows a ketogenic or other low-
carb diet to consume insufficient lutein and zeaxanthin. So the amount
of these two phytonutrients transported in HDL would become highly
significant to dieters' eye health. Therefore, it could be much more important for a person following a ketogenic or other high-fat, low-carb
diet to have a higher HDL cholesterol score than it would be for an Eat-
to-Winner to have a high HDL cholesterol score because the Eat-to-
Winner consumes far more eye-healthy phytonutrients.

For example, in the case of a dieter following the phytonutrient-rich
Eat to Win Diet, which contains ample lutein and zeaxanthin, high HDL
cholesterol scores become less important because the HDL carrier will
regularly contain a more enriched concentration of the two compounds.
Since the Eat to Win Diet is naturally low in cholesterol, trans fats, and
saturated fats, the Eat-to-Winner doesn't require the higher HDL cholesterol score to protect his or her cardiovascular system needed by the
dieter who follows a ketogenic or other high-fat, low-carb diet.

DOES SIZE REALLY MATTER?

Cardiologists are concerned with LDL particle size these days. Smaller
LDL particles are more atherogenic (promoting artery blockages) than
larger ones because they seem to be able to deliver their cholesterol
payload into arterial walls with greater ease than larger particles. As in

the case of HDL cholesterol levels, this becomes important only for people with LDL cholesterol values in the typical ranges seen in Western cultures that eat lots of animal protein and fats. Once you are able to reduce your LDL cholesterol score to 70 and below, LDL particle size loses its predictive significance for heart disease. There is limited and suggestive evidence that shows some dieters who follow a lacto (nonfat dairy)-ovo (egg whites only) vegetarian version of the Eat to Win Diet can actually convert their smaller LDL particle size to the larger and less dangerous size.

Let's let cardiologists debate the merits of measuring LDL particle size. They will discover that LDL particle size doesn't matter in Eat-to-Winners who reduce their total cholesterol levels to 150 and below and their LDL cholesterol to 70 and below.

There is one group of people who can achieve an enviable LDL cholesterol score because of an unenviable health problem: cancer. Don't jump to conclusions: having a low LDL cholesterol does *not* cause cancer, but having cancer can cause a low LDL cholesterol score.

How do you know what your LDL score is? Here's a simple way (called the Friedewald formula) to determine the approximate value of your LDL score based on other values in your blood chemistry profile. In this example, let's assume the following numbers are your blood scores for total cholesterol, HDL cholesterol, and triglycerides:

Total cholesterol (TC)	200
HDL cholesterol (HDL)	50
Triglycerides (TG)	100

The Friedewald formula for calculating your LDL score is:

$$LDL\ score = TC - HDL - (TG \div 5)$$
Calculation:
$$LDL\ score = (200 - 50) - (100 \div 5)$$
$$LDL\ score = 150 - 20$$
$$LDL\ score = 130$$

This formula works only when triglycerides fall below 400. This formula is based on the observation that most of the circulating triglyceride

FIGURE 3.1

EFFECT OF FATS AND OILS ON LIPOPROTEIN CHOLESTEROL LEVELS

Type of fat	Selected food sources	Effects on LDL and HDL
Saturated	Meat, milk, butter, coconut oil, palm oil	Raises LDL Lowers HDL
Monounsaturated	Olive oil and canola oil	Lowers LDL Maintains HDL
Trans	Margarine, baked goods, fast-food French fries, snack chips, potato chips, and other processed foods	Raises LDL Lowers HDL
Omega-3	Oils from salmon, mackerel, sardines, tuna, swordfish, menhaden, lobster, and flaxseed	Lowers LDL Raises HDL
Omega-6	Oils from corn, soybeans, cotton, and sunflower	Lowers LDL Lowers HDL

is carried in the VLDL fraction, the composition of which is relatively constant.

I have counseled a relatively small number of people who were at very low risk of heart disease even though their blood cholesterol scores exceeded 150. This is because they were genetically predisposed to have very high HDL cholesterol scores of 90 and above. HDL cholesterol is part of the total blood cholesterol score, and since the cholesterol carried in the HDL transporter is unavailable to clog arteries, it does not contribute to the risk of premature heart attack. People with HDL cholesterol scores of 90 and above who keep their LDL cholesterol low enjoy exceptional protection against heart disease. This is certainly one time to be grateful for your parents' and your grandparents' genetics.

The body requires a small amount of cholesterol to make steroid hormones, vitamin D, bile acids, and healthy cell membranes, in addition to a number of other biologic functions. The liver and intestine, the largest contributors to the body's own manufacture of cholesterol, make between 500 to 1,000 milligrams of the compound each day—more than we need. Therefore, cholesterol is not an essential nutrient. When you consume foods that contain saturated fat, the liver actually makes more cholesterol and loses some of its ability to remove cholesterol from the blood. That's one reason why diets high in saturated fats *and* cholesterol play havoc with blood cholesterol scores.

WHAT TRIGLYCERIDES DO

Triglycerides are the ordinary fats found in our adipose tissue. They are the fats that make us look fat. Triglycerides are also the form of fat commonly found in the foods we eat. The level of triglycerides carried in the blood reveals much about our diets. Consumption of sugar, fat, alcohol, and excess calories, as well as a sedentary lifestyle all raise triglyceride levels, which can increase the risk of cardiovascular disease, diabetes, and high blood pressure. A high level of triglycerides in the blood deprives arteries and cells of oxygen and can thereby promote artery damage and plaque formation. A low-calorie diet will lower triglyceride levels in the blood and in the fat cells; it doesn't matter if the diet is high in carbohydrate or high in fat.

You can divide your blood triglyceride score by five to calculate its approximate contribution to your total blood cholesterol score. For example, a triglyceride score of 50 means that it contributes about 10mg of cholesterol to your total blood cholesterol score.

When some people switch from a low-carb diet to a high-complex-carbohydrate diet, their triglyceride scores may increase. This is no cause for concern if the diet is low in calories, simple sugars, low in fat (not more than 25 percent of total calories as healthy fats and oils), and high in natural high-complex-carbohydrate foods. This type of diet lowers both total and LDL cholesterol levels, so it doesn't matter if your triglyceride score increases, provided it stays within normal limits. Your overall lipid profile and risk of cardiovascular disease will be those of a much healthier person, and especially when compared to someone who follows a ketogenic or high-protein/high-fat diet with a lower triglyceride score.

GLUCOSE (BLOOD SUGAR)

The level of sugar carried in your blood can affect your mood, appetite, and energy levels, especially during exercise and sports. A high level of sugar in the blood can also prematurely age your body, because sugar combines with amino acids to form products that accelerate aging. If the level of blood sugar falls below the normal fasting level (usually below 50mg for every 3.5 ounces of blood) you can become dizzy. This is one reason why diabetics must carefully monitor their glucose levels and regulate their blood-sugar-lowering medications. Since glucose is the brain's preferred fuel (the brain cannot store glucose as muscles and the liver can), severe hypoglycemia can "starve" the brain, leading to dizziness and unconsciousness. A fasting blood sugar level above 110mg per 3.5 ounces of blood may indicate the presence of diabetes.

URIC ACID

Uric acid is a two-edged sword: This compound, in small amounts, acts as an antioxidant, helping to quench harmful free radicals in the blood. Once the level of uric acid exceeds safe levels, it can increase the risk of cardiovascular disease and may precipitate an attack of gouty arthritis. King George III and Benjamin Franklin are among the most well-known historical figures who suffered from the agonizing pain of gout. Ketogenic diets can raise the level of uric acid in the blood and trigger gout in unsuspecting dieters. Excess uric acid may also precipitate kidney stones.

During fat loss, uric acid levels might temporarily rise irrespective of type of diet. In general, only people following a ketogenic or high-protein/high-fat diet need worry about elevating their uric acid scores.

If you're susceptible to gout, you probably already know it and also know that it can be controlled with diet and prescription medications. Check with a physician before attempting to lose weight on any diet if you suffer from this condition.

YOUR "BEFORE" AND "AFTER" BLOOD CHEMISTRY TEST

I believe it's important to have a blood chemistry profile done prior to beginning the Eat to Win Diet and four weeks after starting the diet. By doing so you will not only have a "baseline" blood chemistry for you and your physician to track your progress, but you will also know, beyond any shadow of a doubt, that the Eat to Win Diet is working for you. Just as important, you will know which level of the Eat to Win Diet to begin and when you should switch to the next level.

The Eat to Win Diet will de-age your blood if you faithfully follow the diet's guidelines. Barring significant laboratory error (this does occur on rare occasions), the numbers in your blood chemistry profile will tell the truth.

Fad-diet doctors can promise you anything, but a blood chemistry profile test reveals the truth. It is the hard-core scientific verification that tells you the Eat to Win Diet is working to bring you better health.

WHICH LEVEL OF THE EAT TO WIN DIET IS RIGHT FOR YOU?

Most people who exercise infrequently and are a bit overweight probably will have vital values that require them to begin the diet at level one—the strictest level of the Eat to Win Diet.

Those who enjoy a regular sports or exercise program and wouldn't mind losing a few pounds in order to be fitter and healthier probably will have values consistent with level two.

Serious competitive amateur athletes and professional athletes who eat a healthy diet may have one or more blood chemistry values associated with level three.

Your goal is level three, the peak-performance level that also reduces the risk of many diet-related diseases. You will be amazed to find how rapidly you can achieve it. After just one month on the Eat to Win Diet, you will be able to measure your progress by comparing your initial five vital values with a second blood chemistry profile taken four weeks after beginning the diet.

In Chapter 4, you will learn which level of the Eat to Win Diet to begin based on your personal blood chemistry values. If you decide not to take a blood chemistry test, you should begin at level one of the diet and remain there at least four weeks. This is will give your blood values a chance to drop into a safer range before continuing on to level two.

In any event, you will be able to measure the results of your new diet on your bathroom scale and with a tape measure. You will also be able to measure your improvement by noting your increased levels of energy and stamina and your improved performance at the job, on the court, and in the bedroom.

Your Personalized Eat to Win Diet

O n the Eat to Win Diet, one size does not fit all.

The Eat to Win Diet differs from all popular high-protein, low-carb diets and other fad diets in many ways, but most significantly, it is the only lifelong eating plan that is personalized to your individual blood chemistry values. Knowing your blood chemistry values is the only rational and scientifically reliable way to begin a diet and to monitor your progress over time.

As the world-champion athletes whom I've helped dominate their sports already know, this is the most scientific, safest, and most effective strategy for success. No other popular diet provides this degree of personalization.

My Eat to Win scoring system, developed after years of analyzing the blood chemistry values of very healthy to very sick people, will help you pick the proper foods, whether dining in or outside of the home, to get you to the highest level of health and fitness possible.

At the start of your diet, your personal physician can be your best coach, because he or she will know if you have any special concerns. Perhaps you're already taking a medication that should not be consumed during the same meal as nonfat dairy. If you are a diabetic taking insulin or oral drugs, or if you are a cardiac patient taking antihypertensive medications or beta-blockers, your physician can help you adjust the dosages of your medications as your blood chemistry and health status improve on the Eat to Win Diet.

I strongly urge everyone to visit his or her physician to have a complete physical and blood chemistry profile before beginning an exercise program or this or any other diet.

Success, like beauty, is in the eye of the beholder. A weekend warrior may define success as simply *finishing* a twenty-six-mile marathon or perhaps beating a regular tennis or golf opponent for the first time. A world-class athlete may define success as winning an Olympic gold medal, the Tour de France, or the Wimbledon finals. The Eat to Win Diet can help athletes and active people at all levels reach their fitness and professional goals. If you are sedentary, the Eat to Win Diet can give you the almost limitless energy to embrace a daily exercise plan.

EATING MEDITERRASIAN STYLE

The Eat to Win Diet for the 21st century emphasizes combining the healthiest foods from the world's two healthiest diets—the Mediterranean and Asian diets.

How do you eat MediterrAsian style?

It's simple—and delicious. The Eat to Win Diet can be as gourmet and sophisticated as you care to make it. It can also be as simple and inexpensive as you wish. Pasta, potatoes, rice, vegetables, tea, and fruits are relatively inexpensive supermarket items, and these are the foods that contribute the most calories on the Eat to Win Diet.

The Eat to Win Diet offers plenty of dining-out options. The reason is that most national cuisines provide ample complex-carbohydrate foods from which to pick. Here a few examples:

Italian: Pasta, vegetables, fruit
Chinese: Rice, noodles, vegetables, soy foods, fruits
Japanese: Rice, noodles, vegetables, soy foods, fruits

Mexican: Beans, tortillas, corn, salsa, vegetables, rice
Thai: Noodles, rice, vegetables, soy foods, fruit
Barbecue: Beans, corn, potatoes, sweet potatoes, bread
Indian: Basmati rice, nan, vegetables, fruit
American: Potatoes, rice, vegetables, fruit

Combine these complex-carbohydrate-rich foods with the pre-
scribed servings and portion sizes of animal-protein foods and fats on
levels one, two, and three of the Eat to Win Diet.

Figure 4.1 shows you how easy it is to construct a MediterrAsian-
style Eat to Win meal. Whenever possible, use these guidelines to combine the foods of each cuisine. By doing so, you will be eating the
healthiest diet possible.

Even fast-food chains make it easy for Eat-to-Winners to stick with
their diet. Figure 4.2 gives you a few examples of how to eat quickly
and cheaply at most fast-food restaurants.

Whether you're dining in or out, Eating to Win MediterrAsian style
is easy, fun, and healthy!

THE EAT TO WIN DIET LEVELS

There are three levels of the Eat to Win Diet, and one of them is right
for you with your personal blood chemistry profile.

The Eat to Win Diet is personalized to your unique, individual biochemical needs because it is based on your own blood chemistry score.
This is the most rational and scientific way to begin your lifelong eating
plan. Moreover, the numbers on your blood chemistry report don't lie.
These scores will be the scientific proof that your new diet is working
when you have a follow-up blood chemistry test just four weeks after
you begin the Eat to Win Diet.

Level one of the Eat to Win Diet is the strictest because it's designed to bring you as quickly as possible to the next two levels of the
diet. It will also improve your level one blood chemistry scores that will
reduce your risk of getting such diet-related diseases as atherosclerosis,
high blood pressure, and type 2 diabetes.

As you move from one level to the next, the Eat to Win Diet be-

FIGURE 4.1

HOW TO CONSTRUCT AN EAT TO WIN MEDITERRASIAN MEAL

Food or beverage	Serving	Mediterranean	Asian
Entrée	1 cup or bowl of whole-wheat pasta with marinara sauce with a 2-oz. serving of clams or lobster	X	
Topping for marinara sauce	1-tablespoon of soy "Parmesan cheese" topping for pasta sauce	X	X
Side salad	Mixed green salad made with a variety of fresh vegetables	X	X
Salad dressing	4 tablespoons balsamic vinegar + 1 teaspoon extra-virgin olive oil	X	
Spirits	Demitasse of saki		X
Spirits	3.5-oz glass of red	X	
Beverage	Green tea with lemon		X
Evening snack	Hot cocoa made with 1%-fat soy milk	X	X

This sample dinner shows how to construct a MediterrAsian-style Eat to Win meal. The gray blocks indicate whether each food or beverage is classified as Mediterranean or Asian or both.

Asian foods and beverages common to the American diet experience include seafood, soy foods and drinks, soy cheese, soy-based mayonnaise (Nayonaise), such vegetables as ginger, daikon root, soybeans, adzuki beans, and such beverages as green tea and saki. Mediterranean foods include seafood, tomato sauce, balsamic vinegar, extra-virgin olive oil, coffee, black tea, cocoa, pasta, and such vegetables as zucchini, squash, and

FIGURE 4.2

EAT TO WIN DINING-OUT SUGGESTIONS

Chinese: grilled tofu; stir-fried mixed vegetables; chow mein; hot and sour soup

Indian: chicken or shrimp tandoori; nan; raita; basmati rice; lentil soup

Italian: any pasta with marinara sauce; chicken cacciatore; pasta e fagi-oli; shrimp or lobster fra diavolo; minestrone soup; mixed garden salad with low-fat dressing; fresh fruit

Japanese: kappa maki roll; California roll; tekka maki roll; grilled tofu; mixed salad with miso dressing; shrimp and vegetables; teriyaki salmon; miso soup; edamame (steamed soybeans); steamed spinach; cucumbers in vinegar

Taco Bell and other Mexican restaurants: bean burritos; beef tacos (lettuce, tomato, and no cheese); pinto or black bean soup; shrimp or chicken fajitas; grilled salmon or mahi-mahi

Pizza Hut: thin-crust pizza (made with tomato sauce, hold the cheese); mixed garden salad with low-fat dressing

Red Lobster and other seafood restaurants: broiled wild salmon; tuna; mahi-mahi; spiny lobster (no drawn butter); steamed vegetables; baked potato; salad with low-fat dressing

Steak house: 4-ounce serving of filet mignon or another lean meat (split one dinner with another person or take the leftover steak home); broiled chicken breast; broiled salmon; steamed broccoli; mixed garden salad with low-fat dressing

Wendy's: mixed green salad with chickpeas; carrot; lettuce, red cabbage, low-fat Italian dressing; baked potato; chili; chicken sandwich with lettuce and tomato (hold the mayo)

Subway: Any low-fat six-inch sub sandwich made with low-fat dressing

comes easier and more permissive. For example, a level one Eat-to-Winner can enjoy up to two fruits each day, with one being a citrus fruit. A level three highly active individual can enjoy up to five fruits each day or a food or condiment with a small amount of added sugar. Steak-and-egg lovers will want to get to level three as quickly as possible to enjoy these foods.

LEVEL ONE: THE GET-IN-SHAPE PLAN

When you want to lose the maximum amount of body fat safely and quickly, this is the plan for you. It's also the plan you must begin if your blood chemistry scores fall in the level one range listed below.

If these are the values reported in your fasting blood chemistry profile, start the Eat to Win Diet at level one:

FIGURE 4.3

Blood chemistry component	Score
Total cholesterol	200 or higher
HDL cholesterol	30 or lower
Triglycerides	150 or higher
Glucose	100 or higher
Uric acid	6 or higher (women) 7 or higher (men)

If any one of your blood chemistry scores matches these numbers, start the Eat to Win Diet at level one.

On the next page are the Eat to Win guidelines for level one. These guidelines include portion sizes, recommendations, and suggestions, which have proven to be quite successful in getting your blood chemistry scores to levels two and three of the diet. These guidelines will get you where you want to go only if you faithfully follow them. They are the result of over twenty years of experience; do not take them lightly.

After only four weeks on level one, you will see a significant improvement in your five vital values, and you will have lost an appreciable amount of body fat. On a ketogenic/high-fat, low-carb diet, much of your weight loss would be due to dehydration and you would walk around glycogen-depleted. Peak physical performance would be impossible.

The Eat to Win Diet is a hydration-based diet, which means that

EAT TO WIN FOOD GUIDELINES: LEVEL ONE

Food group/servings	Examples	Examples	What counts as a serving?
Seafood, meats, egg whites, legumes: 2–4/day Divided between animal and vegetable food sources **Recommended:** At least one serving omega-3 seafood/week **Suggestion:** Enjoy three meatless days each week by choosing legumes or legume-based recipes or entrées	**Omega-3 seafood** Wild salmon, tuna, mahi, mackerel, sardines (avoid farm-raised seafood) **Shellfish** All shellfish except shrimp and Maine lobster (choose spiny lobster)	**Lean meats** Turkey, chicken, buffalo, lean cuts of beef **Eggs** Egg whites; commercial egg substitutes **Legumes** Beans, peas, and lentils	• 2 ounces seafood, lean meat, or white meat poultry • One serving soy-based meat-replacement products • ½ cup peas, beans, lentils • 1 egg white
Vegetable Unlimited Recommended: Have five servings of cruciferous vegetables and five servings of tomato sauce each week; choose at least two vegetables from each category every day	**Carotene-rich** Tomatoes, carrots, sweet potatoes, yams, yellow squash, corn, spinach, tomato sauce	**Cruciferous** Broccoli, cabbage, cauliflower **Organo-sulfur** Garlic, leeks, onions, shallots	• ½ tomato sauce • ½ cup other vegetables (cooked or raw) • 1 cup raw, leafy vegetables such as lettuce
Fruits: 1–2/day Recommended: One serving of citrus every day	**Citrus** Oranges, lemons, limes, grapefruit	**Berries** Blueberries, raspberries, cranberries, strawberries **Other** Apples, cherries, kiwi, melon, papaya, mango, etc.	• 1 medium apple, orange • ½ grapefruit • ½ cup berries or chopped, cooked, or canned fruit (no syrup) • ½ cup diced fruit (e.g., melon)

Grains, cereals, potatoes: 2/day
Recommended: One baked potato w/topping each day as a lunch entrée

Oatmeal
Three- to five-minute whole oats

Russet baking potatoes
1 medium

Rice
Brown is preferred but white is permitted when dining out at sushi bars and Asian restaurants

Bread and pasta
Whole-grain breads, crackers, pasta, etc. White pasta okay when dining out. Avoid pasta made with egg yolks

- 1 slice whole-grain bread
- ½ cup whole-grain cereal, cooked

Dairy: 1–2/day
Recommended: Choose nonfat when possible

Nonfat milk

Low-fat yogurt
No sugar added; choose 1 to 2 percent fat

Low-fat cottage cheese
Uncreamed preferred; choose 1 to 2 percent fat

- ½ cup nonfat milk
- ½ cup low-fat yogurt
- ½ cup low-fat cottage cheese

Added fats and oils: 1–2/day
Recommended: Use extra-virgin olive oil when possible
Suggestion: Limit consumption of all oils as much as possible

Monounsaturated-rich
Olive oil, canola oil, sesame oil

Polyunsaturated-rich
Tofu-based mayonnaise or reduced-fat mayonnaise

Other
Consume no added vegetable fats other than monounsaturated oils; avoid all foods that contain trans fats (check ingredient labels)

- 1 teaspoon oil
- 1 tablespoon tofu mayonnaise (Nasoya Nayonaise brand) or reduced-fat regular mayonnaise

Beverages
Recommended: 3 cups of green tea each day; up to 3 cups of coffee each day if desired (decaffeinated preferred); all sugar-free drinks (Splenda sweetener is okay)

Green tea
With or without caffeine; if decaffeinated, consume as desired, up to 5 cups per day

Hot cocoa
Use sugar- and fat-free brands or use homemade with Splenda sugar substitute
Dark bittersweet chocolate, ½ ounce, three times per week

Coffee
With or without caffeine. Avoid French-press method due to excess caffeine. Limit consumption to 3 cups of caffeinated coffee per day

- 1 cup

FIGURE 4.4

LEVEL ONE

**Average Daily Percent of Total Calories for
Protein, Fat, and Carbohydrate**

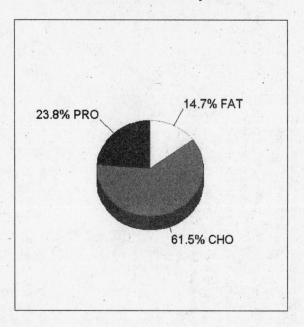

23.8% PRO

14.7% FAT

61.5% CHO

your cells will contain a healthy supply of water and glycogen, ready to fuel your muscles in an emergency or during your next round of golf or game of tennis. The extra water and glycogen you will carry within your muscles will *not* add fat to your body.

You will weigh a bit more than if you were dehydrated and glycogen depleted, but it's healthy and desirable to carry this weight within the body—this is the kind of weight you do not wear. And just like the sports champions you admire, this reserve of water and glycogen will help you go faster, higher, and farther.

In Section II you'll find recipes I have developed for the power meals you will enjoy at every level of the Eat to Win Diet. Professional and weekend athletes alike have tested these recipes and found them delicious and highly effective.

Every recipe contains nutritional information that will tell you how much protein, carbohydrate, fat, cholesterol, sodium, and calories it provides per serving. In this chapter, I've given you a sample week of menus for each of the three levels of the Eat to Win Diet. Even if you dine out more than in, you can still easily follow the Eat to Win food guidelines at most any restaurant, including fast-food chains. Remember Jared Fogel's Subway diet? Jared lost nearly an eighth of a ton of excess body fat eating out exclusively. If he can do it, so can you.

LEVEL TWO: THE STAY-IN-SHAPE PLAN

After you have followed level one for twenty-eight days, you will probably be ready for level two (a second blood chemistry profile test will determine if you meet the criteria for level two). By this time, you will have lost body fat and will have noticed that your energy, endurance, and sports performance have improved.

Level two is designed to help you keep in shape, continue to shed excess body fat, if desired, and continue to move your blood chemistry scores into the healthiest of levels—level three.

If these are the values reported in your fasting blood chemistry profile, move on to level two of the Eat to Win Diet:

FIGURE 4.5

Blood chemistry component	Score
Total cholesterol	160–190
HDL cholesterol	45 or more
Triglycerides	90–149
Glucose	85–95
Uric acid	5 or less (women) 6 or less (men)

If any one of your blood chemistry scores matches these numbers, start the Eat to Win Diet at level two.

EAT TO WIN FOOD GUIDELINES: LEVEL TWO

Food group/servings	Examples	Examples	Examples	What counts as a serving?
Seafood, meats, egg whites, legumes: 2–4/day Divided between animal and vegetable food sources **Recommended:** At least one serving omega-3 seafood/week **Suggestion:** Enjoy three meatless days each week by choosing legumes or legume-based recipes or entrées	**Omega-3 seafood** Wild salmon, tuna, mahi, mackerel, sardines (avoid farm-raised seafood) **Shellfish** All shellfish except shrimp and Maine lobster (choose spiny lobster)	**Lean meats** Turkey, chicken, buffalo, lean cuts of beef **Eggs** Egg whites; commercial egg substitutes	**Legumes** Beans, peas, and lentils	• 2 ounces seafood, lean meat, or white meat poultry • One serving soy-based meat-replacement products • ½ cup peas, beans, lentils • 1 egg white
Vegetables: Unlimited Recommended: Have five servings of cruciferous vegetables and five servings of tomato sauce each week; choose at least two vegetables from each category every day	**Carotene-rich** Tomatoes, carrots, sweet potatoes, yams, yellow squash, corn, spinach, tomato sauce	**Cruciferous** Broccoli, cabbage, cauliflower	**Organo-sulfur** Garlic, leeks, onions, shallots	• ½ tomato sauce • ½ cup other vegetables (cooked or raw) • 1 cup raw, leafy vegetables such as lettuce
Fruits: 1–3/day Recommended: One serving of citrus every day	**Citrus** Oranges, lemons, limes, grapefruit	**Berries** Blueberries, raspberries, cranberries, strawberries	**Other** Apples, cherries, kiwi, melon, papaya, mango, etc.	• 1 medium apple, orange • ½ grapefruit • ½ cup berries or chopped, cooked, or canned fruit (no syrup) • ½ cup diced fruit (e.g., melon)

Grains, cereals, potatoes: 2–3/day
Recommended: One baked potato w/topping each day as a lunch entrée

Oatmeal
Three- to five-minute whole oats

Russet baking potatoes
1 medium

Rice
Brown is preferred but white is permitted when dining out at sushi bars and Asian restaurants

Bread and pasta
Whole-grain breads, crackers, pasta, etc. White pasta okay when dining out. Avoid pasta made with egg yolks

- 1 slice whole-grain bread
- ½ cup whole-grain cereal, cooked

Dairy: 2/day
Recommended: Choose nonfat when possible

Nonfat milk
Three- to five-minute whole oats

Low-fat yogurt
No sugar added; choose 1 to 2 percent fat

Low-fat cottage cheese
Uncreamed preferred; choose 1 to 2 percent fat

- ½ cup nonfat milk
- ½ cup low-fat yogurt
- ½ cup low-fat cottage cheese

Added fats and oils: 1–3/day
Recommended: Use extra-virgin olive oil when possible
Suggestion: Limit consumption of all oils as much as possible

Monounsaturated-rich
Olive oil, canola oil, sesame oil

Polyunsaturated-rich
Tofu-based mayonnaise or reduced-fat mayonnaise

Other
Consume no added vegetable fats other than monounsatureated oils; avoid all foods that contain trans fats (check ingredient labels)

- 1 teaspoon oil
- 1 tablespoon tofu mayonnaise (Nasoya Nayonaise brand) or reduced-fat regular mayonnaise

Beverages
Recommended: 3 cups of green tea each day; up to 3 cups of coffee each day if desired (decaffeinated preferred); all sugar-free drinks (Splenda sweetener is okay)

Green tea
With or without caffeine; if decaffeinated, consume as desired, up to 5 cups per day

Hot cocoa
Use sugar- and fat-free brands or use homemade with Splenda sugar substitute
Dark bittersweet chocolate, ½ ounce, three times per week

Coffee
With or without caffeine. Avoid French-press method due to excess caffeine. Limit consumption to 3 cups of caffeinated coffee per day

- 1 cup

On pages 82 and 83 are the Eat to Win guidelines for level two. You will notice that you can enjoy an extra fruit serving each day, an additional grain, cereal, or daily potato serving, and one additional daily fat/oil serving.

Just four weeks after beginning level two, you will see continued improvement in your five vital values, and you will have lost additional excess body fat. Your tastes will have undergone a change and the diet will have become much easier to follow.

FIGURE 4.6

LEVEL TWO

Average Daily Percent of Total Calories for Protein, Fat, and Carbohydrate

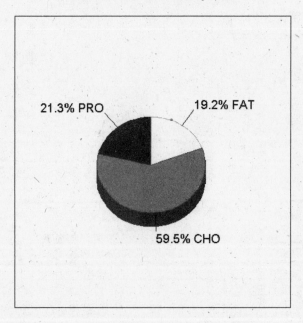

LEVEL THREE: THE PEAK-PERFORMANCE PLAN

When you reach level three of the Eat to Win Diet, you will reach the highest degree of health and wellness possible. Your blood chemistry scores will be superb, you will have reached or be very close to your weight-loss goal, and you will feel the level of energy enjoyed by the sports champions I have helped learn how to eat to win. You'll be at the top of your game, too.

Level three is designed to keep you in peak shape and help you lose the last few pounds of excess body fat (if you still have any to lose).

If you find you are losing too much weight, add one additional fruit serving and one or two servings of whole grains, cereals, or potatoes to your daily menu.

Endurance athletes can add 1 to 2 servings of fats/oil, up to two additional fruit servings, one or two additional servings of nonfat dairy, and additional servings of such complex carbohydrates as pasta, potatoes, rice, bread, and cereals each day as required to maintain body weight.

If the first three components in your fasting blood chemistry profile match these values, *congratulations!* It's time to move up to the highest level of the Eat to Win Diet—level three.

FIGURE 4.7

Blood chemistry component	Score
Total cholesterol	160 or less
HDL cholesterol	60 or more
Triglycerides	75 or less
Glucose	85 or less
Uric acid	4 or less (women) 5 or less (men)

On the next two pages are the Eat to Win guidelines for level three. This level allows you to enjoy an extra fruit serving each day and additional servings of grains, cereals, potatoes, dairy, and animal-protein foods. As with all levels of the diet, vegetables, with few exceptions as noted, can be consumed according to appetite.

EAT TO WIN FOOD GUIDELINES: LEVEL THREE

Food group/servings	Examples	Examples	Examples	What counts as a serving?
Seafood, lean meats, egg whites, legumes: 2–3/day **Recommended:** At least one serving omega-3 seafood/week **Suggestion:** Enjoy three meatless days each week by choosing legumes or legume-based recipes or entrées	**Omega-3 seafood** Wild salmon, tuna, mahi, mackerel; sardines (avoid farm-raised seafood) **Shellfish** All shellfish except shrimp and Maine lobster (choose spiny lobster)	**Lean meats** Turkey, chicken, buffalo, lean cuts of beef	**Legumes** Beans, peas, and lentils	• 2 ounces seafood, lean meat, or white meat poultry • One serving soy-based meat-replacement products • ½ cup peas, beans, lentils • One egg white
Vegetables: Unlimited **Recommended:** Five servings of cruciferous vegetables and five servings of tomato sauce each week; choose at least two vegetables from each category every day	**Carotene-rich** Tomatoes, carrots, sweet potatoes, yams, yellow squash, corn, spinach, tomato sauce	**Cruciferous** Broccoli, cabbage, cauliflower	**Organo-sulfur** Garlic, leeks, onions, shallots	• ½ tomato sauce • ½ cup other vegetables (cooked or raw) • 1 cup raw, leafy vegetables such as lettuce
Fruits: 1–5/day **Recommended:** One serving of citrus every day	**Citrus** Oranges, lemons, limes, grapefruit	**Berries** Blueberries, raspberries, cranberries, strawberries	**Other** Apples, cherries, kiwi, melon, papaya, mango, etc.	• 1 medium apple, orange • ½ grapefruit • ½ cup berries or chopped, cooked, or canned fruit (no syrup) • ½ cup diced fruit (e.g., melon)

Grains, cereals, potatoes: 2–4/day Recommended: One baked potato w/topping each day as a lunch entrée	**Oatmeal** Three- to five-minute whole oats **Russet baking potatoes** 1 medium	**Rice** Brown is preferred, but white is permitted when dining out at sushi bars and Asian restaurants	**Bread and pasta** Whole-grain breads, crackers, pasta, etc. White pasta okay when dining out. Avoid pasta made with egg yolks • 1 slice whole-grain bread • ½ cup whole-grain cereal, cooked
Dairy or dairy substitute: 2–3/day Recommended: Choose nonfat when possible	**Nonfat milk or low-fat soy or rice milk** Use homogenized nonfat milk only; use soy or rice beverages with added calcium	**Low-fat yogurt** No sugar added; choose 1 to 2 percent fat	**Low-fat cottage cheese** Uncreamed preferred when possible; choose 1 to 2 percent fat • ½ cup nonfat milk • ½ cup low-fat yogurt • ½ cup low-fat cottage cheese
Added fats and oils: 1–6/day Recommended: Use extra-virgin olive oil when possible **Suggestion:** Limit consumption of all oils as much as possible	**Monounsaturated-rich** Olive oil, canola oil, sesame oil	**Polyunsaturated-rich** Tofu-based mayonnaise or reduced-fat mayonnaise	**Other** Consume no added vegetable fats other than monounsaturated oils; avoid all foods that contain trans fats (check ingredient labels) • 1 teaspoon oil • 1 tablespoon tofu mayonnaise (Nasoya Nayonaise brand) or reduced-fat regular mayonnaise
Beverages Recommended: 3 cups of green tea each day; up to 3 cups of coffee each day if desired; all sugar-free drinks (Splenda sweetener is okay)	**Green tea** With or without caffeine; if decaffeinated, consume as desired, up to 5 cups per day	**Hot cocoa** Use sugar- and fat-free brands or use homemade with Splenda sugar substitute Dark bittersweet chocolate, ½ ounce, three times per week	**Coffee** With or without caffeine. Avoid French-press method due to excess caffeine. Limit consumption to 3 cups of caffeinated coffee per day • 1 cup

FIGURE 4.8

LEVEL THREE

**Average Daily Percent of Total Calories for
Protein, Fat, and Carbohydrate**

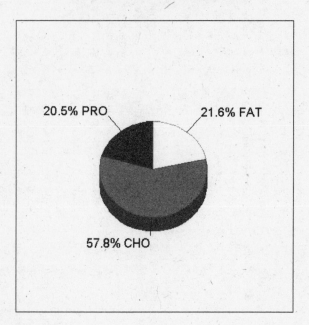

20.5% PRO   21.6% FAT

57.8% CHO

THE EAT TO WIN VEGETARIAN DIET

Most people are only one step away from enjoying a meat-free version of the Eat to Win Diet. Simply replacing the meat, seafood, fowl, pork, and beef with legumes, peas, beans, and lentils turns the Eat to Win Diet into an ovo (egg white)-lacto (nonfat/low-fat dairy) vegetarian diet. Strict vegetarians, or vegans, can simply eliminate the nonfat/low-fat dairy and egg whites to follow the Eat to Win Diet. Since eliminating dairy could mean consuming insufficient calcium, be sure to include calcium-rich vegetables including legumes, broccoli, kale, and other leafy greens.

The body did not evolve in a strict vegetarian diet, a fact made evident by the body's absolute requirement for vitamin B_{12}.[1] The vitamin is found only in foods of animal origin. Some health faddists believe that intestinal bacteria can synthesize enough of the vitamin to sustain human life. I wouldn't want to bet my life on it. That's why I recommend that vegans obtain this vitamin from meat substitutes like soy burgers and tofu dogs that are fortified with vitamin B_{12}, zinc, and iron. Fortified soy beverages will help vegans meet calcium and vitamin D needs. Rice beverages and those made from oats and nuts aren't an adequate substitute for soy milk. Vegans can also take a vitamin B_{12} supplement every two weeks or use the MediterrAsian Maxi-Blend supplement (available at the MediterrAsianDiet.com Web site) to be certain they are meeting their daily nutritional requirements.

For convenience, I have created an Eat to Win Food Guide Pyramid for Vegetarians to help vegetarians make wise food choices and stay within the Eat to Win nutritional guidelines.

Legumes and soy foods make excellent protein-dense food choices for vegetarians. Vegetarians can also enjoy the maximum amount of fat servings per day because the Eat to Win Vegetarian Diet is very low in total fats and saturated fats and cholesterol.

In order for vegetarians to consume sufficient alpha-linolenic acid (ALA), an essential fatty acid that the body can convert into the omega-3 fatty acids eicosapentaenoic acid (EPA) and docosahexaenoic acid (DHA), they must consume such foods as flaxseed oil, walnut and perilla oils, and purslane, a wild plant.

I recommend that carnivores also use the Eat to Win Diet Food Guide Pyramid for Vegetarians (Figure 4.9) to go "meatless" three days each week. This will result in more rapid fat loss and a faster decline in LDL cholesterol levels.

NEXT: THE EAT TO WIN DIET EXPLAINED

Chapter 6 contains all of the rules and guidelines you'll need to begin the Eat to Win Diet. You'll learn why controlling your body's glycogen—

---

1. Although the liver can store vitamin B_{12} for years, many dietary and environmental factors can interfere with the vitamin's absorption and bioavailability.

FIGURE 4.9

THE EAT TO WIN DIET FOOD GUIDE PYRAMID

for Vegetarians

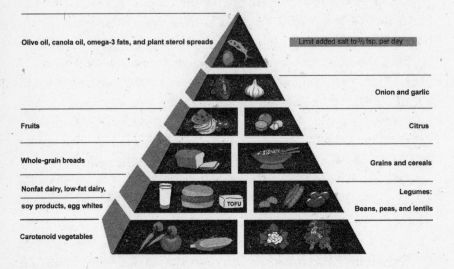

Olive oil, canola oil, omega-3 fats, and plant sterol spreads

Limit added salt to ½ tsp. per day

Onion and garlic

Fruits

Citrus

Whole-grain breads

Grains and cereals

Nonfat dairy, low-fat dairy,
soy products, egg whites

TOFU

Legumes:
Beans, peas, and lentils

Carotenoid vegetables

the storage form of carbohydrate in your body—is vital to lasting fat loss.

I'll tell you how to use the healthiest seafood, nonfat dairy, legumes, slimming carbs, and friendly fats to help you reach your fitness and weight-loss goals safely and quickly. You'll learn which vegetable groups provide the highest phytonutrient protection and how to use alcohol as part of your new diet. I'll even tell you how to enjoy chocolate and not jeopardize your weight-loss or fitness goals.

Q & A

Q. Reading about mercury makes me wonder: Is seafood really a healthier alternative than red meats and poultry?
A. Seafood poses its own health risks—like most other food groups—unless you know from whence the seafood came. People who switch from beef to fish for health reasons (including avoiding mad cow

disease) now have their own worries. Eating a healthy diet has become tricky business.

Although such fish as salmon, mackerel, sardines, shark, tuna, and trout contain friendly omega-3 fats, there are some potential risks that you can avoid by picking the proper fish. Here's the scuttlebutt on seafood safety, matey:

Recent press coverage on methylmercury contamination of seafood, especially swordfish and shark, sent people searching for alternatives to their favorite fish. These fish tend to contain more mercury than other seafood, but unless you are pregnant or have a medical condition that would be aggravated by trace amounts of mercury in your diet, you probably don't have to worry about enjoying this seafood on occasion. The health benefits of enjoying omega-3-rich seafood far outweigh the health risks of ingesting methylmercury (mercury is also found in many vegetables as well). Thus far, there are no published scientific studies showing that consuming moderate amounts of seafood leads to anything but better health. There are a few precautions you can take to minimize any risk.

A new and more relevant concern with seafood safety relates to eating *farm-raised* fish, not wild fish that swim freely in oceans. A recent U.S.–Canadian study reported in *Science* magazine, which sampled seven hundred wild and farmed salmon, found that farm-raised fish contains alarming levels of toxic contaminants. The seafood industry scrambled to allay public fears that salmon could cause cancer if consumed with regularity. Government officials in Norway, Scotland, Sweden, and the United States dismissed the report as meritless.

While we await further scientific investigation, it would be prudent to avoid consuming seafood laced with assorted environmental toxins; select wild fish and avoid farm-raised seafood.

Farmed salmon in Scotland and the Faroe Islands in the North Atlantic had the most contaminated samples, followed by fish from North American farms. Although the study doesn't conclusively demonstrate why that occurs, the commercial feed used at all the salmon farms appears to be the source of contamination, according to Jeffrey Foran, an environmental scientist and one of the authors of the study. Salmon raised in the waters off Chile appear to contain lower levels of industrial pollutants than anywhere else in the world, according to the study.

In fairness to the farmed fishing industry, these same contaminants are present in meat, poultry, and milk. But rendering plants, which boil down animal carcasses, including those infected with mad cow disease, sell the nutrient-rich residue to animal-feed manufacturers whose products may then be fed not only to cattle but also to farm-raised fish, farm livestock, and even to companion animals. This means that the abnormal proteinlike compounds that cause mad cow disease could be lurking in farm-raised fish, dog and cat food, milk and cheese, and even vitamin supplements (ever wonder where those gelatin capsules come from?).

Choosing wild fish over farm-raised fish makes better sense not only because of its higher omega-3 fatty acid content but also because there's almost no chance it will be infected with mad cow prions. One note of caution: If your waiter tells you that the salmon on the menu is "Atlantic" or "Pacific" salmon, this does not ensure that it swam in those oceans. These labels only describe a type of fish and not where it was caught. The salmon has to be designated as "wild" salmon, which means that it lived and was caught in an ocean or stream.

If you're still in doubt about salmon, you can order arctic char, a fish that looks like and tastes similar to wild salmon but doesn't contain the same high levels of environmental toxins. It has a light, delicious taste.

Fish-oil supplements are generally free of such environmental contaminants as mercury, lead, cadmium, arsenic, PCBs, and dioxin, but their safety has been called into question by a number of studies that link them to raising blood cholesterol and blood sugar scores. Fish-oil supplements will also raise the fat content of your diet. Check with a physician to see if they're right for you before using fish-oil supplements.

Q. I've heard that using flaxseed can replace the need to eat seafood to obtain healthy omega-3 fats. Is this true?

A. It is true that flaxseed and purslane, a wild plant, contain a rich supply of alpha-linolenic acid, which the body can convert into EPA and DHA, the friendly fats in seafood. We cannot assume that linolenic acid confers the same health benefits as EPA and DHA because it is structurally different and enjoys only limited conversion to these two fatty acids in people.

The health benefits of alpha-linolenic acid have not been as widely studied or firmly established as EPA and DHA. If you have no reason to avoid seafood (i.e., you are not a vegetarian or allergic to seafood), I recommend eating fish rather than relying exclusively on flaxseed or other sources of alpha-linolenic acid to obtain a healthy dose of EPA and DHA.

Q. Is it healthier to switch from eating red meats to eating chicken?

A. The ordinary supermarket bird is nothing to cluck about. It's the main source of the poison arsenic in the human diet. Researchers at the National Institutes of Health found that Americans who consume 12 ounces of chicken a day consume about 15 percent of the "tolerable" daily limit for arsenic. (I'll bet you didn't know the government has decided that there is actually a safe amount of arsenic you can ingest each day.)

Scientists don't really know how much arsenic people can tolerate over the long-term before they become ill. Arsenic is actually an approved animal-feed supplement used to control the growth of intestinal parasites in chickens. Even if the government's standard for the allowable arsenic content of chicken meat is safe, there are still thousands of cases of food poisoning each year in people who eat tainted chicken, which casts doubt on the desirability of switching exclusively to chicken as your main source of animal protein. The good news for chicken lovers: As long as you select organic free-range chickens and remove the skin before eating the white meat only, you probably won't run the risk of consuming dangerous levels of environmental toxins or getting a food-borne illness (provided you cook the bird thoroughly). More good news: There is no documented case of anyone having died of arsenic poisoning from eating chicken. Now that's something to crow about.

Q. Some health experts claim eggs are too high in fat and cholesterol; others claim eggs are a healthy food. What's the truth?

A. Many Americans are frying up a new breed of egg produced by chickens fed flaxseed and other sources of omega-3 fats. These eggs contain fewer grams of fat and less cholesterol than regular eggs. Many consumers report they taste better than regular eggs and are willing to pay a premium price for better health and perceived taste.

Consumer demand for designer eggs is fueled more by the desire to follow a low-carb diet than by the need for better-tasting eggs. Chickens that lay reduced-fat/cholesterol eggs are fed canola oil and other types of vegetable oil along with flaxseed and kelp. Hens raised on a special-diet produce eggs with fewer saturated fats and more omega-3 fatty acids, iodine, vitamins A and E, and B vitamins B_6, B_{12}, folic acid, and vitamin E. If marigold extract is added to their diet, they lay eggs high in lutein, a nutrient linked to eye health.

A compound in egg yolks called lecithin (phosphatidylcholine) reduces the absorption of cholesterol by the intestine. Because eggs provide about half the dietary cholesterol in a typical Western diet, health experts have advised people to cut back on egg consumption. Even though designer eggs are healthier than regular eggs, eating too many eggs each week will raise your blood cholesterol score to dangerous levels if it is already 150 or below (the healthiest score). Only a person with the extremely rare genetic capacity to handle excessive dietary cholesterol can eat several egg yolks every week and enjoy a cholesterol score below 150.

On level three of the Eat to Win Diet, you could enjoy one whole egg each week—provided your blood cholesterol score does not increase as a result. Egg whites are a wonderful fat- and cholesterol-free alternative to whole eggs. They contain fewer calories and just as much protein.

Q. I know fat has twice the calories of protein and carbohydrate and that it increases the risk of heart disease. Are there any other health issues associated with a high-fat diet?

A. Fatty foods have also been declared a health hazard for conditions as varied as gallstones, age-related maculopathy, glaucoma, hearing loss, and several types of cancer. Now a new book suggests that a high-fat diet could be responsible for migraine.

According to Zuzana Bic, author of the book *No More Headaches, No More Migraines,* the elevated levels of free fatty acids in the blood that result from a high-fat diet can prompt a chain of events that culminate in the pounding headache characteristic of migraine.

"By reducing fat intake, you can reduce the severity and frequency of migraines, if not eliminate them altogether," said Bic, who is a professor of hematology and oncology and a preventive medicine specialist at the University of California at Irvine.

Migraines occur when the arteries to the brain narrow and widen, which activates nearby pain receptors. It is generally believed that abnormally low levels of a chemical substance called serotonin trigger these contractions.

Bic's research indicates that fat in the bloodstream promotes changes in blood-vessel walls and platelets, the cell-like particles in the blood. These changes cause serotonin levels to fall, prompting a migraine.

Research shows that reducing fat can lower the frequency and duration of migraines, according to Bic. In a study she led a few years ago, fifty-four migraine patients were told to record food consumption in a diary and keep a record of their headaches. After keeping track of this information for four weeks, participants were then given a further twenty-eight days to make the adjustment to a new diet that limited fat intake to 20 grams per day. In the final twenty-eight-day period participants recorded their headaches and food consumption.

Bic found that a reduction in dietary fat by an average of 60 percent was associated with a 71 percent drop in migraine frequency, a

66 percent decrease in headache intensity, a 74 percent decrease in the duration of the headache, and a 72 percent reduction in quantity of treatment medications.

Q. Is it important to maintain as high an HDL cholesterol score possible? What is a healthy HDL cholesterol score?

A. Cardiologists associate a low HDL cholesterol score with an increased risk of coronary artery disease. In general, this is a valid cause for concern in people and populations that consume cholesterol-rich, moderate- to high-fat diets.

Restricting dietary fat to 25 percent and below tends to cause HDL cholesterol levels to drop. For one reason, such a diet is usually both low in fat and cholesterol; as total cholesterol blood levels decline, HDL cholesterol levels tend to decline as well because they are part of the total cholesterol level.

In countries that consume very-low-fat diets (5 to 20 percent fat and 0 to 100mg cholesterol/day), the incidence of coronary artery disease is much lower than in the United States, despite significantly lower HDL cholesterol scores. For example, the Tarahumara Indians of Mexico have total cholesterol scores of 125, on average, and HDL cholesterol scores of 25, on average. This tribe enjoys great stamina and endurance because of hard work and their favorite sport of kickball that sometimes lasts more than twenty-four hours! Heart disease is extremely rare among the Tarahumaras.

Laboratory studies have shown that reverse cholesterol transport (the job of the HDL carrier molecule) is not impaired by fat restriction even when a low-fat diet leads to a 50 percent drop in HDL cholesterol scores.

Some scientists have mistakenly assumed that feeding a high-complex-carbohydrate, low-fat diet can lead to a downward shift in not only HDL cholesterol but also in the size of LDL cholesterol particle size. This is a cause for concern, since smaller particle size leads to increased atherosclerosis. There is no research, however, to show that this occurs with any regularity, but there is suggestive evidence that such a diet can convert smaller LDL particle sizes to larger ones. One study has shown that a low-fat diet can reduce the oxidation of LDL cholesterol even though the LDL particle size did not change. This would by itself exert a cardiovascular-protective role.

Irrespective of HDL cholesterol and LDL cholesterol levels, we know that participants in the Framingham Heart Study who were able to reduce their total blood cholesterol score to 150 or below didn't die of heart disease. It didn't matter what diets they followed.

In theory, it's best to have the lowest possible LDL cholesterol score and the highest possible HDL cholesterol score. In the real world, the only diet that can achieve sustained blood levels of total cholesterol below 150 (and low levels of LDL cholesterol) is a very-low-saturated-fat, very-low-cholesterol, high-complex-carbohydrate diet. People who follow high-protein, low-carbohydrate diets will not, as a rule, be able to achieve this highly protective blood cholesterol score or sustain it. All evidence to date has shown that people following a ketogenic diet have little to no hope of achieving this heart-healthy score.

Q. If vegetable oils are harmful, then why do you allow extra-virgin olive oil on the Eat to Win Diet?
A. Olive oil has long been touted as heart-healthy oil. Recent studies reveal new evidence why: extra-virgin olive oil helps reduce the oxidation of LDL, or "harmful," cholesterol, linked to the hardening of the arteries.

Replacing other oils in your diet with olive oil can lead to better health provided you follow the Eat to Win guidelines for fats and oils. Daily use of olive oil:

- Improves fluidity of cell membranes
- Diminishes the hazard of lipid peroxidation that affects polyunsaturated fatty acids
- Scavenges free radicals and affords protection against peroxidation of blood fats.
- Decreases plasma levels of LDL cholesterol and increases levels of HDL cholesterol
- Controls the hypertriglyceridemia accompanying diabetes

- Renders circulating lipoproteins less sensitive to peroxidation and thereby diminishes the development of atherosclerosis
- Reduces the risk of breast cancer and colorectal cancer
- Improves inflammatory and autoimmune diseases, such as rheumatoid arthritis, by modifying inflammatory cytokines production
- Enhances gallbladder emptying, thus reducing gallstone risk
- Helps heal gastric ulcers and affords a higher resistance against nonsteroidal anti-inflammatory drug–induced gastric ulcers
- Reduces LDL or "bad" cholesterol levels with consumption of only 25ml of extra-virgin olive oil a day
- Raises levels of antioxidants in the blood, including vitamin E and phenols.

While all types of olive oil are sources of heart-healthy monounsaturated fat, the fact that extra-virgin olive oil is less processed than others means that it also contains higher levels of antioxidants. Other types of phenols—notably those found in products such as red wine and onions—have also been shown to help control cholesterol in a similar fashion. As a bonus, certain compounds in olive oil called UCPs speed up fat metabolism, thus helping counterbalance the fat calories in this heart-healthy oil.

Even though olive oil and another oil rich in monounsaturates, canola oil, don't seem to raise LDL cholesterol levels, the Eat to Win Diet allows only one tablespoon of these oils per day because they are very calorically dense and can upset the healthy chemical balance of the diet. Endurance athletes or those who exercise strenuously can consume a bit more of these oils, but regardless of exercise intensity, too much of these oils can add fat to your body and stop weight loss cold.

A recent study published in a respected medical journal has found that mice bred especially to have high blood levels of LDL cholesterol developed a greater amount of atherosclerosis on these oils than on other vegetable oils. This does not mean this will happen in people, but it does point to the fact that we don't know enough about the effects of oils to recommend them in any but the smallest quantities.

Q. Why is alcohol consumption limited to seven servings of wine or beer each week on the Eat to Win Diet? Can alcohol consumption be a part of a healthy diet?

A. Alcohol can be a source of significant calories in the diet. It supplies 7 calories per gram, compared to fat, which contains 9 calories per gram, and protein, which has just 4 calories per gram. It should be considered a food group because it contains calories and nutrients. Of course, alcohol is toxic to the body and therefore its consumption must be closely regulated. Despite its classification as a toxic substance, alcohol does provide some documented health benefits when consumed in moderation. No one knows if someone who follows the Eat to Win Diet will enjoy the benefits of alcohol because the diet is already so healthy.

A large new long-term Harvard study reported in the *New England Journal of Medicine* reveals it's okay to enjoy daily servings of beer, wine, or spirits because alcoholic consumption protects against heart attacks.

The study, which tracked the drinking habits of nearly forty thousand men over a twelve-year period, provides an important clue as to how alcohol protects against coronary heart disease. It also found that men who drank moderate amounts of alcoholic beverages three or more times a week had a risk of heart attack 30 to 35 percent lower than nondrinkers.

Alcohol can raise levels of HDL cholesterol and improve the body's sensitivity to insulin, platelet function, and other blood-clotting factors. Alcohol improves how the body metabolizes blood sugar while it helps prevent the development of blood clots, which can lead to a heart attack. Since the anti–blood clotting effect is brief, frequent alcohol intake appears to be of greatest benefit.

It's premature to apply these findings to women or to individuals, especially those with a tendency toward alcohol dependency and abuse. Published studies have shown that alcohol can raise the level of a harmful type of estrogen in the body, which could increase the risk of hormone-related cancers. The overall effect of the diet becomes critical: The Eat to Win Diet, which emphasizes cruciferous vegetables, could theoretically negate the undesirable estrogen-raising properties of alcohol, thus allowing women to enjoy a glass of red wine without increasing their risk of breast cancer. Another potential benefit of enjoying wine: Some studies link regular alcohol consumption to increased bone density in women. There is also new research that suggests that long-term consumption of white wine can improve lung function.

The benefits of wine drinking don't stop with the heart: According to new research from Denmark, people who regularly enjoy a glass or two of wine each day are less likely to develop dementia. The new Danish study revealed that the intake of wine, on a monthly or weekly basis, was significantly associated with a lower risk of dementia. They noted that the results did not vary between men and women.

Scientists have identified a compound in red wine that could be just as important as the antioxidant resveratrol in fighting cholesterol. The new family of compounds, known as saponins, seems to be just as healthful as resveratrol, the phytonutrient in red wine thought to be responsible for the so-called French Paradox—the association between red wine and decreased risk of heart disease. There is credible research to cast doubt on the ability of resveratrol to contribute to health. Most wines contain barely detectable levels. A few wines, such red wines from upstate New York, contain small amounts of the substance, but most people don't consume these wines exclusively.

Saponins, located in grape skins, dissolve into wine during the fermentation process. Scientists estimate that the average dietary saponin intake is 15mg per day; one glass of red has a total saponin concentration of about half that, making red wine a significant dietary source. Red wine contains significantly higher saponin levels than white—about three to ten times as much. Among the red wines tested, red zinfandel contained the highest levels. Syrah had the second highest, followed by pinot noir and cabernet sauvignon, which had about the same amount. The white varieties tested, sauvignon blanc and chardonnay, contained much less. Although merlot was not analyzed in this study, researchers believe it contains significant amounts of saponins at levels comparable to the other red wines.

The study also revealed a positive correlation between alcohol content and saponin levels. The red zinfandel tested, which contained the highest level of saponins among all the wines tested, also had the highest level of alcohol, at 16 percent. Other foods containing significant amounts of saponins include olive oil and soybeans.

Alcohol, when consumed as part of the Eat to Win Diet, doesn't seem to add fat to the body, despite what many carb-bashing diet-book authors claim. While studies remain inconclusive at this time, there is evidence to suggest that alcohol may be metabolized in a different manner from other macronutrients. Many alcohol-dependent people consume excessive calories from alcohol yet remain remarkably thin. What is clear is that moderate consumption of alcohol—up to seven servings of wine, beer, or sake each week—will not jeopardize your weight-loss goals.

Q. What are the healthiest beverages to drink on the Eat to Win Diet?

A. Research by Penn State University shows that the average cup of tea brewed for two minutes contains about 172mg of flavonoids. Drinking one cup could be expected to cause an immediate antioxidant protective effect in the body, and about three and a half cups could possibly produce a continuing effect throughout the day.

Tea, cocoa, and chocolate attenuate the inflammatory process in atherosclerosis by reducing the tendency of blood to clot prematurely and by promoting normal endothelial function in the arterial wall. Studies have shown that consuming three to five cups of green tea (decaffeinated is best because it won't keep blood sugar levels elevated as caffeinated tea would do) can accelerate body-fat loss and may help protect against viral infection, cancer, and heart disease.

Consuming moderate amounts of cocoa and dark chocolate,

which are rich in flavonoids, can help cut the risk of cardiovascular disease and may accelerate calorie burning similar to the way green tea increases fat burning.

Coffee (decaffeinated is recommended to stabilize blood sugar levels) contains powerful antioxidants and cancer-fighting phytonutrients. Caffeinated coffee can improve sports performance and endurance, but diabetics must avoid caffeine from all sources because it can keep blood sugar levels dangerously elevated.

Green tea is a special case unto itself because it contains phytonutrients that can stimulate fat burning, reduce the risk of cardiovascular disease, and strengthen the immune system. In addition, these compounds repair cellular damage by neutralizing harmful oxygen molecules, called free radicals. Green tea, with a higher content of the compound EGCG, is not fermented like black tea, which helps preserves the antioxidants in the tea leaf. Black tea is recognized for its ability to protect against heart disease, but green tea may possess some unique cancer-fighting properties. Recently, Australian researchers discovered that drinking green tea could reduce the risk of developing ovarian and prostate cancer. A Dutch study has also revealed that drinking green tea reduces the risk of heart attack.

Studies show that a maximum benefit comes from drinking four to five cups a day. Adding milk or sugar to tea diminishes some of its antioxidant power and slows down the absorption of antioxidants.

Q. Do I have to give up my favorite indulgence—chocolate—on the Eat to Win Diet?

A. Dieters are always eager to find scientific evidence that tells them that their favorite foods are healthy foods. Here's some good news for chocolate lovers: A small amount of chocolate several times a week can be part of your weight-loss diet and provide a healthy dose of disease-fighting phytonutrients. Be sure to choose only dark, bittersweet chocolate with a cocoa content of 60 percent or greater.

- *Cocoa and chocolate contain powerful disease-fighting phytonutrients.* Chocolate contains the same type of phytonutrients found in grapes, tea, and vegetables known to protect against cancer and heart disease.

- *Cocoa and chocolate contain saturated fats but do not raise serum cholesterol levels.* A recent study revealed that feeding several ounces of chocolate per day to young men actually led to a drop in their blood cholesterol levels. No one really knows why, but the major fatty acid in cocoa butter—stearic acid—may be handled differently by the body than other saturated fats because its melting point is above body temperature. The fat in chocolate is a major exception to the rule that eating saturated fats raises blood cholesterol levels.
- *Cocoa and chocolate are tooth-friendly.* Despite the fact that it contains sugar, chocolate contains phytonutrients that create an unfriendly environment for the type of bacteria that causes dental caries. Sorry—you still have to brush and floss!
- *Cocoa and chocolate make you feel good.* Chocolate can behave as a stimulant in some people yet exerts a calming effect in others. How chocolate affects you depends upon your diet, sleep patterns, gender (it seems to elevate mood in women more than in men, but additional research is needed to confirm this anecdotal observation), and genetics.
- *Cocoa and chocolate help you stick to your fat-loss plan.* Indulging in a delicious and healthful treat like chocolate or a warm cup of hot cocoa can keep you from feeling deprived while cutting calories.

5

Eat to Win Diet Rules

Despite what you may have read in fad diet books, you must consume fewer calories than you burn each day (or burn off more calories during physical activity) in order to lose excess body fat.

A ketogenic diet will burn a bit more body fat than a high-carb diet due to energy spent converting protein to sugar, which in turn floods the body with ammonia, urea, and acidic keto acids. The buildup of toxic products forces the body to dehydrate in an attempt to rid itself of these poisons. Dehydration and concomitant loss of glycogen creates the impression that such a diet leads to profound and rapid weight loss when in fact it doesn't. Such diets carry such steep health risks that they simply aren't worth losing a few extra pounds in the short run. Studies have shown that dieters simply can't stick with these diets and begin to regain weight at a much faster rate than they lost it.

You've already learned that your body first must store every morsel of fat you eat before it can be burned for energy. You've also learned that the protein in beef can be converted to fat and sugar and that it causes a larger insulin spike than pasta. Unlike fat and protein, the body uses dietary carbohydrates directly as fuel for energy.

The most scientifically safe and effective strategy for losing excess body fat is to follow a high-complex-carbohydrate diet that is low in fats and oils (but not so low that the diet loses its taste appeal) and walk five or six hours each week. That's a blueprint for lasting fat loss.

The key to this strategy is to empty part of your body's glycogen reserves each day. By doing so, you will have plenty of room to store the complex carbs you eat that the body doesn't use for energy.

Carbs stored as glycogen don't add fat to your body. They simply wait in line to be used as fuel during your next walk or recreational activity.

Since all dietary fat is stored immediately as body fat (carbohydrate and protein are not), it is apparent that the amount of fat you consume becomes the controlling factor in how fat you will look.

The Eat to Win Diet, combined with regular walking or other activity, forces your body to surrender its fat. At the same time, the food chemistry of the Eat to Win Diet lowers your LDL cholesterol and your blood pressure, and normalizes your blood sugar level. Calorie for calorie, it supplies more disease-fighting phytonutrients than any popular high-protein, low-carb diet.

CEREALS

Nothing can keep you from losing weight faster than eating sugary, fat-soaked breakfast cereal. When you mix Mr. Fat with Mr. Sugar, you set the stage for a host of biochemical processes that quickly and easily add fat to your body or keep you from losing additional body fat. Use only whole-grain cereals without added fats, oils, or sugars.

There are many commercial brands of whole-grain cereal from which to select, but I will give you a short list of the tried-and-true cereals that have nourished my world-champion clients:

- Oatmeal
- Shredded Wheat
- Wheatena
- Quaker 100% Whole Wheat

As I've mentioned, oatmeal is *the* breakfast of champions.

LOSE THESE FOODS TO EAT TO LOSE

Peanut and other nut butters

Tahini and other seed butters

Egg yolks

Ice cream

Butter

Mayonnaise

Margarines made with hydrogenated oils (trans fats)

Cheeses

Fatty cuts of meat (e.g., T-bone, porterhouse, pork chops, lamb chops, veal)

Granola and other fatty and sugary cereals

Anything deep-fat fried

Nonfat cookies, cakes, pies

Conventional high-fat salad dressings

Avocado (avoid during weight loss)

Olives (avoid during weight loss)

Hearts of palm (too high in unhealthy fats)

Movie theater popcorn (some chains are now serving reduced-fat popcorn made without trans fats)

Most commercial "energy" bars (satiety value is too low for the calories)

The good news is that many food manufacturers now make low-fat/low-sugar versions of some these food items. Check the nutrition label to make certain that these ersatz products do not contain hydrogenated oils, or added fats or sugars. Some ice-cream manufacturers make low-fat frozen yogurts and ice-cream substitutes that you can enjoy. Use common sense and follow the Eat to Win Diet guidelines when making such choices.

EAT TO WIN BASIC MARINARA SAUCE

28-ounce can of crushed tomatoes
4 cloves garlic, minced
1 tablespoon fresh basil
1 tablespoon low-sodium tamari soy sauce
Parsley

1. Spray a nonstick pan with olive oil cooking spray
2. Place a small amount of water in a frying pan. Sauté garlic.
3. Add crushed tomatoes. Cook for 1 minute.
4. Add basil and tamari. Add parsley to taste.
5. Heat through. Serve over pasta.

Those on levels two and three of the Eat to Win Diet can add 1 teaspoon of extra-virgin olive oil to this recipe. Without the added oil, this recipe has only 50 calories and no fat or cholesterol. Even with the low-sodium soy sauce, it contains less than 400mg of sodium.

THE THREE RULES OF THE EAT TO WIN DIET

1. Select your foods from the Eat to Win guidelines in Chapter 4.
2. Follow the recommended portion sizes to meet your daily calorie requirements.
3. Enjoy a 60-minute walk or its caloric equivalent in exercise at least five days each week. Your goal is to burn at least 300 extra calories each day through exercise (walking is fine) or sports. (Chapter 10 contains a simple and effective exercise plan for beginners.)

Protein
- **Seafood**. Such seafood as salmon, tuna, mackerel, sardines, and anchovies contain health-promoting omega-3 fatty acids. These fats can help reduce muscle and joint inflammation and reduce the risk of degenerative diseases. Studies have shown that people who eat just one serving of fish each week have less body fat and

enjoy reduced risk of cardiovascular disease compared to those who eat a meat-based diet.

- **Nonfat and very-low-fat dairy.** The Eat to Win Diet recommends two servings each day of nonfat milk and other very-low-fat dairy products. Such fermented very-low-fat products as 1-percent-fat yogurt and 1-percent-fat buttermilk are also acceptable. If you don't eat dairy, use a calcium-fortified soy or rice beverage or take a MediterrAsian Multivitamin & Phytonutrient Supplement (available at the MediterrAsianDiet.com Web site).

- **Legumes.** The Eat to Win Diet emphasizes all types of beans, peas, and lentils. Legumes are protein-dense and contain cholesterol-lowering fiber and phytonutrients that can prevent cancer, heart disease, and diabetes. Legumes are also a low-fat and cholesterol-free food source of iron and calcium. Dozens of scientific studies have shown that legumes can reduce the risk of plaque buildup in arteries and normalize blood sugar in diabetics.

- **Soy foods.** Inconclusive research has linked soy consumption to lower rates of disease. Japanese men and women, who eat traditional diets rich in seafood, legumes, and such fermented soy foods as tofu and miso, enjoy much lower rates of prostate and breast cancer than do Americans. When Japanese men migrate to the United States and adopt a high-fat, meat-based Western diet, their rate of prostate cancer approaches that of American men. Native Japanese women, who enjoy a breast cancer rate nearly five times lower than American women, suffer higher rates of the disease when they move to the United States and embrace the ordinary American diet.

Friendly fats

With all the health risks associated with high-fat diets, you may be surprised to learn that there are a few oils that can be a part of a healthy diet. The Eat to Win Diet uses only friendly fats and oils that provide disease-fighting phytonutrients and fatty acids that promote good health, fitness, and fat-burning fats:

- **Extra-virgin olive oil** (derived from the first pressing of olives, which maintains the highest phytonutrient content of any other type of olive oil) is not only a healthy oil but it also promotes fat burning because it contains compounds called UPCs that boost the body's metabolic rate. When extra-virgin olive oil replaces other fats and oils in your diet, the inflammation potential of your diet decreases, allowing joints and muscles to recover faster and with less damage after vigorous physical activity or injury. Olive oil can also help reduce the risk of heart disease when it supplants the saturated fats and trans-fatty acids (found in meat, milk, butter, and many commercially prepared baked goods) in your diet.

- **Canola oil** contains healthy monounsaturated fatty acids and omega-3 fatty acids. Don't get too excited: It still contains far too many calories to be used in anything but single-teaspoon quantities.

- **Soy "mayonnaise"**: Nasoya's Nayonaise brand is sold in most natural foods markets and in supermarket chain stores. This mayonnaise-type spread makes an excellent replacement for real mayonnaise in all Eat to Win recipes. It contains no cholesterol, has less than half the fat of regular mayonnaise, and contains powerful soy isoflavones that lower blood cholesterol levels and reduce the risk of cancer and heart disease.

Slimming carbs

- You can enjoy two servings of starchy, whole-grain breads or cereals each day, but most of your carbs will come from vegetables and one to two servings of low-carb fruits.

- The fiber found in vegetables and oatmeal helps provide satiety and regularity as well as lower blood lipids.

- The secret to enjoying carbohydrate-rich foods while burning fat is to enjoy the carbs found in most vegetables, whole grains (including brown rice), and legumes.

- I recommend choosing at least one citrus fruit each day if you enjoy this type of fruit.[1]
- If you enjoy breakfast cereal, I would like to recommend that you make oatmeal your breakfast cereal of choice. It stands heads and shoulders, nutritionally speaking, above all other breakfast cereals because it contains essential fatty acids, disease-fighting
- phytonutrients, and cholesterol-lowering soluble fiber that also helps maintain stable blood sugar levels.

Don't use instant oatmeal. If you enjoy oatmeal, avoid instant oatmeal, which usually contains added sugar and salt. Instead, use oats that require some cooking. The best-tasting oatmeal is steel-cut oatmeal, which takes about 45 minutes to prepare. If you don't have the time, use oats that require about 3 to 5 minutes to prepare. Oatmeal is the true breakfast of champions because it contains cholesterol-lowering fiber, a full day's ration of essential fatty acids, protein, and trace minerals, and B-complex vitamins.

USING FATS AND OILS ON THE EAT TO WIN DIET

There's an old saying that was never truer than in the 21st century: *You wear all of the fat you eat.*

Many people are surprised to learn that the fat they eat is not burned directly for energy.

When you consume any fat or oil, it goes directly to your hips, thighs, butt, and belly. Dietary fats and oils cannot be burned for energy until your body first stores all of the fat. It's not fair but it used to confer a survival advantage to our forebears who could store enough fat to last through famine and food shortages.

Remember that the next time you eat a fatty food or add fat to your

---

1. Citrus contains potent anticancer compounds—so potent, in fact, that a recent study revealed that people who eat citrus fruit daily may enjoy *more than a tenfold lower* cancer risk than those who rarely eat citrus.

diet. Every gram of the fat in the food you eat will be stored in your problem areas first, so be prepared to wear it proudly.

Now you understand why it's so important to eat a low-fat diet. It's the only healthy way to stay lean for life. The Eat to Win Diet is designed to burn the fat your body stores for energy. When you add regular daily exercise, such as walking, to your lifestyle, you have a winning formula for lasting fat loss.

The Eat to Win Diet allows the use of small amounts of extra-virgin olive oil (derived from the first pressing, and the most acidic) and canola oil in recipes and on salads. Olive oil contains disease-fighting phytonutrients. One tablespoon provides 8 percent of recommended daily intake for vitamin E (about 1.6mg, or 2.3 IU). Olive oil is unique compared to other oils because it can be consumed directly in crude form without refining. This helps reduce oxidation and conserve vitamins and phytonutrients.

Canola oil, like olive oil, is high in monounsaturates and contains the omega-3 fatty acid ALA (alpha-linolenic acid).[2] This is the same omega-3 fatty acid found in high concentrations in flaxseed and in walnuts and leafy vegetables. ALA tends to reduce both beneficial and harmful prostaglandins—hormonelike chemicals made by the body that help regulate immunity and control such vital bodily functions such as inflammation and healing. A third oil—sesame—is okay to use on *rare* occasions when dining on Asian cuisine. Sesame oil contains monounsaturates in addition to sesamin, a compound that possesses anti-inflammatory and cholesterol-lowering properties.

Although not technically an oil, you may use soy-based "mayonnaise" (Nasoya's Nayonaise is my first choice). This makes an excellent replacement for real mayonnaise in recipes and on sandwiches. It contains no cholesterol, has half the fat of regular mayonnaise, and contains disease-fighting soy isoflavones that could reduce the risk of certain cancers and heart disease. Since it contains 4 grams of fat per

2. Scientists at the National Cancer Institute and the departments of Epidemiology and Nutrition, Harvard School of Public Health, have questioned the safety of consuming oils high in ALA. These researchers believe that "increased dietary intakes of ALA may increase the risk of advanced prostate cancer. In contrast, EPA and DHA intakes may reduce the risk of total and advanced prostate cancer."

tablespoon, you must use it wisely to avoid exceeding your fat quota for the day.

ARE MONOUNSATURATED OILS HEART-FRIENDLY FATS?

Many health experts believe that such monounsaturated fats as those found in olive and canola oils may protect against heart disease. This is primarily because these oils contain a smaller percentage of heart-unfriendly saturated fats than butter and because olive oil is the main source of vegetable fat on the highly venerated Mediterranean diet.

This view is misleading. To begin with, all oils tend to raise triglyceride levels in the blood and can easily add fat to the body because they are calorically dense. Oils have poor satiety value, so it's easy to overeat foods laced with them.

Laboratory studies show that feeding unsaturated oils to lab animals promotes atherosclerosis. Scientists have long known that feeding peanut oil, another oil with a high degree of monounsaturates, causes rampant atherosclerosis in lab animals.

Published studies suggest that olive oil and other monounsaturates lower blood cholesterol levels. Published studies link olive oil consumption to lower rates of heart disease, breast cancer, colon cancer, and stroke. One study suggests that the omega-9 fatty acids found in olive oil seem to help reduce body fat by appetite regulation and increased thermogenesis. Although omega-9 fatty acids haven't yet enjoyed the notoriety of monounsaturated and omega-3 fats, you will begin to read more about them because they may play an important role in health and obesity prevention.

Research on the safety of olive oil, canola oil, and other vegetable oils remains inconclusive but it makes sense to limit consumption of these because of their caloric density. Of course, the more you exercise, the more oil your body can handle. Until the 1960s, the natives of Crete consumed a diet of 40 percent fat (much of which was from olive oil). They were very athletic, worked hard, walked great distances each day, and consumed only small amounts animal protein just a few times each week. They enjoyed excellent health and fitness, and didn't become obese.

FOODS DERIVED FROM THE SOYBEAN

Miso	A fermented paste made from cooked, aged soybeans, salt, water, and *koji*, a cultured grain from rice or barley that contains *Aspergillus oryzae* or *Aspergillus sojae*; miso is rich in friendly bacteria and digestive enzymes.
Natto	Made from whole cooked soybeans fermented with *Bacillus natto* until it has a sticky consistency and a pungent odor; natto can be used in place of ordinary cheese.
Soy flour	Made from finely ground roasted soybeans; contains a rich supply of protein; available in a defatted version.
Soy grits	Made from coarsely ground, whole, dried soybeans.
Soy milk	A creamy, milklike beverage made from whole soybeans by grinding soaked, cooked soybeans and pressing soy "milk" out of the beans; commercial soy milks have added ingredients such as sugars, oils, and salt.
Soy sauce	Made from a mixture of whole roasted soybeans, wheat flour, and fermenting agents (e.g., yeast, mold).
Soy yogurt	Made from soy milk fermented by active bacterial cultures.
Tempeh	Made from whole cooked soybeans infused with a culture (a mold called *Rhizopus oryzae*) and left to stand for twenty-four hours; forms a dense cake with a chewy meatlike texture.
Textured vegetable protein	Made from defatted soy flakes that are compressed until protein fibers change structure; must be reconstituted with water before it can be used in recipes to replace ground beef
Tofu	Made from dried soybeans that have been soaked in water and then crushed and boiled. A coagulant (calcium sulfate, vinegar, or lemon juice) is added to separate curd from whey; curds are poured into molds and let sit.

Perhaps this is inducement enough for you to stick with your six-hours-a-week Eat to Win exercise plan!

No vegetable oils, regardless of their source, should be eaten in great quantities. When it comes to added fats and oils, less is better for everyone. You will obtain all of the essential fatty acids required by the body for excellent health from such foods as oatmeal, whole grains and small amounts of olive oil.

SELECTING AND STORING OLIVE OIL

Many major-brand-name olive oils sold in the United States contain only a fraction of "extra-virgin" olive oil—the most desirable and healthiest of all varieties of olive oil. High-quality extra-virgin olive oil is rich in polyphenols and antioxidants. I recommend using only olive oil designated as "cold-pressed extra virgin." You may have to shop around to find it because not all supermarkets carry this type of olive oil. Specialty shops and online catalogs are a good place to look if you can't find this oil in your local market.

I strongly recommend storing olive oil and canola oil in a dark glass container. Research has shown that that olive oil stored in clear or opaque bottles exposed to light can develop unacceptable amounts of peroxides—compounds that can damage health tissues—within three weeks. Olive oil stored in a cool, dark environment can last 120 to 190 days without significant oxidation. Exposure to light and heat increase oxidation and rancidity. Never store olive oil near a stove but rather store it in a cool, dark cupboard, pouring only a small amount into a dispenser for daily use. You may also store olive oil in a refrigerator or freezer without harm; this will actually extend its shelf life. Cloudiness or precipitation may occur with chilling, but letting the oil reach room temperature will clear it and reliquefy it.

Use the chart in Figure 5.1 to figure out how to replace butter and margarine with olive oil or canola oil in recipes.

FIGURE 5.1

BUTTER-TO-OLIVE-OIL CONVERSION FOR USE IN RECIPES

Butter	Olive oil
1 teaspoon	¾ teaspoon
1 tablespoon	2¼ teaspoon
2 tablespoons	1½ tablespoons
¼ cup	3 tablespoons
⅓ cup	¼ cup
½ cup	¼ cup plus 2 tablespoons
⅔ cup	½ cup
¾ cup	½ cup plus 1 tablespoon
1 cup	¾ cup

FIGURE 5.2

GOOD VEGETABLE SOURCES OF OMEGA-3 FATS

Alpha-linolenic acid content of vegetables from highest to lowest:

- Legumes
- Tofu
- Walnuts
- Flaxseed
- Broccoli, cauliflower, spinach

EAT TO WIN VEGETABLE GROUPS

Various vegetables and vegetable groups provide different types of phytonutrients that you will need for optimal health and fitness. Through years of research, I have determined that we require a full spectrum of phytonutrients to achieve maximum protection from the diet-related diseases that stalk most Americans. Here is a summary of the four Eat to Win vegetable groups and why they are important:

1. **Carotenoid**: These vegetables and fruits (e.g., tomatoes, tomato sauce, carrots, yams, watermelon, pink grapefruit, guava) provide the full spectrum of carotenoids, so important in preventing cancer and heart disease and promoting good lung function and eye health.

2. **Cruciferous**: This category of vegetables, which includes broccoli, cauliflower, and cabbage, helps the liver deactivate environmental carcinogens and helps prevent certain types of estrogen-related cancers by helping the body convert the hormone into its benign form. Cruciferous vegetables also contain important carotenoids.

3. **Organo-sulfur**: These pungent vegetables (onions, garlic, shallots, leeks, etc.) contain important trace minerals and sulfur compounds that protect against various types of cancer and heart disease. Researchers at the National Cancer Institute recently reported in a new study that a diet rich in organo-sulfur vegetables group reduces the risk of prostate cancer by about half.

4. **Phytoestrogen**: This category includes all types of beans, peas, and lentils. In addition to providing high-quality protein, this group is rich in phytoestrogens and antioxidants, which may exert a protective effect against several types of cancer. This group also provides the type of fiber that will lower your risk of cardiovascular disease and colon cancer. Phytoestrogen-rich vegetables are a good source of iron and B-complex vitamins, calcium, magnesium, and such trace minerals as manganese and selenium.

PEAK-PERFORMANCE SUGGESTIONS

Eat a combination of raw and cooked vegetables. Cooking can rob vegetables of such water-soluble nutrients as B-complex vitamins and vitamin C, and such minerals as calcium and magnesium. Some vegetables release their powerful vitamins and phytonutrients only when cooked. The ly-copene in a tomato tends to become concentrated in cooked tomato sauce and becomes more bioavailable, which means your body will absorb more of the lycopene. Thus, it makes good sense to eat raw tomatoes and tomato sauce.

Never add salt to the water in which you boil pasta or vegetables. Conventional cookbooks call for salt in the cooking pot. The only reason for this is that water boils faster when you add salt to it, but this also means unnecessary sodium in your diet. Less added salt is better for everyone except those with medical conditions (e.g., neurocardiogenic syncope, which causes dizziness upon standing) that may require some additional sodium in the diet. Check with your physician to determine if there is any medical reason you should avoid added salt in your diet.

Use a microwave oven to prepare crisp and nutritious vegetables. Microwave ovens cook vegetables without sacrificing their essential nutrients. Vegetables come out crisp and tender and more nutritious when prepared this way.

EAT TO WIN–STYLE STIR-FRY COOKING

Slice vegetables of choice as thin as possible. Heat a nonstick pan until a drop of water "dances" on it. Measure 2 teaspoons of olive or canola oil into the pan. Stir vegetables in rapid and continual motion with a nonmetal spatula until they become bright green or translucent (one to two minutes). Reduce heat to low. Add 2 tablespoons of lemon or lime juice and ¼ teaspoon of low-sodium soy sauce plus 1 tablespoon of water. Cover the pan with a tight-fitting lid and cook for two to three minutes. Use any additional spices you enjoy to taste. The vegetables will be crisp-tender, deliciously flavored, and will retain most of their vitamin and mineral content.

Potatoes and other root vegetables (beets, turnips, parsnips, etc.) are not suitable for the stir-fry method. Bake them or steam them without peeling before cooking. A vegetable steamer is inexpensive and easy to use, but a colander placed in a small amount of unsalted boiling water and closely covered will do the trick.

Make the ordinary baked potato into a meal. I have many enviably thin clients who have used this healthy weight-loss strategy to stay lean and fit for the last twenty years. The trick is to turn an ordinary russet baking potato into a meal. You can have a bowl of vegetarian vegetable soup or a salad made with a nonfat or very-low-fat dressing with it as well. Use such low-fat toppings for your baked potato as Benecol or other heart-healthy butter substitute, low-fat yogurt, low-fat cottage cheese, or even barbecue sauce. You can add a small amount of soy bacon bits or chips and pepper or vegetable seasoning. If you make this a lunchtime habit, you will be quite satiated (recall that the ordinary baking potato provides the highest satiety of any food thus far tested) and well nourished. You will also shed excess body fat faster.

WHAT ABOUT SUGAR AND SALT?

When it comes to sugar and salt, less is better for everyone. I recommend that you do not use added salt in cooking or at the table. There is no reason to add sugar to foods because of the availability of the relatively safe sugar replacer sucralose (Splenda). All herbs and spices ordinarily used in cooking are permitted on the Eat to Win Diet.

Sugar

More than three decades ago, John Yudkin, MD, author of the book *Sweet and Dangerous*, asked, "Is there a link between sugar and cancer?" Yudkin had studied the health effects of sugar for decades and found that a high sugar intake was linked to serious health problems such as leukemia in men and women, rectal cancer in men, and breast cancer in women. Yudkin also suspected that sugar intake was associated with heart disease. Now, more than twenty years later, it seems Yudkin asked the right question.

How harmful is sugar? In the past, nagging nutritionists warned that sugar is devoid of all nutrients except calories, and dentists have decried sweets as a risk for tooth decay. Now health experts have issued a third caution that can't be sugarcoated: two recent reports, one from the Netherlands and the other from Italy, suggest that a high sugar intake might, indeed, be a risk factor for certain types of cancer.

When researchers at the National Institute of Public Health and Environmental Protection in the Netherlands studied more than a hundred cases of gallbladder cancer and biliary tract cancer, they discovered that sugar intake was linked to an increase in biliary tract cancer. Previous studies had shown evidence that high sugar intake was associated with gallstone formation, which itself is linked to biliary tract cancer, along with obesity.

In the other study, conducted in Italy, researchers studied food intake data between 1985 and 1992 from a variety of dietary factors of people with colorectal cancer. Compared to patients who added no sugar to their beverages, the sugar users showed an increased risk of colon and rectal cancers. The risks increased proportionally with amounts used.

How much sugar is too much? Some scientists would argue that any refined sugar in the diet is a risk factor for cancer, heart disease, obesity, gallstones, hypoglycemia, depression, and gout.

Most people enjoy the taste of sugar but should limit its intake because it is a highly concentrated food stripped of its fiber and nutrients. Americans consume, on average, over two pounds of sugar each week— about 25 percent of their total calories. The average American woman eats nearly her weight in sugar every year. Three-fourths of the sugar we eat comes in processed foods, one-fourth from pure tabletop sugar.

I've found that by limiting the use of tabletop sweeteners, such as white or brown sugar, honey, molasses, and syrups, you can reduce your sugar intake to a reasonably safe level. This allows for the use of sugar-containing foods and condiments, such as ketchup, and an occasional sweet dessert. Whole fruit—which contains sugar—is acceptable because it contains disease-fighting phytonutrients and fiber, which helps slow the release of carbohydrates into the blood during digestion. That's why fruit and not the sugar bowl should be your primary source of sugar. If you must add sugar to coffee, tea, or other beverages, limit consumption to two teaspoons a day for all tabletop sweeteners.

Use Splenda brand sweetener in place of sugar. If you like to sweeten your coffee, tea, or other beverage, use this sweetener above all others. Splenda is made from ordinary sugar, but its molecular structure prevents the body from absorbing it and breaking it down into calories. You can also use Splenda to sweeten a particularly tart fruit such as grapefruit. It tastes great on strawberries as well. Many commercial presweetened beverages, such as those made by Ocean Spray, now use Splenda as a sweetener. You still have to be careful with these commercial drinks because they do contain appreciable calories from other carbohydrates. I suggest that you limit your intake to one 8-ounce serving per day.

Salt

Many health experts now believe that salt in the American diet does not contribute substantially to hypertension for the majority of Americans. While some people who are sodium-sensitive must drastically curtail their intake of salt, most of us don't get hypertension as a result of eating it. Why, then, is salt restricted on the Eat to Win Diet?

Salt causes edema (swelling) in the body, depriving cells of oxygen. The ratio of sodium to potassium is also adversely affected, creating an unhealthy environment inside cells.

Salt, when consumed in excess, increases calcium losses through urine and may decrease bone density. Studies have shown that at sodium intakes above 2,100mg a day (slightly less than what's in 1 teaspoon of salt), women lost calcium each day in their urine. Women who ate the most sodium lost the most bone in their hips. If your diet is high in sodium you'll need to increase your calcium intake significantly.

Cancer cells thrive in an oxygen-poor (anaerobic) environment. Excess salt in the diet fosters this cancer-promoting milieu by blocking oxygen transfer between blood vessels and cells. Too much dietary salt disrupts the delicate sodium/potassium ratio inside cells, creating a cancer-friendly environment.

There is some added salt permitted in the Eat to Win Diet. For example, some recipes use canned tomatoes, tomato sauce, ketchup, and mustard. All of these products generally contain some salt (salt-sensitive individuals can choose low-sodium and sodium-free versions of these products). I discourage adding salt to foods or to the cooking pot, but most healthy adults can safely use up to ½ teaspoon of added salt to recipes and foods. Even limiting salt in this way, people may overconsume salt if they use too many canned or frozen foods. That's why your new way of eating should include one-third to one-half of its calories from fresh fruits and vegetables.

I suggest monitoring the amount of salt you can tolerate with a home blood pressure kit, sold in most drugstores. As with sugar, less is better for most people.

FIGURE 5.3

PICKING THE SAFEST SEAFOOD ON THE EAT TO WIN DIET

No seafood is 100 percent contamination-free but this list will allow you to select your favorite seafood and enjoy the health benefits of omega-3 fats and reduce the risk of methylmercury contamination. Clams, mussels, oysters, salmon, sardines, shrimp and tilapia contain methylmercury levels so low that they are undetectable. Try to consume only fresh seafood whenever possible.

Albacore tuna	Pollock
Atlantic cod	Salmon, Atlantic, wild
Calamari	Salmon, Coho, wild
Clams	Sardines (water-packed)
Dungeness crab	Scallops
Spiny lobster	Shrimp
Flounder	Sole
Halibut	Stone crabs
Mahi-mahi	Tilapia
Mussels	Tuna (light meat, water packed)
Oysters	

Avoid these fish, because they contain the highest levels of methylmercury contamination.

Bass	Marlin
Chilean sea bass	Shark
King mackerel	Swordfish

A CAUTION ABOUT ALCOHOL

Wine contains phytonutrients that can help fight cancer and heart disease. If you enjoy drinking wine, there's no reason to stop, provided that you consume no more than a glass each day (I believe one glass each week provide a healthy dose of phytonutrients). If you don't enjoy drinking wine, you can obtain a wealth of disease-fighting phytonutrients from eating the fruits and vegetables on the Eat to Win Diet.

On a high-fat, low-carb diet, alcohol can help convert the hormone estrogen into a more toxic form that can raise the risk of certain types of cancer. The rich phytonutrient content of the Eat to Win Diet offers protection against the conversion of estrogen into its harmful form. The bottom line: If you enjoy alcohol, continue to do so in moderation on the Eat to Win Diet. If you don't drink, don't start.

ENJOYING CHOCOLATE

Chocolate? On a healthy diet?

Yes. Chocolate. Pure, rich, dark, bittersweet chocolate, that is.

Most of my clients are surprised to learn that they can cheat with chocolate and "get away with it." The truth is, chocolate is a respectable "cheat." Here's why:

Chocolate—in the recommended amounts—won't make you fat. A ½-ounce serving of dark chocolate contains only 75 calories. No one ever got fat eating 75 calories of anything.

Chocolate makes you feel good. Chocolate can behave as a stimulant in some people yet exerts a calming effect in others. How chocolate affects you depends upon your diet, sleep patterns, gender (it seems to elevate mood in females more than in men, but additional research is needed to confirm this anecdotal observation) and genetics.

Chocolate helps you stick to your fat-loss plan. Indulging in a delicious and healthful cheat like chocolate can keep you from feeling deprived while dieting. In my clinical experience, people who rely on chocolate to satisfy their urge to enjoy a tasty treat seem to find it easier to stick with their weight-loss plan.

As long as you don't exceed the recommended amount of dark, bittersweet chocolate per week (½ ounce up to four times a week), you will be able to enjoy the taste and health benefits of this unique food product on the Eat to Win Diet. Dark, bittersweet chocolate contains less sugar and more phytonutrients than regular milk chocolate because of its higher cocoa content.

There are many fine chocolates on supermarket shelves to pick from, such as Godiva and Lindt brands. Some manufacturers make dark chocolate with 70 percent cocoa butter. This type of chocolate has a high phytonutrient level. If you can't find the 70 percent cocoa version of your favorite chocolate, you can use Lindt semisweet chocolate in a pinch.

Here's an even healthier way to get your chocolate fix: Hot cocoa

FIGURE 5.4

SUGGESTED FOOD SUBSTITUTIONS ON THE EAT TO WIN DIET

Replace these foods:	With these foods:
Regular mayonnaise	Nasoya's Nayonaise
Whole egg	Egg white
Conventional candy bars	Dark chocolate (70 percent cocoa)
Ice cream	Sugar-free frozen yogurt
Margarine, butter	Benecol spread
Vegetable oil (corn, safflower, sunflower)	Olive or canola oil
Full-fat milk	Nonfat milk or low-fat soy beverage
Peanut butter and jelly sandwich	Oil-free tuna salad sandwich made with Nayonaise
Full-fat cheese	Veggie low-fat "Parmesan" cheese (0.5g fat/serving)

made from pure cocoa powder also contains the same powerful phytonutrients as chocolate and contains negligible fat. Preparing hot cocoa made with nonfat or low-fat soy milk or cow's milk makes a
delicious and healthful treat, especially for people (your children, perhaps?) who don't consume enough phytonutrients from vegetables. Be
aware that white chocolate has no phytonutrients because it's not made
from cocoa beans and is not an acceptable food on the Eat to Win Diet.

Sport-Specific Diet Guidelines

6

Different sports make different demands on your body. Jogging, recreational skiing, skateboarding, surfing, and dancing are endurance sports that require *aerobic* metabolism. Competitive running, swimming, cycling, and martial arts often call for *high-energy anaerobic activity*; such sports as tennis, basketball, soccer, and football demand both types of metabolism.

I have counseled champion athletes in almost every field of competition, and I have leaned that each type of sport (depending upon whether it demands aerobic metabolism, anaerobic metabolism, or both) requires different diet chemistry. To my knowledge, no other sports nutritionist has developed the detailed instructions that will enable you to eat to win in your favorite sport or activity.

Only when you have completed level one—the get-in-shape level of my program—when your blood chemistry values meet or surpass the standards I have established for entering level two, the stay-in-shape level, should you follow the sport-specific eating plans that follow.

I am going to show you how to easily adjust the Eat to Win Diet to meet the varying metabolic demands of the following sports:

Aerobic dancing	Martial arts
Baseball	Performance car racing
Basketball	Racquet sports
Cycling	Skiing
Football	Soccer
Golf	Strength training
Jogging	Swimming
Long-distance cycling	Triathalon
Marathon running	

But first I want to give you my recommendations for the all-important pregame meal and tell you what and how to eat after competition in order to replenish everything you lost during physical activity.

RECOMMENDATIONS FOR COMPETITORS IN ALL SPORTS

Your Precompetition Meal

Locker-room lore abounds with fact and fiction surrounding the best foods to eat just prior to competition. Collegiate and professional football coaches and trainers still provide plenty of steak and eggs to fuel the fires of ferociousness in their players; professional boxers wolf down lots of red meat; triathlon competitors load up on carbohydrates. Tennis players? Each player has his or her own special pregame meal based more on superstition than science (e.g., "I won my last match eating bacon and eggs, so I'll eat the same way").

There is no single precompetition meal that is best or right for every athlete in every sport. Whenever I work personally with an athlete, I devise the optimal breakfast, lunch, or pregame meal to suit the athlete's individual needs. But there are some very helpful scientific principles I can give you to help you select the best precompetition meal to suit your chosen sport and your personal tastes, as well.

Don't eat a large meal before competition or exercise. Your body cannot perform at its best if your stomach is overloaded. Since physical activity severely retards digestion, you should go into battle with that lean and hungry look. Keep food intake to a minimum to satisfy hunger (no more than 250 calories, if possible). This is equivalent to about 4 slices of whole-grain bread or ¼ cup of whole-grain cereal with ½ cup of nonfat milk and one fresh fruit. Wait at least two hours after eating before beginning your favorite sport or exercise.

Eating fat or protein at this time provides no metabolic advantage to an athlete, because neither can be used directly as energy during imminent competition. Your precompetition or preexercise meal should consist primarily of complex carbohydrates (about 60 to 80 percent of the kilocalories in your pregame meal should come from whole grains, cereals, fruits, breads, pasta, and vegetables). You body will quickly process this type of pregame meal and be able to meet its energy demands.

Drink 1 cup (8 ounces) of water beyond what your thirst requires. Insufficient hydration (lack of water) is the single most frequent fatal flaw in the diet of almost every athlete I've studied or advised. During competition, if possible, drink 1 cup of water for every fifteen minutes of physical activity.

Your Postcompetition Meal

This meal must do three things for you: (1) give you the nutritional building blocks to restore the glycogen your muscles have burned during exercise; (2) replace the fluid, vitamins, minerals, and protein your body needs every day; and (3) replenish amino acids to repair and rebuild muscle tissue. Carbohydrate and protein play a vital role in restoring and rebuilding after sports or exercise.

Athletes in all sports need to replenish their competition-weary muscles with the same basic nutrients. Although each athlete's nutritional needs vary from sport to sport, day to day, I have created an ideal postcompetition meal to meet the metabolic requirements of the most demanding sports and physical activities.

No matter what level of the Eat to Win Diet you follow, enjoy this ideal postcompetition meal after your match.

- 4 ounces of fish or poultry (strict vegetarians should eat 2 cups of beans, peas, or lentils; lacto-vegetarians should eat 1 cup of low-fat cottage cheese and 1 cup of beans; lacto-ovo vegetarians should eat two egg whites [no fatty, cholesterol-laden yolks, please], ½ cup of low-fat cottage cheese or yogurt, and ½ cup of beans)

- One medium baked potato with low-fat topping or two small boiled potatoes or 1 cup of cooked pasta with plain tomato or marinara sauce
- 1 cup of green, yellow, or orange steamed or raw vegetables such as broccoli, hard yellow squash, or carrots
- Two fresh tropical or citrus fruits
- Water according to thirst

People who enjoy noncompetitive physical activities such as aerobic dancing, weight or machine training, or calisthenics require the same special pre- and postperformance nutrition immediately before and after exercise. Many of these popular "solo" or noncompetitive activities still require that you compete against yourself. My pre- and postcompetition guidelines will give you the vital peak-performance nutrition you need to be your personal best during competition or individual workouts.

When you have achieved the blood chemistry values I recommend for entering level two of my peak-performance program, you can follow the sport-specific diets outlined in this chapter, but first it is vitally important that your blood chemistry values meet or exceed the levels I recommend for level two. If you participate in more than one sport, choose the sport-specific diet that provides the highest level of kilocalories from complex carbohydrates. This will ensure that you achieve peak performance levels in the most physically demanding sport you enjoy.

Some Important Secrets of the Champions That Will Help You Eat to Win

Maintain your present body weight. Do not lose more than 2 pounds of body weight in one week if you intend to compete at your peak performance level. This extremely valuable secret has become one of the most important rules of competitive sports. Unfortunate is the athlete who violates this rule and follows a crash weight-loss diet in order to qualify for competing in a specific weight category, such as heavyweight or lightweight. Boxers, wrestlers, and martial arts competitors who attempt drastic weight loss shortly before competing stand to lose not only the weight but the match as well.

Don't drink alcohol after competition if you have to compete the next day. Alcohol dehydrates (robs) your body of its precious water supply, and along with the water go vital nutrients such as B vitamins, calcium, magnesium, and potassium—the very peak-performance nutrients you need to win. You'll enjoy your favorite drink all the more if it's your victory toast.

How soon should you eat after competition? I recommend consuming a protein-rich food and a complex-carbohydrate-rich food within two hours of competing or completing a strenuous workout. Mother Nature in her infinite wisdom has decreed that strenuous physical activity should delay hunger, and for good reason: You need to replace the most vital nutrient lost through athletic competition—water. Your first duty is to replenish your body's water supply before you do anything else. Fortunately, the Eat to Win Diet emphasizes foods that possess high water content, so you won't have to drink more than you feel comfortable imbibing. As an insurance policy, I recommend drinking an additional 8 ounces of water beyond what your thirst tells you to drink.

To sum up:

1. Follow my pre- and postcompetition guidelines for meals that you eat immediately before and after athletic competition or workouts.

2. Return to your regular program level (based on your blood chemistry values) in between competition or workouts.

3. When your blood chemistry values meet or exceed level two standards, you may follow the sport-specific diet programs outlined in the next section.

4. If you enjoy more than one sport, always choose the diet that provides the most kilocalories from complex carbohydrates.

THE EAT TO WIN SPORT-SPECIFIC DIET GUIDELINES

I have created the following sport-specific guidelines to meet the metabolic requirements of professional and amateur athletes in twenty-one of the most popular sports. If you enjoy more than one of these sports, *always choose the sport-specific diet that provides the greatest amount of daily kilocalories from complex carbohydrates.*

These are four sport-specific diet programs that cover all twenty-one sports:

CATEGORY ONE:
CONTINUOUS SPORTS
Aerobic dancing
Cycling
Jogging
Skiing
Swimming

CATEGORY TWO:
INTERMITTENT-ACTIVITY
SPORTS
Baseball
Basketball
Football
Golf
Martial arts
Skating

Skateboarding
Soccer
Surfing
Racket sports
Track

CATEGORY THREE:
POWER SPORTS
Strength training

CATEGORY FOUR:
ELITE ENDURANCE SPORTS
Triathlon
Marathon
Long-distance cycling
Formula One racing

All of these sports require that you use the largest muscles in your body—leg muscles. The amount of muscle glycogen you store and the enzymes you manufacture to burn that glycogen efficiently will determine your level of endurance and performance in these sports.

Each sport can demand a wide range of energy expenditure (in general, according to the duration of the event) from a few hundred kilocalories to a few thousand. Cross-country skiing and marathon running may require 2,000 or more kilocalories in one event.

James and Jonathan DiDonato, the identical-twin long-distance swimmers who breaststroked their way into the *Guinness Book of World Records*, followed my sport-specific swimming diet even though one eats meat and the other is a vegetarian. James is actually a lacto-vegetarian: He eats only nonfat and low-fat milk products and beans, peas, or lentils (which are excellent vegetable sources of protein) as substitutes for such animal-protein sources as chicken, turkey, and fish.

PORTION SIZE

Weekend athletes may be unaware of the enormous physical demands faced by world-class athletes; they may be equally uninformed about the enormous appetites of these competitors—Gene and Sandy Mayer, world-champion tennis professionals during the early 1980s and clients of mine, each ate at one sitting fifteen Big Macs and several orders of French fries (large), and washed it all down with a couple of milk shakes—of course, that was before they came under my wing!

Rather than restrict yourself to a specific portion size (although I have listed suggested portions ranges below), you may want to let appetite rule the portions you eat. Most athletes I've advised discover that this is sound and prudent advice, and I believe that you will too.

Shortly after you begin the program, your appetite will automatically readjust itself. The appetite center in your brain is like the thermostat in your house: Once you set it, it stays there until you reset it. The chemical composition of your diet, as well as the intensity and duration of your exercise or sport, will set your "appestat" (your appetite thermostat located in the hypothalamus) to your own unique peak-performance level. The harder you train, the more in harmony will be your desire for food and your body's need for energy.

Athletes who begin my program report that for the first time they feel more in touch with their body's needs and requirements. A high-complex-carbohydrate diet based on foods with a naturally low-fat content and rich in vitamins and minerals seems to provide the body's sensitive appestat with the right chemical balance to eliminate over- and undereating. The Eat to Win Diet supplies the perfect diet chemistry (based on your own blood chemistry) for appetite control. If your body requires more food, you'll feel hungry; once you meet your body's nutritional needs, you'll feel full and satisfied.

If you want to gain muscular weight, simply eat larger portions of the foods I recommend and follow a strength-training program designed to help you increase muscle mass. Extra daily calories from three food groups—complex carbohydrates, protein, and fats—will make you stronger and larger when you stress your muscles.

SPORT-SPECIFIC GUIDELINES

The American lifestyle has conditioned most of us to regard specific foods as appropriate for breakfast, lunch, or dinner. The Eat to Win Diet does not restrict any food or food group to specific meals or time of day. You may enjoy your favorite breakfast cereal for lunch, or your favorite pasta recipe for breakfast (as many marathon runners do). These peak-performance meals are just as effective whether you eat them morning, noon, or evening.

The Eat to Win recipes you will find in the second section of this book provide you with fail-safe eating regardless of your diet level or the sport-specific diet of your choice. I have created each recipe so that you can enjoy them, as the world champions do, anytime.

My basic eating plan—the foundation for all the sport-specific diet guidelines—divides all the foods you will enjoy into three categories in order of importance: carbohydrate sources; protein sources; and fats and oils. There is also a special section on condiments and beverages.

For your convenience, I have listed suggested portion sizes for an ideal reference athlete. You can judge your own nutritional needs against those of this reference athlete. This imaginary reference athlete weighs 150 pounds, stands 5'11", and burns 600 kilocalories in exercise or sports every day (equivalent to one and a half hours of singles tennis or one hour of slow jogging or regular aerobic dancing). If you weigh more than 150 pounds or expend more than 600 kilocalories per day, you may increase my suggested portions accordingly; if you weigh less than 150 pounds, or burn less than 600 kilocalories per day, you'll need to proportionally decrease these suggested portions.

FOOD CATEGORIES

There are three food categories—carbohydrates, proteins, and fats—that supply peak-performance nutrition for each sport-specific eating plan. Under category one (carbohydrates), you'll find the maximum daily limits listed next to each specific carbohydrate food source—your individual sport-specific diet will tell you the maximum amount of these carbohydrate sources you can choose each day.

You may eat less than the maximum amounts I've listed, but to achieve peak performance in your chosen sport or activity, do not exceed these limits. The same advice applies for category two (protein), and category three (fats and oils). You may use the recommended condiments as desired within reasonable limits. I've listed the maximum allowable amounts for each approved beverage. Only water—the drink of champions—is permitted in unlimited quantities.

Skim and Low-Fat Dairy Products

If you enjoy milk and milk products, you can consume up to two servings each day from this food group. Use nonfat milk or 1 percent soymilk on oatmeal and other cereals, in coffee, tea, or hot cocoa. Use 1-percent-fat cottage cheese and yogurt as snacks but do not exceed two cups per day from this group.

Fresh Fruits

Fresh fruits are a good source of complex carbohydrates. If you limit your fresh fruit intake to the amounts I recommend daily for levels one to three of the Eat to Win Diet and the sport-specific eating plans, you'll consume the optimal level of nutrients from this group. Always consume at least one citrus fruit per day, because citrus supplies vitamin C and powerful disease-fighting phytonutrients called polyphenols.

Fruit Juices

Fruit juices are a concentrated source of sugar—not complex carbohydrates—and you should avoid them whenever possible. If you must consume some fruit juice, choose a brand sweetened with su-cralose (e.g., Ocean Spray Light juice drinks).

Vegetables

Eat as many steamed or raw vegetables as desired. Pick a variety of colors to get a variety of nutrients—red, orange, yellow, and green. Athletes remember which vegetables to choose by thinking of Roy Green—R: red; O: orange; Y: yellow; Green: Consume at least four servings of legumes each week because they provide a rich source of high-quality protein, iron, calcium, and fiber. Bean, pea, and lentil soups count!

Animal Protein

Try to avoid the fatty meats such as lamb, duck, pork, luncheon meats, and well-marbled cuts of beef. Choose lean protein sources such as fish (you may eat two fish that are relatively high in fat, salmon and mackerel, because they are rich sources of EPA and DHA, the "friendly" fat), skinless white-meat chicken, skinless white-meat turkey, and shellfish: lobster (always your first choice), crab, oyster, clams, scallops, and shrimp (always your last choice because of its rela-tively high cholesterol content).

Try to limit total animal protein intake to no more than 1.5 pounds per week. For better health, I prefer that you eat like a lacto-ovo vege-tarian (limiting animal protein to egg whites and nonfat/low-fat dairy, respectively).

Fats and Oils

World-class endurance athletes can enjoy more fats and oils than weekend warriors but both should keep total fat intake to no more than 20 percent of total daily calories.

As you've already learned, you are unique, with unique blood chem-istry and unique nutritional needs, but fats and oils can cause damage to vital organs and tissues without raising blood lipid values. A diet that keeps total fat calories to no more than 20 percent of daily calories will provide more than enough diunsaturated linoleic acid (oatmeal, corn, and brown rice), monounsaturated fats (olive and canola oils), and omega-3 fats (seafood).

A good rule of thumb to follow concerning the use of fats and oils is to include foods rich in these biologically friendly fats that naturally occur in foods. If you add other fats and oils to your foods, use them in the amounts I've suggested in Chapter 4 for each level of the Eat to Win Diet.

WHY I ALLOW THOSE CONDIMENTS ON MY DIET PROGRAM

The Eat to Win Diet permits the occasional use of condiments that contain salt and/or sugar, including ketchup, pickle relish, mustard, steak sauce, barbecue sauce, etc., because of their negligible fat content. If you don't abuse these condiments, they won't abuse you. As always, if you follow a sugar- and/or sodium-restricted diet, check with your physician before using any foods, food products, or condiments that contain these substances.

SPORT SPECIFICS

Published research shows that men and women who participate in daily aerobic exercise (exercise that raises your heart rate above 120 beats per minute) generally are slimmer, fitter, and healthier than their more sedentary friends and relatives. Moreover, when these active people eat a low-fat, low-cholesterol, high-complex-carbohydrate diet, they don't suffer from the diet-related degenerative diseases—heart disease, diabetes, hypertension, obesity, stroke, for example—with nearly the same frequency as sedentary people who eat high-fat, high-cholesterol diets.

Jogging, skiing (and especially cross-country skiing), aerobic dancing, cycling, and swimming are some of the best aerobic physical activities. However, no amount of exercise alone is enough to afford you maximum protection against diet-related diseases. Proper nutrition is essential for optimal health, longevity, and peak performance.

Viki Fleckenstein, a former champion U.S. Ski Team racer and U.S.

Olympic Team competitor, used the sport-specific category-one plan to eat to win. Viki's event, the slalom, demands great strength and endurance and peak effort. Viki visited my sports nutrition clinic in Florida to boost her already excellent stamina to peak performance levels.

Tennis and other racket sports require both aerobic and anaerobic activity. I've developed the category-two eating plan to give you the competitive edge to outlast and wear down your opponents through extraordinary stamina and extra power for explosive bursts of energy.

In contrast to sports such as jogging, cycling, and swimming, where movement is virtually continuous, category-two sports often require athletes to expend bursts of discontinuous, explosive energy, with intermittent periods of reduced physical demand or rest. Football players, basketball players, soccer players, and ice hockey players have time-outs and rest periods at halftime; boxers, wrestlers, and martial arts competitors rest between rounds.

These sports demand endurance, but not exactly the type required for marathon running, long-distance cycle racing, long-distance swimming, or cross-country skiing.

The caloric costs of these sports can be tremendous: a fifteen-round boxing match or typical basketball game requires more kilocalories than jogging or dancing for thirty minutes—so this sport-specific diet guideline provides more kilocalories than category one does.

Golf—really good golf—demands exquisite and elegant neuromuscular coordination, and the pros win or lose based upon the amount of it they can muster. Mental concentration is no less important. The best golfers possess the mental abilities of concentration and focus enjoyed by chess masters and brain surgeons.

Under the stress of competition (or a heavy wager), a golfer's blood sugar can plummet to hypoglycemic levels—along with any chance of winning. Special brain chemicals, which improve concentration and brain-to-muscle communication, must be present in optimal quantities for championship play. Golf demands a constant optimal concentration of these neurochemicals as well as finely tuned muscular movements.

The caloric cost of golfing is, of course, directly dependent upon whether you walk (and how far) the five or six miles of the course or whether you ride in a golf cart, where all the energy is burned by the motor, not your body.

Weight training demands explosive, anaerobic activity that places unique demands on your muscles. Weight training can also be aerobic, if you use the circuit-training technique: highly repetitive lifting and moving to the next weight station or routine as quickly as possible without giving your heart rate a chance to slow down. Research has demonstrated that you must engage in *continuous* lifting for at least twenty minutes for it to become aerobic.

When you follow my category-three diet guidelines and eat the right foods in the right combinations, you will train your muscles to utilize blood sugar and fat efficiently to give you the explosive power you need.

Large amounts of muscle tissue may be torn down during exhaustive weight training, so category-three eating guidelines provide the necessary nutrients for building and rebuilding muscle tissue. Weight lifters do not need the large amounts of muscle glycogen that marathon runners rely on to go the distance. Serious amateur and professional bodybuilders do need a bit more protein each day, but not the amounts that are typically consumed at most training tables. Category-three guidelines for strength training provide ample protein to meet the most demanding of protein needs of a world-champion power lifter.

Emerson Fittipaldi, a Brazilian Formula One racing champion, embraced the Eat to Win Diet in 1984. I never got a chance to work personally with Emerson due to my hectic schedule at the time, but judging from his remarkable accomplishments, he did quite well on his own!

Emerson still holds the record for being the youngest driver to ever win a Formula One championship. In 1984, he joined the Championship Auto Racing Teams (CART) series in the United States and became a household name in this country. He continued his outstanding career by winning the CART Championship in 1989 and the Indianapolis 500 in 1989 and 1993. Emerson Fittipaldi ended his thirty-year racing career in 1996, after thirty-six career wins and twenty-three poles in 339 starts.

Formula One racing is one of the most demanding of all sports. If you think it's anything like driving a car fast, think again. Formula One racing requires exceptional strength, fitness, endurance, focus, and razor-sharp reflexes. A Formula One driver can lose a tremendous amount of water through dehydration. Cramps are common among these athletes. They need plenty of water, electrolytes, and complex carbohydrates. Category-four guidelines for performance racing are designed to meet the metabolic needs of this extreme sport.

CARBOHYDRATES (50 TO 70 PERCENT DAILY KILOCALORIES)

Cereals

Fresh fruits

Dried fruits

Fruit juices

Potatoes

Brown rice

Pasta

Vegetables (raw or steamed)

Whole-grain breads

Whole-grain pancakes

Desserts: original Haas recipes only

PROTEINS (15 TO 25 PERCENT DAILY KILOCALORIES)

Skim milk

Nonfat dry milk, prepared

Low-fat, part-skim cheeses

Grated Parmesan or Romano cheese

Low-fat cottage cheese, ½ to 2 percent fat

Low-fat yogurt, 1 to 2 percent fat

Meats:

    Beef, lean cuts only

    Poultry

    Bison

    Elk

Fish

Ostrich

Shellfish

Venison

Olive oil

Canola oil

Legumes: beans, peas, and lentils, any type

FATS AND OILS (15 TO 20 PERCENT DAILY KILOCALORIES)

Only one portion (up to 1 tablespoon total fats and oils) is permitted per day from the following list:

Sesame oil

Nayonaise (tofu-based "mayonnaise")

SPECIAL CONDIMENTS

The following condiments may be used in reasonable amounts to taste:

Splenda (sucralose) sugar substitute

Any oil-free or low-fat salad dressing

Vinegar (any type)

Mustard (regular or spicy)

Ketchup (Low-sodium, low-sugar varieties are available in the diet section of supermarkets and in most health food stores.)

Steak sauce (Most steak sauces are high in sodium, so use sparingly. If you follow a sodium-restricted diet, check with your physician before using.)

Barbeque sauce (Most brands or those served in restaurants are usually high in sodium and sugar—use sparingly. If you follow a low-sodium, low-sugar diet, check with your physician before using.)

Lemon or lime juice

Bacon bits or chips, soybean type (These usually contain sugar and salt. If you are following a low-sodium or low-sugar diet, check with your physician before using.)

Any other salt-free or sugar-free herb or spice such as cinnamon, nutmeg, paprika, fresh garlic or garlic powder, basil, thyme, pepper

BEVERAGES

Water (tap, bottled, carbonated, salt-free carbonated beverages are available in most supermarkets if you follow a sodium-restricted diet)

Coffee and tea (use water-processed decaffeinated coffee; decaffeinated teas are available in most supermarkets and health-food stores)

Vegetable juices (carrot, tomato, V8, up to 8 ounces per day. These juices contain sodium. If you follow a sodium-restricted diet, check with your physician before using)

Alcoholic beverages:

Light beer

Regular beer

Wine, white or red

Champagne

Hard liquor (vodka, scotch, rum)

Sake

Hot chocolate, reduced-calorie (Swiss Miss No Sugar Added or Carnation brand, for example.)

Diet soda, noncaffeinated (These beverages contain sodium. If you follow a sodium-restricted diet, check with your physician before using.)

APPROVED CEREAL LIST

The cereals listed below will vary from sport-specific diet to diet— some cereals are too high in fat or sugar or both for peak performance in certain sports. In general, the more calorically demanding a sport, the more liberal will be the approved cereal list for that sport.

Shredded Wheat

Grape-Nuts

All-Bran

Quaker 100% Whole Wheat

Puffed brown rice or wheat

Oatmeal

Wheatena

Cereal toppings: Use skim or nonfat dry milk and fresh fruit of choice. Use Splenda sugar replacer for sweetening cereal.

CATEGORY ONE—Continuous Sports: Jogging, Skiing, Aerobic Dancing, Cycling, Swimming

Approved Cereal List

All-Bran

Grape-Nuts

Oatmeal

Puffed brown rice or puffed whole wheat

Quaker 100% Whole Wheat

Shredded Wheat

Wheatena

Eat up to 1 cup per day for each continuous hour of sport or exercise. Top with ½ cup skim or nonfat dry milk and one fresh fruit of choice. Use Splenda sugar substitute if you desire additional sweetener.

Additional fresh fruit: up to three fresh fruits of your choice per day

Dried fruits: up to 1 ounce per day

Potatoes: up to four per day

Brown rice: up to 2 cups (cooked) per day

Pasta: up to 2 cups (cooked) per day

Vegetables: raw or steamed, as desired; avoid avocado, hearts of palm, and olives

Whole-grain breads: up to two slices per day

Whole-grain pancakes (made without egg yolks): up to two 6-inch pancakes per day with approved topping

Fruits: up to five servings

Nonfat dairy: up to 3 cups per day

Low-fat, part-skim cheeses: up to ½ ounce per day

Grated Parmesan or Romano cheese: up to 2 teaspoons per day

Meats: up to 4 ounces any type per day

Legumes: up to 1 cup per day

Nuts and seeds: up to 1 ounce per day, any type

Fats and oils: up to 1 tablespoon extra-virgin olive oil or canola oil

Dietary supplement: MediterrAsian Multi Caps (see: www.Mediterr AsianDiet.com)

See the basic sport-specific eating plan for approved beverages and condiments.

CATEGORY TWO—Intermittent-activity Sports: Baseball, Football, Golf, Skating, Soccer, Basketball, Ice Hockey, Boxing, Wrestling, Martial Arts, Surfing, Racket Sports, Skateboarding, Track

Approved Cereal List

Shredded Wheat

Grape-Nuts

All-Bran

Quaker 100% Whole Wheat

Wheatena

Puffed brown rice and puffed whole wheat

Eat up to 1 cup per day for each continuous hour of sport or exercise. Top with ½ cup skim or nonfat dry milk and one fresh fruit of choice. Use Splenda sugar substitute if you desire additional sweetener.

Additional fresh fruit: up to six fresh fruits of your choice per day

Dried fruits: up to 2 ounces per day

Fruit juices: up to 6 ounces per day

Potatoes: up to four per day

Brown rice: up to 3 cups (cooked) per day

Pasta: up to 4 cups (cooked) per day

Vegetables: raw or steamed, as desired; avoid avocado, hearts of palm, and olives

Whole-grain breads: up to six slices per day

Whole-grain pancakes (made without egg yolks): up to three 6-inch pancakes per day with approved topping

Desserts: up to two servings, original Haas recipe

Skim and nonfat dry milk, prepared: up to 2 cups per day

Low-fat, part-skim cheeses: up to 1 ounce per day

Grated Parmesan or Romano cheese: up to 3 teaspoons per day

Low-fat cottage cheese and yogurt: up to 1 cup per day

Meats: up to 4 ounces per day, any type

Legumes: up to 2 cups per day

Nuts and seeds: up to 2 ounces per day, any type

Fats and oils: up to 2 teaspoons, any type

Dietary supplement: MediterrAsian Multi Caps (see: www.Mediterr AsianDiet.com)

See the basic sport-specific eating plan for specific condiments and beverages.

CATEGORY THREE—Power Endurance Sports: Strength Training

Approved Cereal List

Shredded Wheat

Grape-Nuts

All-Bran

Quaker 100% Whole Wheat

Wheatena

Puffed brown rice and puffed whole wheat

Eat up to 1 cup per day for each continuous hour of sport or exercise. Top with ½ cup skim or nonfat dry milk and one fresh fruit of choice. Use Splenda sugar substitute if you desire additional sweetener.

Additional fresh fruit: up to two fresh fruits of your choice per day

Dried fruits: up to 1 ounce per day

Fruit juices: up to 6 ounces per day

Potatoes: up to two per day

Brown rice: up to 1½ cups (cooked) per day

Pasta: up to 1½ cups (cooked) per day

Vegetables: raw or steamed, as desired; avoid avocado, hearts of palm, and olives

Whole-grain breads: up to two slices per day

Whole-grain pancakes (made without egg yolks): up to two 6-inch pancakes per day with approved topping

Desserts: up to one serving, original Haas recipe

Skim and nonfat dry milk, prepared: up to 1 cup per day

Low-fat, part-skim cheeses: up to ½ ounce per day

Grated Parmesan or Romano cheese: up to 2 teaspoons per day

Low-fat cottage cheese and yogurt: up to ½ cup per day

Meats: up to 4 ounces per day, any type

Legumes: up to 1 cup per day

Nuts and seeds: up to 1 ounce per day, any type

Fats and oils: up to 1 teaspoon, any type

Dietary supplement: MediterrAsian Multi Caps (see: www.Mediterr AsianDiet.com)

See the basic sport-specific eating plan for specific condiments and beverages.

CATEGORY FOUR—Elite Endurance Sports: Triathlon, Marathon, Long-distance Cycling, Formula One Racing

Approved Cereal List

Shredded Wheat

Grape-Nuts

All-Bran

Quaker 100% Whole Wheat

Wheatena

Alpen

Mueslix

Bran Chex

Puffed brown rice and puffed whole wheat

Eat up to 1 cup per day for each continuous hour of sport or exercise. Top with ½ cup skim or nonfat dry milk and one fresh fruit of choice. Use Splenda sugar substitute if you desire additional sweetener.

Additional fresh fruit: up to four fresh fruits of your choice per day

Dried fruits: up to 1 ounce per day

Fruit juices: up to 6 ounces per day

Potatoes: up to six per day

Brown rice: up to 3 cups (cooked) per day

Pasta: up to 4 cups (cooked) per day

Vegetables: raw or steamed, as desired; avoid avocado, hearts of palm, and olives

Whole-grain breads: up to six slices per day

Whole-grain pancakes (made without egg yolks): up to three 6-inch pancakes per day with approved topping

Desserts: up to two servings, original Haas recipe

Skim and nonfat dry milk, prepared: up to 2 cups per day

Low-fat, part-skim cheeses: up to ½ ounce per day

Grated Parmesan or Romano cheese: up to 3 teaspoons per day

Low-fat cottage cheese and yogurt: up to 1 cup per day

Meats: up to 4 ounces per day, any type

Legumes: up to 2 cups per day

Nuts and seeds: up to 1 ounce per day, any type

Fats and oils: up to 1 teaspoon, any type

Dietary supplement: MediterrAsian Multi Caps (see: www.Mediterr AsianDiet.com)

See the basic sport-specific eating plan for specific condiments and beverages.

Do You Eat Like a Rat?

THE DIRTY SIDE OF PROTEIN

If you were a rat, a high-protein diet would be just what the rat doctor ordered.

Since you don't have pointy ears and long tail, you don't need as much protein as a rat, relatively speaking. But protein-pushing diet book authors tell you that you do.

They want you to eat like a rat.

Those who eat like rats come to resemble them. If you've ever noticed an elderly lady or gentleman with a curved back and stooped posture, then you've seen what eating like a rat could eventually do to you. Osteoporosis is just one of the many health hazards of regularly consuming excessive amounts of protein.

The human need for protein is much smaller than protein-pushing diet doctors would have you believe. The amount of protein you need each day is so small that—well, I really can't tell you how small just yet because you wouldn't believe me. You'll have to read on a bit so I have time to prepare you for the sticker shock.

It's possible to eat varying amounts of fats and carbs and not get sick, but when it comes to protein, you don't enjoy the same wide margin of error: if you were to eat too little protein, your hair might start to thin because hair is made from protein. If you were eat too much protein, your hair might also start to thin. This is a side effect seen in studies that examine the effects of ketogenic/high-protein diets in humans.

Too little or too much protein—the results can be unpleasant and unhealthy. In either case, you will exhibit the symptoms of illness.

Protein is trendy—people think it's fashionable to be on a high-protein diet. Everyone else is. It makes you a member of the club—hardly an exclusive one, but a club nonetheless. But a high-protein diet, metabolically speaking, makes a terrible fashion statement.

If you follow a high-protein diet, here's something to contemplate the next time you urinate. Watch as the stream of water leaves your body. It may look like ordinary urine but you are actually watching part of your skeleton go down the toilet. At the same time, your kidneys will be aging at a much faster rate than the vegetarian who lives down the block from you.

We already know that high-protein diets do little to make elite athletes run, cycle, or swim faster or farther. Vegetarian competitors (and winners) of one of the most grueling events in all endurance sports, the Hawaii Ironman Triathalon, have already proven that. Many athletes have set new world records without eating a single gram of beef, poultry, lamb, pork, or fish. Vegetable proteins, not animal proteins, helped these athletes experience the thrill of peak performance.

In my entire career as a sports nutritionist, the hardest task I've ever faced is convincing a world-champion athlete or coach or team physician that when it comes to protein, a bit less can mean more.

While you don't have to swear off animal protein to enjoy a healthy diet, it is worth noting that there is only one major difference between animal and vegetable protein—animal protein is inferior to vegetable protein.

The reason? Animal protein foods contain lots of saturated fats, cholesterol, hormones, and antibiotics. Vegetable proteins, which are "complete" proteins, contain no cholesterol, negligible amounts of saturated fats, and are not injected with growth-stimulating hormones or antibiotics. They come from sources that are much lower on the food chain, and so they don't concentrate environmental toxins as animals do. A steer, a chicken, or a sea bass makes a highly efficient chemical laboratory for concentrating methylmercury, PCBs, dioxin, and other harmful substances.

YOU CAN GET ALL THE PROTEIN YOU NEED FROM WONDER BREAD

I bet that header got your attention. Wonder bread's original "Builds strong bodies twelve ways" claim notwithstanding, you can get all the protein you need even from this refined, nutritionally devalued bread—right down to every last essential amino acid. Essential amino acids—there are nine in all—are those we need to obtain from foods. Our bodies can manufacture the other twenty-plus amino acids we use each day. Bread contains all of them. So does spinach.

Relax; you won't have to fulfill your protein needs from bread on the Eat to Win Diet. I mention this only to emphasize the point that even highly refined plant foods contain complete protein. The body doesn't care which foods supply the essential amino acids we need each day. Chemically, they are all identical, whether they come from highly processed foods like Wonder bread or an expensive porterhouse steak. As Figure 7.1 reveals, athletes can obtain all the high-quality, complete protein they need each day simply by eating spinach.

But as you can see from the two graphs in Figure 7.1, which compare the amino acid "profiles" of spinach and steak, Popeye's favorite vegetable looks almost identical to Wimpy's beloved burger. The difference is, of course, that one would have to eat many more calories from spinach to equal the absolute amount of amino acids in 3.5 ounces of ground beef. Over the course of a day's worth of eating, it's quite easy for any athlete—even an endurance athlete—to meet his or her protein requirements exclusively from plant foods. It's not necessary that they do, but it certainly is easily accomplished.

The key to meeting one's daily protein needs has nothing to do with where the protein comes from and everything to do with how many *calories* one consumes. Once an athlete consumes sufficient calories to maintain body weight, the requirement for protein is only a bit higher than it would be for a recreational sports enthusiast.

FIGURE 7.1

COMPARISON OF ESSENTIAL AMINO ACID PROFILE OF SPINACH AND BEEF

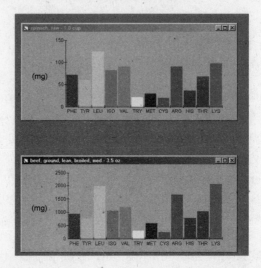

Spinach and beef both contain about 40 percent of their calories as protein. Of course, you have to eat more spinach get the amount of protein in beef. The point of this illustration is to show how a diet based exclusively on plant proteins contains all essential amino acids found in beef as well as a similar amino acid profile. There are no "incomplete" proteins in the plant world, despite what the American Heart Association and popular diet books and newsmagazines tell you.

It doesn't matter whether you're an elite endurance athlete competing in the Hawaii Triathalon or a weekend sports enthusiast: Peak-performance eating has always been fueled by carbohydrate calories. It's *never* been about the protein.

MARTINA'S SECRET

One week after beginning the Eat to Win Diet, Martina Navratilova knew she had discovered one of the best-kept secrets in sports. As soon as she realized this, she asked me not to work with any other woman in professional tennis. Why? She knew the Eat to Win Diet gave her the competitive edge.

Winning often depends on the difference of one or two points or a fraction of a second. Athletes look for any edge to beat the competition. Until I began working with Martina, her competition on the court was Chris Evert.

After Martina embraced the Eat to Win Diet, her rivalry with Chris became just another tennis match. I haven't checked the record books, but to my memory, I can't recall that Chris won a single match against Martina after Martina embraced the Eat to Win Diet. If you happened to be in the Navratilova tennis camp during that time, you would have seen little concern the day before these two champions were scheduled to play each other. You would have found Martina shopping, watching TV, shooting hoops with Nancy Lieberman, the first woman to compete in men's professional basketball, or enjoying a light workout with her coach. After Martina embraced the Eat to Win Diet, it wasn't a rivalry; it was just another tennis match.

Martina was seriously concerned about some of the up-and-coming younger players, but Chris Evert wasn't on that short list. Don't get me wrong; Chris is one of the all-time great tennis champions in history, and until Martina began training on the Eat to Win Diet, Chris Evert literally defined women's professional tennis as only a truly great world champion could. I used to watch Chris train as a child with her father, Jimmy, at Holiday Park in Fort Lauderdale, Florida, and marveled at her precision and near-perfect ground strokes. I run into Chris at her tennis academy whenever I train there, and her precision form on the court is as good as it's ever been.

As John McEnroe discovered when his archrival, Ivan Lendl, began the Eat to Win Diet, when two athletes of roughly the same talent compete, the athlete who enjoys the Eat to Win advantage will prevail. McEnroe followed the Häagen-Dazs diet; Ivan followed the Haas diet and went on to dominate McEnroe and men's professional tennis for the next five years, just as Martina Navratilova did in women's professional tennis.

Martina's diet consisted of a mix of vegetable and animal proteins only because it suited her tastes at the time. Since then, Martina has become a vegetarian. She can still hold her own on center court against much younger competitors even as she approaches her half-century birthday! Vegetable proteins take Martina where she wants to go, and they will do the same for you.

A LITTLE TRICK WITH NICK

Nick Saviano, who is now the president of the Association of Tennis Professionals (ATP), walked into my office twenty years ago with two problems: He suffered from hypoglycemia, a condition in which blood sugar can drop so low that physical activity becomes impossible, and he wanted to lose a few pounds to reach his ideal weight.

Nick had been told that a high-protein diet would correct his hypoglycemia and help boost his endurance and stamina. This is an example of how locker room lore can hamper an athlete's career.

I said, "Nick, let's try an experiment for one day. I'd like you to carry a bag of bread with you all day long during your next training day. Whenever you start to feel hungry, eat as much bread (I suggested whole-grain) as hunger dictates. There's no limit on how many slices you can eat in a day. Come back and tell me how you felt after training all day and eating nothing but bread."

"But eating all that bread will make me fat and will cause my blood sugar to plummet!" Nick retorted.

"Nick, it won't do either of those things, but I'd like you to prove it to yourself. Just try it for a day and see what you think," I requested.

Three days later Nick walked into my office with a huge grin on his face. Here's what he told me:

"I've never felt so good in my life. I trained six hours yesterday, and for the first time, I didn't have an episode of hypoglycemia. What I did have was unlimited energy, stamina, and incredible alertness on the court. I ate bread slices all day and all evening. I never felt the slightest bit hungry. I was completely satisfied."

I explained how a high-complex-carbohydrate diet could help him achieve greater energy, endurance, and blood sugar stability over a high-protein diet. Nick agreed to follow the Eat to Win Diet.

Two weeks later, I walked over to the court where Nick was training like a maniac. He saw me and yelled, "I've lost six pounds and I feel incredible!"

"What about your hypoglycemia?" I asked.

Nick looked at me like I had just asked him to tell me the square root of pi.

"Wow, I forgot all about it!"

Nick had learned three important lessons about protein:

1. Eating only vegetable proteins doesn't hamper athletic performance—it helps it. Eating vegetable protein relieved Nick's body of the task of handling the high-acid load that would have coursed through his blood as a result of following a high-protein, meat-heavy diet. Relying solely on the protein from bread— hardly an ideal way to eat—Nick was able to train hard and avoid hypoglycemia. On the Eat to Win Diet, you'll enjoy meals with far superior nutrition than Nick Saviano's bread diet, but the results will be the same: For the first time, you'll feel what it's like to eat like a champion.

2. Carbohydrate, not protein, is the "cure" for simple hypoglycemia. Since complex carbohydrate foods enjoy lower caloric density and greater nutrient density than animal protein foods, they will fill you up without filling you out. Instead of making you feel heavy or sluggish, they'll help you feel lighter and more energetic.

3. Carbs will fill you up and slim you down. Ounce for ounce and pound for pound, carbohydrate-rich vegetables, grains, and fruits provide the most nutrition and satiety for the fewest calories. If you want to lose weight and keep it off permanently, a diet based on vegetable protein and nutritious carb-rich foods will do that. Any scientist at the National Weight Registry will confirm this.

TOXIC BY-PRODUCTS OF PROTEIN METABOLISM

Your Body's Enzymes Make the Same Toxic Products as a Chemical Factory!

Urea is the final waste product of protein metabolism. Chemical companies must use very high temperature and pressure to manufacture the toxic compound urea, but your body can easily make urea out of ammonia and a few enzymes. In order to neutralize ammonia and urea, the body draws calcium and other minerals from bones, along with water from muscle cells. The more protein you eat, the more ammonia and urea you make. High-protein diets thin your bones, predisposing you to osteoporosis later in life; they also dehydrate your body, crippling athletic performance and endurance.

ANIMAL PROTEIN MAKES A DIRTY FUEL

Actually, I'm being a bit disingenuous, because all proteins, whether from animals or vegetables, make a dirty fuel. But animal protein is *especially* dirty. Blame it all on sulfur.

Of all the amino acids we consume each day, methionine and cysteine and related amino acids contain the element sulfur, which is essential for life.[1] Like everything else, too much of a good thing can be a bad thing, and sulfur is no exception.

Animal proteins contain an unusually large amount of sulfur-containing amino acids when compared to most vegetable proteins. This is an important distinction between the two types of protein because excessive amounts of sulfur-containing amino acids can stress the body in a number of ways:

All sulfur-containing amino can create sulfuric acid in the body. An excess of this strong acid, derived from eating too much protein from animal or vegetable sources, leads to bone loss, osteoporosis, and kidney-stone formation.

The body converts methionine to homocysteine, a compound that

---

1. A number of other sulfur-containing amino acids are derived from these two primary sulfur-containing amino acids: cystathionine, cysteic acid, cystine, homocysteine, keto-methionine, and taurine.

has been linked to cognitive impairment and, perhaps, Alzheimer's disease, depression, and cardiovascular diseases that affect the heart and the veins in the legs.

Animal-protein foods are the major source of this amino acid. In general, the more animal protein one consumes, the higher one's blood level of homocysteine. A diet high in fruits and vegetables helps reduce levels of homocysteine in the blood.

PROTEIN MAKES AN INEFFICIENT BODY FUEL

Protein has more important jobs to do in your body than supply energy; if you force your body to use it for energy, as you would on a ketogenic diet, you would rob your body of peak performance. When you need to go the extra mile—whether it's keeping up with your kids at a shopping mall or finishing a 10k race—protein provides scant energy compared to carbohydrate. The reason is that your body has to expend more energy to convert protein into energy than it does for carbohydrates. And needlessly wasting energy is the last thing you want or need. High-protein diets defeat peak physical performance in two ways:

1. By reducing an athlete's carbohydrate intake, they actually *increase* the daily requirement for protein. The reason is a little-appreciated biochemical fact: *Carbohydrate spares protein.* During exercise and long periods of exertion your body craves carbohydrate—not protein—and it will do whatever it takes to get it, including cannibalizing your own muscle tissue. Protein from muscles can be converted to glucose, but it is an inefficient and dirty process. This slows the rate of protein synthesis and accelerates the loss of protein from muscles.

2. They literally cramp an athlete's style because a reduced carbohydrate intake drains the body's supply of glycogen (a reserve of carbohydrate stored in muscles and liver), thereby limiting the amount of time an athlete's muscles can perform to exhaustion. As you will learn, glycogen is the key to achieving permanent fat loss.

Protein in—garbage out; that's how the human body handles the protein you eat.

Consuming extra protein, as all popular ketogenic/high-fat, low-carb diets require you to do, does not create larger and stronger muscles. Rather, these diets deprive your mind and body of the carbohydrate they require to reach peak performance levels in the office, at school, and on the court.

To make up for this loss of carbs, the body struggles to convert protein in the diet to carbohydrate. It's a dirty process:

1. First, the body must detoxify the ammonia that results from protein breakdown. This puts undue strain on the kidneys and the bones.
2. Next, the body converts the remainder of the protein molecule to sugar in a series of steps that wastes energy.
3. After the body's sugar needs are met, the rest of the protein molecule is converted to fat where it is stored around internal organs and under the skin.

Unlike carbohydrates and fats, protein contains nitrogen. And therein lies the problem. Instead of producing such clean metabolic by-products as carbon dioxide and water (as carbohydrates do), protein produces two toxic waste products, ammonia and urea, a less toxic form of ammonia that all humans excrete in an attempt to rid their body of toxic protein waste.

On a ketogenic diet, excess protein creates large amounts of ammonia and urea that force the kidneys and bones to work together, first to neutralize the acids in the blood and then to form urea, the final product of protein metabolism.

Active people and professional athletes, who already lose tremendous amounts of water through sweating and evaporation, must take great care to avoid dehydration. If they lose enough body water, they can suffer heatstroke, seizure, and even sudden death from cardiac arrest.

The acidity created by a ketogenic or high-fat, low-carb diet causes the body to release the stress hormone cortisol. Cortisol causes acute and chronic loss of bone minerals in the same way prescription steroid medications lead to osteoporosis.

So a high-protein diet is a metabolically dirty diet that weakens the skeleton as it robs it of its structural minerals. If you double your ordinary intake of protein, as protein-pushing diet doctors would have you do, you might double the loss of calcium from your bones each day.

The Eat to Win Diet protects your skeleton and doesn't rob it of vital calcium. It also doesn't lead to kidney stones caused by ketotosis and high-animal-protein foods.

As you learned previously, the American Heart Association's Nutrition Committee believes that plant proteins are "incomplete" proteins and that they are inferior to "complete" animal proteins. Such misinformation can send you down a dangerous path that could predispose you to heart disease! Somehow, I don't think that goal is listed in the health organization's bylaws and public health goals.

As muscle mass increases, so does the need for protein to support the additional growth. Obviously, an overweight couch potato would require fewer grams of protein each day than an active person of the same weight would require because the couch potato is not rebuilding muscle tissue after exercise. Even so, Mr. Couch Potato's protein requirement is only a bit less—about a tenth of a gram of so per kilogram of body weight.

Now you can understand why most people are in little danger of suffering from a protein deficiency. In fact, many inactive Americans eat excessive protein—beyond 150g of protein a day—on popular high-protein, low-carb diets. For most sedentary and mildly active people, this is far more than their bodies can safely use. When you follow the Eat to Win Diet, you will safely consume an adequate but not excessive amount of protein each day.

HOW MUCH PROTEIN DO PROFESSIONAL BODYBUILDERS NEED?

Recent studies indicate that professional bodybuilders require additional protein to meet their bodies' needs.

Most ordinary people don't need more protein than they could obtain on the Eat to Win Diet. Studies show that people require only a short adaptation period to adjust to a lower and healthier rate of protein intake. Even on a moderate training program, it takes only a few weeks to reach new protein equilibrium. People who exercise regularly require only a bit more protein than nonexercisers. The Eat to Win Diet contains a large margin of safety to account for a wide variety of situations and needs. This range is more than adequate for most people, except, perhaps, professional bodybuilders.

A number of studies involving very small numbers of subjects indicate that some bodybuilders may require in excess of 2.0g/kg of body weight per day. In one study, five adult bodybuilders whose diets consisted of 0.8g/kg per day of protein and whose total calorie intake was adequate experienced a decreased muscle cell mass over six weeks of strength training. With continued training and an increase in protein intake to 1.6g/kg of body weight per day, their muscle cell mass increased. Several recent studies have found greater nitrogen retention (a measure of protein sufficiency) and greater gains in muscle mass during four weeks of strength training when bodybuilders consume 2.4 grams of protein per kilogram of body weight per day compared to those consuming 0.8 grams of protein per kilogram body weight per day. One study that examined elite endurance athletes found that 1.6g/kg of body weight was more than sufficient to meet their protein needs.

These studies suggest that extreme stresses increase the need for protein. While bodybuilders await more definitive dietary recommendations, many continue to consume upward of 2.0g/kg of body weight per day.

Professional bodybuilders are the exception to the rule. They force their bodies into a hypermetabolic state due to chronic muscle injury and inflammation. Their protein needs become chronically elevated, as do their levels of such growth hormones as IGF-1. Studies have linked chronically high IGF-1 levels in the body to an increased risk of cancer, so it behooves professional bodybuilders to remain hypervigilant about their health and have regular physical examinations.

Eating large amounts of protein, especially protein from such animal foods as eggs, seafood, and beef, puts enormous stress on the kidneys. Once an athlete retires from professional bodybuilding, it's important for that athlete to reduce the amount of daily protein to much safer levels in order to stop the rapid aging of organs and to reduce the amount of IGF–1 and other anabolic and anticatabolic hormones in their bodies.

Here's the final Eat to Win protein rule you should commit to memory: *If you eat like a rat, you'll die like a rat.*

Rats have much higher protein requirements and much shorter maximum life spans than do people. Even rats die prematurely on a very-high-protein diet (Figure 7.2). It should come as no surprise that professional bodybuilders who eat high-protein diets are not recognized for their great longevity.

FIGURE 7.2

EFFECT OF HIGH-PROTEIN DIET ON LIFE EXPECTANCY

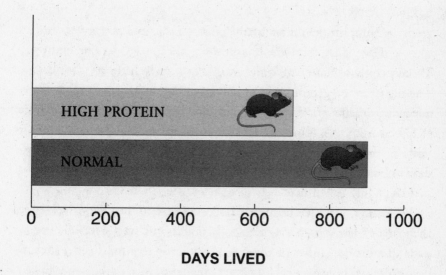

DAYS LIVED

Rats need more protein proportionally than do humans, but even rats shorten their life expectancy on a high-protein diet. The graphic above represents a summary of the research data published on the effects of high-protein diets in the rodent.

My Beef with Beef and Other Meats

Bart Simpson had it right all along—*"Don't have a cow!"*
Ever since McDonald's brought the burger to our embrace, it's been only a matter of time until beef's dirty little secret got out: The next bite of ground round you enjoy might harbor a malevolent molecule, called a *prion*, that could reduce your brain to a pathetic mass of quivering protoplasm. No one knows how many of the 100 million cattle in the United States might be carrying prions, which can arise spontaneously within an animal's cells. And that's no bull.

Commonly called mad cow disease, or BSE (bovine spongiform encephalopathy), this 21st-century plague, when found in humans, is referred to as "new variant Creutzfeldt-Jakob disease" (vCJD). Unfortunate souls who eat beef infected with the pesky prion that most scientists believe causes vCJD can expect their gray matter to turn to the neurological equivalent of Swiss cheese. This leads to uncontrollable tremors, dementia, paralysis, and death. There's no cure. Clearly, this is one Big Mac attack no one wants.

In the early 1990s BSE ravaged the United Kingdom's beef industry with thirty-seven thousand clinical cases of BSE and about sixty thousand of the highest-risk animals entering the food supply, compared with less than one a year today. In December 2003, U.S. health officials identified a BSE-infected cow in the state of Washington, leading to a ban by more than twenty countries on imports of U.S. beef.

Beef-pushing diet doctors are scrambling to revise their eating plans in light of the risk that dieters might encounter deadly prions in their next T-bone or taco. But once you take the beef out of a low-carb diet, you have to cut a lot of pages out of your recipe book, so to speak. Dining out becomes a disappointing event for hard-core beef lovers and presents new challenges to staying on such a diet.

We could all do better with less saturated fat in our diets, mad cow disease notwithstanding. When you add the risk of becoming infected with a terminal brain-wasting disease with no known cure to the well-documented health risks of eating a beef-heavy diet, the choice is clear: Eat fewer burgers to lower your risk of getting mad cow disease.

Mad cow disease may be just one of a number of life-threatening diseases that lurk in loin and chop. Several studies suggest the possibility that a virus that causes leukemia in cattle may be responsible for infecting humans as well.

The risks of mad cow disease and other infectious diseases, small as they may be at the moment, gives many dieters pause. No one is yet certain about the safety of the world's beef supply since scientists discovered mad cow disease on both sides of the Atlantic Ocean. If you're concerned about mad cow disease, you can follow a no-beef version of the Eat to Win Diet or embrace the Eat to Win vegetarian diet until the day arrives that scientists give the nation's cattle herd an unconditional clean bill of health.

U.S. MAD COW TESTING PROBLEMS REVEALED

The U.S. Department of Agriculture is responsible for monitoring the nation's cattle herds for possible mad cow disease. The USDA has admitted that at times it has permitted slaughterhouses to select which animals should be tested.

Consumer watchdog groups say the practice raises doubts about the validity of the testing program. A USDA spokesman confirmed that the department sometimes asks meatpackers to choose the cattle whose brains will undergo screening for mad cow disease at federal laboratories in order to determine whether the fatal disease is present in U.S. cattle. Critics complain that such a role by companies could have tainted the testing program because the companies' officials had an incentive to send only the brains of cattle that appeared to be healthy.

Many nations are reluctant to reopen their borders to U.S. beef since the first U.S. case of mad cow disease was announced on Dec. 23, 2003. The USDA is resisting calls for widespread testing of U.S. cattle, and defends the accuracy of its surveillance methods. The USDA, which tested just one out of every seventeen hundred cattle slaughtered in 2003, targeted about 10 percent of the cattle that arrived at plants unable to walk. This stands in stark contrast to the mad cow testing program used in Japan. The Japanese government tests 100 percent of all cattle marked for human consumption. The Japanese strategy is the only plan that can eliminate mad cow disease from a country's food supply. The USDA refuses to adopt it.

In summer 2004, U.S. livestock investigators found that the USDA wasn't testing adult cattle that died while on the farm and that it had failed to test hundreds of cattle condemned due to possible contamination with mad cow disease as well as many other diseases.

The USDA's Office of Inspector General reported: "The problems identified during our review, if not corrected, may . . . reduce the credibility of any assertion regarding the prevalence of BSE [mad cow disease] in the United States."

The report also said the USDA failed to test 518 of the 680 cattle condemned at slaughter for central nervous system symptoms between 2002 and 2004. Such symptoms can indicate that an animal could be suffering from mad cow disease or one of several other illnesses.

In April 2004, the USDA admitted that it had violated its own regulations when federal inspectors in Texas failed to test a twelve-year-old cow for mad cow disease even though it was exhibiting symptoms of the central nervous system disorder.

"The new BSE surveillance plan appears to have major deficiencies," said California Representative Henry Waxman, the top Democrat on the House Government Reform Committee.

U.S. BEEF SPECIAL INTERESTS: BEEF FIRST, SAFETY LAST?

Since the discovery of the first mad cow in the United States, the American beef industry has lost two-thirds of its $3 billion export market, primarily to Japan, Korea, and Mexico. Two dozen nations, including China, have since banned the importation of U.S. beef.

The lobbying arm of the National Cattlemen's Beef Association (NCBA) packs a lot of muscle, and they intend to fend off calls for stricter regulation of their industry while at the same time reassuring the public about the safety of U.S. beef. Prior to the discovery of the first case of BSE in this country, NCBA lobbyists helped defeat legislative attempts to ban injured, crippled, and immobilized animals—the so-called "downers" that pose a greater risk for mad cow disease than other animals.

The lobby, with the help of Senate Democratic leader Tom Daschle of South Dakota, also helped reverse requirements that beef be labeled with its country of origin. The NCBA argues that the discovery of the mad cow case in Washington State shows the current system is working. Opponents and critics of the NCBA counter that if such a ban had been implemented, the mad cow found in Washington State would never have entered the food supply. In what amounts to a case of "a day late and a dollar short," the NCBA has softened its position on downer cattle, reluctantly agreeing to a ban on allowing them to enter the U.S. food supply.

John McDougall, MD, a health writer and an antimeat activist, wonders whether it is coincidental that USDA Secretary Ann M. Veneman chose Dale Moore, former chief lobbyist for the National Cattlemen's Beef Association, as her chief of staff, or Alison Harrison, former director of public relations for the Cattlemen's Association, as her official spokeswoman, or that one of the new mad cow committee appointees is William Hueston, who was paid by the beef industry to testify against Oprah Winfrey in hopes of convicting her of beef "disparagement."

Dr. McDougall notes: "After a similar conflict of interest unfolded in Britain, their entire Ministry of Agriculture was dissolved and an independent Food Safety Agency was created, whose sole responsibility is to protect the public's health."

OTHER HEALTH CONCERNS

I'm concerned with the potential to overconsume saturated fats and cholesterol that naturally occur in beef and other meats, but I'm equally concerned with other problems that many dieters may not yet know about.

A high beef intake increases the body's output of a bile acid called deoxycyclic acid, which promotes unregulated cell turnover and growth in large-intestine lining (olive oil, on the other hand, reduces the amount of bile acid produced and slows down cell turnover and growth in the large bowel).

Published studies have linked consumption of red meat with higher rates of large bowel cancer, prostate cancer, and breast cancer. Two recent studies, for example, found that meat consumption was also linked to the growth of uterine fibroid tumors. In one study of 843 women with uterine fibroids, comparing them to 1,557 women without any uterine symptoms, scientists found that women with the benign tumors reported on average eating more beef, ham, and other red meat and fewer vegetables, fruits, and fish than women without the tumors. Frequent beef consumption raised the risk for fibroids 1.7 times higher than normal. Researchers also found that consumption of green vegetables cut the risk of developing fibroids in half; consumption of fish lowered the risk by around 30 percent.

Researchers also speculate that meat consumption could raise estrogen levels in women, a risk factor for developing fibroids and reproductive cancers. According to the University of Michigan Women's Health Program in Ann Arbor, half of the 550,000 hysterectomies performed nationwide every year are due to fibroids, a type of benign tumor that grow in the uterus (fibroids cause abdominal pain, bleeding, infertility, and increase the risk of miscarriage).

CAN YOU ENJOY BEEF WITHOUT THE RISK?

Many dieters cannot imagine life without beef. I understand this, and I wouldn't want anyone to steer clear of the Eat to Win Diet because of a weakness for the taste of meat. Accordingly, I have developed guidelines to minimize, to the extent possible at this time, the risk of becoming infected with mad cow disease, bovine leukemia virus (this infects the majority of the nation's beef supply), *E. coli* infection, or other contaminants typically found in beef, poultry, and other farm livestock.

Here are a few simple precautions to follow that can minimize the health risks linked to beef consumption:

- Choose certified 100 percent organic beef that has been grass-fed. Grass-fed beef (when possible, choose beef fed purslane, a wild, green, leafy plant) has a much higher ratio of healthy omega-3 fats to omega-6 fats than beef from grain-fed cattle. Grass-fed beef is leaner than grain-fed beef and has not been fed antibiotics. In addition, it contains more CLA (conjugated linoleic acid), a compound known to reduce the risk of certain types of cancer, obesity, and autoimmune diseases. Though grass-fed (sometimes called *natural* beef) is safer and healthier than grain-fed beef, unfortunately there are no laws or regulations governing what can be called grass-fed, and rules about the use of the term *natural* applied to animal products does not cover animal feeds.

- Check with your butcher or supplier before purchasing grass-fed beef. One potential risk is whether or not grass-fed animals were slaughtered in the same place as conventional cattle. Ask the supplier before purchasing.

- If you can't purchase grass-fed beef, choose such whole cuts of beef such as boneless steaks and roasts, rather than ground and chopped beef or processed beef products such as sausages and hot dogs. Ground beef is more likely to come from older cows (such as dairy cows that no longer produce enough milk). Ground beef and processed beef products are also more likely to become contaminated with central nervous system tissues due to the way meat is removed from all parts of the animal.

- Make your own ground beef from whole cuts of beef in your food processor or a meat grinder. Home-ground meat is less likely to become contaminated with such food-borne pathogens as *E. coli*,

MAD COW FACTOIDS

- 5,200 people die each year of food-related illnesses unrelated to mad cow disease.
- Some scientists estimate that between 1 and 12 percent of all deaths attributed to Alzheimer's disease are actually due to vCJD. Most people who die of Alzheimer's never undergo autopsy and have their brain tissue analyzed by a laboratory that tests for the disease. Based on all available evidence, it's likely that more people are infected with mad cow disease in the United States than has been reported.
- Prions, the cause of mad cow disease and the human form, vCJD, are impervious to all known methods of destruction: heat, irradiation, and antibiotics. Even incineration can't kill the pesky prion.
- The Japanese have 4 million cattle and slaughter 1.2 million of them each year. The United States has 100 million cattle and kills 35 million a year.
- Japan tests each and every cow slaughtered before it can enter the food supply. Last year, the United States tested only twenty thousand cows out of 35 million.
- The only way to stop mad cow disease in the United States is to test every animal. Early this fall, the Japanese surveillance found two new cases of the disease in animals ages twenty-one and twenty-three months. Under no testing regime except Japan would these cases have been found.

- The United States spends about $2.5 billion each year on HIV/AIDS research. About fourteen thousand people die each year from HIV/AIDS in the U.S. Research dollars spent on vCJD totals $27 million. An estimated 250 people die each year from vCJD (unrelated to mad cow disease).

- A new, highly sensitive test can detect the presence of extremely small amounts of the disease in very young animals with no symptoms. A single testing site could process eight thousand samples each day. If adopted in the United States, such testing would raise the price of a pound of beef no more than six to ten cents, a price most concerned beef lovers would gladly pay for piece of mind, not to mention avoiding the deadly disease.

Listeria, and *Salmonella.* Avoid ordering hamburger and other ground beef products while dining out.

PORK: THE OTHER INFECTED MEAT?

Although not widely discussed, pork is a potential source of BSE infection. Rendered cattle carcasses can be legally fed to pigs and other livestock in the United States. The FDA allows this exemption because, at present, there is no evidence that pigs spontaneously become infected with spongiform encephalopathy, as do cows. The problem is that pigs are generally slaughtered very early in life, at about six months of age, which is well before the disease can cause symptoms.

Thus far, we do know pigs can become infected with the disease. Researchers point to the fact that pigs fed cow brains from infected animals acquire the disease just as cows and people do. An untold number of "downer" pigs—those too crippled to walk—find their way into U.S. slaughterhouses each year.

Although the evidence is not yet robust enough to cause widespread alarm, researchers have linked the sporadic outbreak of vCJD to pork consumption. By analyzing the diet histories of people infected with the disease, researchers found that some cases of vCJD were related to eating hot dogs, pork chops, ham, and scrapple—a mélange of pork parts cooked together in a stew. The association is weak but suggestive nevertheless.

PROTEIN: ANIMAL OR VEGETABLE?

Nutritionists who defend the eating of animal protein correctly point out the following:

- The human body is physiologically and structurally equipped to eat, digest, and assimilate animal protein.
- The human body evolved on a mixed diet of animal and vegetable foods.
- Animal protein foods contain important nutrients, including vitamin D, B-complex vitamins, and minerals, including iron and calcium.
- Animal protein contains all the essential amino acids required to support life.

These are all accurate statements. But there's a scientifically sound rebuttal for each of them:

- The human body is physiologically and structurally equipped to eat, digest, assimilate, and thrive on a diet whose only source of protein comes from plants.
- The human body can thrive solely on a vegetarian diet. An ovo (egg white)-lacto (nonfat and low-fat dairy) vegetarian version of the Eat to Win Diet is an exceptionally healthy diet.
- Vegetable-protein foods contain all nutrients required by the human body except vitamin B_{12}, which the liver can store for five years.
- Vegetable protein contains all the essential amino acids required to support life.

Thus far, it's a draw—but here's the real dish on why you shouldn't eat animal protein, or at least why you should minimize your intake of it:

Mad cow disease is coming to a neighborhood near you. In fact, it may already be there. After examining all available research, I have concluded that the U.S. government has not adequately tested the nation's beef supply to insure against an outbreak of the disease. Even if all infected cows from other countries are prevented from entering the U.S. food supply, it can't stop the spontaneous mutation that occurs in the U.S cattle herd. It doesn't happen with great frequency, but it does happen. Since the government has refused thus far to test every cow, as the Japanese government does, the possibility exists that people will become infected with the disease unless they avoid consumption of beef and other meats.

Various forms of the disease can be found in swine, poultry, and other livestock. It could be just a matter of time before scientists uncover the first case of mad pig and mad lamb disease. This is a disease that spontaneously occurs in all animals, including humans.

Other things being equal, a diet consisting of vegetable proteins is a healthier and safer diet than one consisting of animal protein foods. An all-plant-protein diet contains minimal amounts of saturated fats, and no cholesterol.

A plant-protein diet will lower your LDL cholesterol far below levels that can be achieved on a meat-heavy diet. A diet composed mainly of plant foods improves blood pressure and minimizes the risk of the diseases that stalk most Americans: heart disease, stroke, type 2 diabetes, and colon, breast, and prostate cancers. Your kidneys will function better for longer on a plant-based diet, as will your liver, pancreas, gallbladder, and intestines. In fact, every organ system in your body would perform better on a scientifically devised predominantly plant-protein plan like the Eat to Win Vegetarian Diet.

If you eat a vegetarian diet or would like to discover the health benefits of this type of diet, Chapter 4 will help you get started. You can achieve superb health and outstanding fitness on the standard Eat to Win Diet, but the vegetarian version removes the health risks associated with eating beef and other meats.

Phytonutrients:
21st-century "Vitamins"

⑨

If we could all just pop a few pills each day to beat back cancer, heart disease, and diabetes, life would be wonderful. Regrettably, such is not the case, even with the ever-growing body of evidence that indicates that specific nutritional supplements can wage war against obesity and the diseases of aging.

In kitchens across the country, millions of Americans take their morning once-a-day-type multivitamins as "health insurance" to atone for their dietary sins. But do such pills actually forestall disease and help any of us live longer?

Researchers at the Centers for Disease Control and the American Cancer Society followed the health of nearly 1 million men and women for seven years to discover whether people who took low-dose, garden-variety multivitamins suffered fewer deaths due to heart attacks and strokes. Those who took them regularly died from heart disease and stroke at about the same rate as those who didn't. There were no measurable differences in deaths from other causes. No studies to date show that taking once-a-day-type multivitamins improve the survival of well-nourished people.

The reason, as my research indicates, is that scientists have been focusing on the wrong nutrients. The real "vitamins" of the 21st century are *phytonutrients*—the disease-fighting compounds found in fruits and vegetables. These are the nutritional factors that really make the difference between health and disease.

The Eat to Win Diet is based on a MediterrAsian nutritional profile that contains the most powerful disease-fighting and antiaging phytonutrients from the diets of the two healthiest and most long-lived populations on the earth: the traditional Mediterranean and Asian diets.

If we lived in a perfect world, ate perfect diets free from contamination by environmental toxins and carcinogens, few people would need to rely on phytonutrient supplements to enjoy ultimate protection against such diseases as cancer and heart disease. Due to the imperfect nature of diets and the people who follow them, no one can or does eat perfectly at all times. Most of us expose ourselves to UV radiation, and we breathe polluted air and consume contaminated foods and drinks.

The Eat to Win Diet, as good as it is, can be made even better by supplementing it with additional phytonutrients that have withstood the scrutiny of scientific study. I'm not talking about the questionable and unproven "remedies" one finds while surfing the Internet or the nutritional nostrums hawked on TV infomercials.

There are a number of credible studies that suggest taking additional phytonutrients can make a good diet even better. For example, we know that naturally occurring relatives of vitamin A in the plant world, called carotenoids, can effectively treat age-related maculopathy (ARM), a leading cause of poor vision and blindness in the United States. Twenty percent of individuals over the age of sixty-five have early signs of ARM, which affects the natural pigments concentrated in the retina, even though many may not know they have it yet.

Scientists who study the disease have discovered that giving supplements containing lutein and zeaxanthin (found in corn, green vegetables, fruits, broccoli, green beans, green peas, Brussels sprouts, cabbage, kale, collard greens, spinach, lettuce, kiwi, and honeydew) can restore a degree of health to the macula and protect the retina and the crystalline lens of the eye. These phytonutrients filter out phototoxic blue light and near-ultraviolet radiation from the macula, and by doing so they protect the lens and retina against UV radiation and oxygen. Some scientists believe it may put the disease on hold—leading to a permanent remission. These two phytonutrients may also help protect against cataract formation.

Research has shown this to be the case for many other phytonutrients, including the ability of soy isoflavones to reduce blood cholesterol scores, the ability of selenium to prevent prostate cancer and slow its progression, and the ability of grape polyphenols to reduce LDL cholesterol oxidation, which means less damage to arteries.

Even people undergoing plastic surgery can benefit from a combination of vitamins and phytonutrients. Researchers from the University of Texas found that patients taking a supplement that contained a mixture of the fruit phytonutrients bromelain (papaya), rutin (oranges), grape-seed extract, and vitamin C recovered from a face-lift three days faster than those taking a placebo.

I have been helping my clients recover from surgery and sports injuries faster by using various phytonutrients and other nutrients. Surgeons have remarked that they have never seen their patients heal as quickly as when they use these nutritional supplements. I recently used phytonutrients to help Gregor Fucka, the basketball star from Barcelona, heal from a serious tendon injury that might have sidelined him for four to six months. Instead, Gregor returned to competition within two months and led his team, FC Barcelona, to victory and to win the 2004 Spanish League Championships.

What about apparently healthy people? Do they need to take phytonutrients?

WHAT THE EVIDENCE SHOWS

Such studies as the ones I mentioned are far from conclusive, but some suggest that certain phytonutrients, taken in quantities beyond those available in ordinary foods, may provide powerful protection against disease and may treat diseases and prevent them from worsening. Some nutrients may help place a disease in a long-term or permanent remission, a term I coined in 1991 to describe the process of holding degenerative diseases in check using diet, phytonutrients, and medical treatments.

Phytonutrient supplements can play an important albeit ancillary role in preventing and reversing disease. That's why they are called supplements: They are meant to complement and augment a healthy diet, not supplant it. Always consult with a physician before taking any dietary supplements, including those that contain phytonutrients.

EAT TO WIN PHYTONUTRIENTS

Why didn't Mother Nature just put disease-bashing phytonutrients in our bodies instead of sending us to the supermarket for them? Why did she give them to plants but not her two-legged creatures?

One reason is that we have legs and plants do not. We can run from predators. Plants, on the other hand, can't run from danger. Plants rely on phytonutrients to discourage insects and animals from eating them (many phytonutrients are distasteful to predators; others render predators sterile and thereby reduce the predator population). Plants also lack an immune system, so nature has given them the ability to manufacture phytonutrients that protect them against bacteria and viruses. And, since plants can get cancer too, phytonutrients play an important role in keeping them disease-free.

Plants must also make their own antioxidant phytonutrients such as polyphenols and carotenoids to protect their delicate cellular structures from the sun's ultraviolet radiation. Photosynthesis, a process by which plants use sunlight, carbon dioxide, and water to manufacture carbohydrates and oxygen, generates a large number of free radicals, which would kill the plants were it not for the presence of protective phytonutrients. Phytonutrients also protect young seeds, guarding their ability to germinate.

More than twenty classes of phytonutrient compounds found in plant foods exert anticancer activity in animals and humans. Compounds in garlic, onions, and cruciferous vegetables such as broccoli and cabbage detoxify carcinogens and prevent them from doing their dirty work. Retinoids, indoles, isothiocyanates, polyphenols, and trace minerals found in cabbage alone can inhibit breast cancer in rats. Scientists at the National Cancer Institute believe that phytonutrients are active against human cancer as well.

Researchers at the NCI's Diet and Cancer branch and at the American Heart Association have just begun to understand how phytonutrients can halt and even reverse the growth of cancerous cells and cholesterol-filled tumors, called plaque, that cause a heart attack or stroke. And scientists have recently discovered that phytonutrients can help adult-onset diabetics reduce or eliminate their need for insulin injections and oral medications.

Many phytonutrients come packaged in a variety of familiar containers: broccoli, tomatoes, strawberries, oranges, lemons, grapefruit, watermelon, grapes, carrots, cabbage, garlic, and onions, to name just a few. Nearly all of them sport tongue-twisting names such as isothiocyanates, allylic sulfides, and isoflavonoids. Fortunately, you don't have to know how to pronounce them, but you do have to know where to find them and how to use them. Highly concentrated phytonutrients have been incorporated into biodesigned food products, sometimes called functional foods or nutraceuticals. These high-tech food and beverage products are currently the focus of investigation by the NCI's Diet and Cancer branch.

For the last decade, I have been developing phytonutrient formulas that combine the most powerful disease-fighting phytonutrients in the Mediterranean and Asian diets. This MediterrAsian line of phytonutrient supplements may be available in the marketplace by the time you read this book. Check the MediterrAsianDiet.com Web site for availability.

But never underestimate the healing power locked inside a tomato, onion, orange, or cantaloupe. Food is the most chemically complex substance you will ever encounter. The phytonutrient-rich foods that you will enjoy on the Eat to Win Diet contain more than half a million naturally occurring compounds, many of which are active against cancer, heart disease, and diabetes.

FIGURE 9.1

SELECTED PHYTONUTRIENTS IN THE EAT TO WIN DIET

Phytonutrient	MediterrAsian foods	Activity
Carotenoids	Broccoli, Cantaloupe, Carrots, Mandarin Oranges Papaya, Pumpkin, Spinach, Yellow Squash, Sweet Potatoes	A powerful family of antioxidants that suppress or reverse cancer, reduce risk of atherosclerosis
Catechins	Green and Black Teas	Quench free radicals involved in cancer formation and atherosclerosis
Flavonoids	Broccoli, Cabbage, Carrots, Citrus Fruits, Cucumbers, Soy Foods and Beverages, Tomatoes, Yams	Block sex hormones that promote the growth of cancer cells
Indoles	Broccoli, Brussels Sprouts, Cabbage, Cauliflower, Kale, Kohlrabi, Mustard Greens, Rutabagas, Turnips	Activates the body's enzymes that detoxify carcinogens; help metabolize estrogen into its harmless form
Isoflavones	Beans, Peas, Lentils	Block the cancer-promoting effects of sex hormones; inactivate enzymes produced by cancer cells
Isothiocyanates	Broccoli, Brussels Sprouts, Cabbage, Cauliflower, Kale, Kohlrabi, Mustard Greens, Rutabagas, Turnips	Activates the body's enzymes that detoxify carcinogens; help metabolize estrogen into its harmless form
Lignans	Nuts and Seeds	Quench free radicals, block sex hormones from promoting tumor formation and growth

Limonoids	Citrus Fruits	Stimulate the body's enzymes that detoxify carcinogens
Monoterpenes	Broccoli, Cabbage, Carrots, Citrus, Fruits, Eggplant, Parsley, Peppers, Squash, Tomatoes, Yams	Quench free radicals, activate the body's enzymes that detoxify carcinogens, reduce risk of atherosclerosis
Omega-3 Fatty Acids	Flaxseed, Walnuts, Purslane	Block estrogens from promoting cancer, reduce inflammation that leads to cancer and atherosclerosis
Organo-sulfur Compounds	Garlic, Leeks, Onions, Shallots	Block carcinogen formation and suppress tumor formation
Protease Inhibitors	Soy Foods and Beverages	Block the enzymes made by cancer cells that help them spread, limit the rate of cell division, give cells time to repair DNA damage that can lead to cancer
Sterols	Broccoli, Cabbage, Cucumbers, Eggplant, Peppers, Soy Foods and Beverages, Tomatoes, Whole Grains and Cereals, Yams	Help cells that have taken a step toward cancer revert to a normal state, help block the body from absorbing dietary cholesterol
Triterpenes	Licorice Root	Block sex hormones and prostaglandins from promoting cancer

PHYTONUTRIENTS AT ANY AGE

A 2004 study by researchers in Hong Kong, reported in the scientific journal *Menopause*, shows that postmenopausal women taking 80mg of isoflavones daily enjoyed positive benefits on bone mineral content, particularly if they were more than four years into menopause, had lower body weights, or had a lower calcium intake.

"Many studies have shown that soy isoflavones have an effect in preventing estrogen-related bone loss, but no data reported whether such an effect could be influenced by other important factors affecting bone loss," noted the researchers.

The results of this study stand in stark contrast to one also reported during 2004 in the *Journal of the American Medical Association*. The results of these conflicting studies can be explained by the fact that certain factors important to bone health are so powerful that they overpower any potential benefit seen from eating or taking supplemental isoflavones.

SOY FOR MENOPAUSE?

The team from the Chinese University of Hong tested isoflavones in women ages forty-eight to sixty-two years old. These women received either a placebo with 500mg calcium and 125 IU of vitamin D, a mid-dose (40mg isoflavones with 500mg calcium and 125 IU of vitamin D), or a high-dose (80mg isoflavones with 500mg calcium and 125 IU of vitamin D) supplement every day for one year.

The researchers found significant benefit of high-dose soy isoflavone supplementation on bone mineral content in the hip compared to those women on low-dose isoflavones or placebo. There was no significant improvement in bone mineral density.

Women who had been postmenopausal for more than four years, as well as those with a lower body weight, benefited from taking isoflavones with calcium and vitamin D. Women who consumed less than 1,095mg of calcium per day, on average, also benefited from taking the combined nutrients, although in those with a high calcium intake, soy isoflavones seemed to make no difference to their bone health.

The researchers concluded "body weight is a much stronger predictor of bone mass than many other factors, including menopause status."

They also note "soy isoflavones at current doses may not have any additional benefits to bone mass among women with a high body weight. Our findings suggest that the *beneficial effects of isoflavone supplementation could be potentiated in women with lower body weight* or in women with low dietary calcium intake" (my italics).

ANTICANCER BENEFITS OF RESVERATROL

Resveratrol is a natural substance made by grapes and other plants in response to fungal infection. Grapes sprayed with pesticides that prevent fungal infection contain little, if any, resveratrol. How much resveratrol is in your favorite glass of *vino* depends on a number of factors. Many wines contain either no resveratrol at all or very little (less than a milligram per glass).

In addition to resveratrol's well-known health benefits, researchers have recently discovered resveratrol's ability to augment cancer chemotherapies. For example, vitamin D_3 converts to a steroid in the body that inhibits the growth of breast-cancer cells. Researchers at the University of Notre Dame have shown that resveratrol increases the anticancer effects of vitamin D. Other research shows that it causes drug-resistant non-Hodgkin's lymphoma cancer cells to become more susceptible to such chemotherapeutic drugs as gemcitabine, vinorelbine (Navelbine), cisplatin, and paclitaxel. Researchers in Austria have conducted studies showing that resveratrol blocks the ability of cancer cells to metastasize to bone.

RESVERATROL: THE FOUNTAIN OF YOUTH?

Harvard Medical School researchers have demonstrated that resveratrol activates a longevity gene in yeast that extends life span by 70 percent. The effects mimic those of calorie restriction, the only proven way of extending maximum life span. Resveratrol activates one of the same longevity genes as calorie restriction. Although the research has been conducted only on yeast, flies, and worms so far, humans have their own version of the same life span–extending gene, and there is no reason to believe that humans respond differently to resveratrol than other species.

SHOULD YOU TAKE RESVERATROL SUPPLEMENTS?

Resveratrol supplements are typically derived from an extract of the plant *Polygonum cuspidatum*. Resveratrol is extracted from grape skins to retain other compounds such as quercetin that naturally occur with it. Some resveratrol supplement labels claim they contain 15mg per serving or higher. Although there is no typical dosage, most commercial products list their resveratrol content between 5mg to 20mg per serving.

Don't be too eager to start taking resveratrol supplements just yet; scientists who study resveratrol say that the phytonutrient is so susceptible to oxidation that ordinary resveratrol supplements are probably useless. That warning doesn't stop dietary supplement companies from selling resveratrol-labeled products, however. Check with the Mediterr AsianDiet.com Web site to stay abreast of the latest developments on this powerful disease-fighting phytonutrient.

Caution: Anyone who suffers from a platelet deficiency or blood-clotting problems or anyone taking blood-thinning drugs should use resveratrol supplements only under medical supervision. The similarity in structure between resveratrol and diethylstilbestrol (a synthetic estrogen) has prompted investigations into resveratrol's potential as a phytoestrogen (a plant compound that produces estrogenlike effects). Resveratrol is contraindicated in those hypersensitive to any component of a resveratrol-containing product. Those who are pregnant or breast-feeding should avoid using dietary supplements unless advised to do so by a physician. Always check with a physician before changing your diet or taking any supplements, including those mentioned in this book.

The Eat to Win Exercise Plan

A SIMPLE GUIDE TO HELP YOU DETERMINE HOW MANY CALORIES YOU NEED TO BURN EACH WEEK

Permit me to jog your memory.

I'd like to take you back to the early 1980s, when the running fad swept the nation.

Jim Fixx, the fifty-two-year-old patron saint of running enthusiasts in the late 1970s and early 1980s, had discovered a new runner's high—writing about running. Jim was an avid jogger and marathon runner who wrote a best-selling book that recounted, in diarylike fashion, his life as a runner and author. Nine months prior to his untimely demise from a heart attack while jogging, I had lunch with Jim. I couldn't help but notice that he consumed two large servings of roast beef smothered in gravy. While this would have been an Atkins Diet–approved lunch, I don't think Jim was specifically following any special diet at that time.

I asked Jim to get a blood chemistry profile test and send it to me. He agreed and had his physician perform one. The test showed his cholesterol was dangerously elevated but Jim and his personal physician were not concerned. I strongly advised Jim to follow the Eat to Win Diet but he felt that his daily long-distance running protected him from cardiovascular disease.

During that time, one outspoken physician-runner claimed that anyone who could complete a marathon in fewer than four hours could not possibly have serious heart problems. He also believed that following a very-low-fat, high-complex-carbohydrate diet would disable or kill a marathon runner within eighteen months. Why? He claimed that such a diet doesn't contain sufficient linoleic acid—an essential fatty acid that cannot be made by the body.

In a study published at least a decade before this physician-runner made his view public, researchers compared the essential fatty acid intake of Japanese men to American men. Japanese men, who eat a very-low-fat, high-complex-carbohydrate diet, consumed about 9g of linoleic acid each day; American men consumed up to 12.5g per day of the fat. This apparent difference in intake actually represents no difference at all because Japanese men weigh about twenty percent less than American men of the same height. On a per-weight basis, both groups actually consume about the same amount of linoleic acid.

When researchers analyzed the adipose tissue of both groups of men (adipose tissue reflects the proportion of essential fat to nonessential fats in the diet), they found that the fat cells of the Japanese men contained about 17 percent linoleic acid; the fat cells of the American men contained only 10 percent of the fat.

Published studies reveal that despite claims to the contrary, marathoners do die from cardiovascular disease. In fact, a 1982 study published in the *New England Journal of Medicine* revealed that the more vigorous exercise you do, the greater will be your chance of dying with your running shoes on.

Recently, Edmund Burke, PhD, who was as popular among serious endurance cyclists as Jim Fixx was among running enthusiasts, died on a training ride in 2003 at age fifty-three. You may not have heard of Dr. Frederick Montz, Dr. David Nagey, or Dr. Jeffrey Williams, three physicians at Johns Hopkins University who died while running. The oldest of the three was fifty-one. The cause: heart disease.

Today's diet doctors promote high-fat, low-carbohydrate diets for active people. They don't believe as I do that a low-fat, complex-carbohydrate-rich diet confers superior protection for active people against cardiovascular disease. In fact, they hold the polar opposite view. The difference is that I can point to thousands of published studies to support my position (interested readers will find hundreds of them in the research bibliography at the end of this book). I don't believe they could do the same for theirs.

When it comes to exercise, none of the carbophobic cardiologists who write popular diet books insist that their readers embrace a regular program of heart-healthy sports or physical activity. Perhaps it's fortunate that they don't! You can exercise and die while following a high-fat, high-cholesterol diet. The autopsy reports of highly conditioned marathon runners prove this beyond any doubt.

Exercise alone confers no protection against cardiovascular disease when you overwhelm your arteries with excess calories, especially when they're from fat and sugar. Once you add large amounts of dietary cholesterol to the mix, you have a recipe for sudden death while exercising. When you follow the Eat to Win Diet, you can be certain that you are enjoying optimum protection against cardiovascular disease, at home or on the track.

A LITTLE EXERCISE MAKES A BIG DIFFERENCE

Most people can prevent weight gain without changing their diets. Just walking forty-five to sixty minutes on most days can prevent weight gain. *New York Times* health columnist Jane Brody discovered this and now takes nightly walks to prevent middle-age spread.

The more you exercise, the easier it is to prevent weight gain. Even walking as little as five miles per week (that's less than fifteen minutes each day) can prevent weight gain with no dieting at all. For lasting weight loss and better health, you should trade walking five miles per week for walking at least five hours per week.

Aerobic exercise—the type that makes your heart race and your skin sweat—can harm your body if you follow a diet rich in fats and cholesterol. People on such diets would do well not to engage in endurance training. Some physical exertion, however, can be beneficial, even on a high-fat, high-cholesterol diet. An often-quoted study published in 1970 that looked at death rates in San Franciscan longshoremen found that those who were promoted to management positions and no longer lifted heavy items developed 25 percent more heart disease than those engaged in heavier labor. None of the longshoremen were doing endurance exercise. Their exercise was intermittent and involved walking, lifting, and stopping.

Another well-known Harvard study that tracked the health and exercise habits of alumni found that cardiovascular disease declines when people burn between 500 to 2,000 calories each week. They study found that beyond the 2,000-calorie mark, exercise didn't improve heart disease risk.

I recommend using the number of calories burned as a starting point in planning your exercise program. There's also the question of intensity. Some studies show that moderate-intensity exercise is heart-healthy; others show that this level doesn't provide much benefit; rather, it isn't until you run instead of walk that heart disease risks go down.

What is clear is that populations who follow a low-fat, phytonutrient-rich diet and enjoy moderate exercise live much longer and healthier lives, on average, than do Americans. It's the combination of a low-fat, phytonutrient-rich diet with moderate exercise no more strenuous than walking four miles in an hour that provides superb protection against heart disease. If you follow a high-fat, low-carb diet, all bets are off.

BURN GLYCOGEN TO GET THIN AND STAY THIN

It doesn't matter if you take a walk, climb some stairs, mow the lawn, or play a round of golf. As long as you move enough to burn off at least 1,500 extra calories each week from exercise and follow the Eat to Win Diet, you will stay lean and fit. It works like magic, but it's nothing more than simple biochemistry.

As a rule of thumb, you can assume that half of the calories you burn during such moderate physical activity as walking burn off stored carbohydrate (glycogen) calories. The remaining calories you burn come from fat.

People who follow an ordinary American diet can store about 1,000g of glycogen. Glycogen is stored in the muscles and the liver; liver glycogen provides the most readily available store of glycogen. The liver normally stores about 300 to 500 calories of glycogen that it uses to replenish low blood sugar levels as needed. Endurance athletes can store nearly double that amount.

What is the benefit of partially emptying your stored glycogen reserves? Let's say you have burned about 300 calories during an hour's walk, half of them from glycogen. The next 150 calories you consume as carbs—the two slices of whole-grain bread you used to make a sandwich, for example—will be stored as glycogen by the body to make up the 150-calorie carbohydrate deficit created by exercise. It actually amounts to a bit more because it costs additional calories to form and store glycogen.

Glycogen calories are not fat calories and therefore do not add fat to your body. With respect to body-fat loss, this means that the next 150 carbohydrate calories you consume are, in a sense, *free calories.* The more you exercise, the more you can enjoy pasta and potatoes and not add fat to your body.

After your morning walk, you will continue to burn fat and carbohydrate throughout the day. The carbohydrates you consume will help feed your brain and muscles the optimal fuel mix they need to function properly. That's why daily exercise is a natural partner to the Eat to Win Diet. It burns off stored body fat and glycogen at the same time. By partially emptying your body's glycogen "storage tank" you will make room for the carbohydrate calories in the bread, pasta, rice, and potatoes you'll get to enjoy without adding any fat to your body.

THE CALORIE MYTH

Most diet experts will tell you that exercise is not a very efficient way to lose weight. They point out that you have to burn 3,500 calories to lose a pound of fat and you'll have to walk thirty-five miles to accomplish this. As it turns out, both statements are inaccurate. Here's why:

You'd have to walk seventy miles to burn off a pound of body fat—not thirty-five miles, as the experts claim. The reason is quite simple. On average, most people burn a fuel mixture of about 50 percent fat and 50 percent carbohydrate while walking. Depending upon the type of exercise you do (aerobic or anaerobic), the amount of time and level of intensity you spend exercising, and the type of diet you eat, this mixture will vary. But as a rule of thumb, you can use the 50:50 ratio to calculate that the practical caloric cost of burning a pound of body fat is actually closer to 7,000 calories than to 3,500 calories:

Walking 1 mile burns 100 calories (50 fat calories + 50 carbohydrate calories)

3,500 (usable calories in 1 pound of fat) ÷ 50 fat calories burned/ 1 mile = 70 miles

While this seems to support the argument that exercise is not an efficient way to lose weight, it actually upholds my contention that daily exercise is essential to permanent fat loss. Why? As I previously mentioned, burning calories from stored glycogen allows you to make room in your body for "free" carbohydrate calories—the calories that won't add fat to your body. In addition, you'll burn off about 150 calories of body fat.

Compounded over the course of a year, the caloric cost of a daily one-hour walk will add up to quite a few calories. This translates into a loss of *15 pounds of pure body fat,* the ability to enjoy potatoes and pasta without gaining fat, and a healthier cardiovascular system. To me, that's a terrific deal.

Evidence for the importance of emptying your glycogen tanks with exercise each day comes from laboratories the world over. When researchers allow unexercised lab animals to eat at will from a smorgasbord of high-fat and low-fat foods, the animals consume over 50 percent more calories from fat than do exercised animals. So we know that *exercise blunts the drive to gorge on fat.*

Exercise plays an essential role in getting you to lose excess body fat permanently. You already know this because you've seen that when you partially empty your glycogen storage tanks each day, you also burn off body fat. People who don't exercise each day can't store as many dietary carbohydrates as exercisers, because their muscles stay loaded with glycogen.

FIGURE 10.1

CALORIES BURNED DURING SELECTED ACTIVITIES*

Activity	Calories per hour	Glycogen calories per hour
Running 10 mph (six-minute miles)	1,200	600
Jogging 5.5 mph (eleven-minute miles)	700	350
Cross-country skiing	700	350
Bicycling 12 mph	400	200
Bicycling 6 mph	220	110
Swimming 25 yards/min	250	125
Swimming 50 yards/min	500	250
Tennis—singles	400	200
Walking 2 mph (thirty-minute miles)	220	110
Walking 3 mph (twenty-minute miles)	300	150
Walking 4.5 mph (13.3-minute miles)	420	210

*All values are approximate. Differences will depend on body weight, gender, exercise intensity, and percent of fat and carbohydrate in the diet.

TEN-WEEK AEROBIC PROGRAM FOR BEGINNERS

If you are not a regular exerciser or sports enthusiast (an active one, not a sports spectator), this plan will help you ease into the wonderful world of exercise.

Begin with short workouts and gradually lengthen them as you become fitter. By week ten, you'll be walking, cycling, or doing some other aerobic activity for forty-five to sixty minutes at a time, five to six days a week. Always check with a physician before starting an exercise plan if you've been leading a sedentary existence.

Begin every workout with five minutes of slow and easy walking or its equivalent. If you exercise at moderate intensity, allow yourself an additional five-minute cooldown period when the workout is over to allow your circulation to normalize.

How hard should you push yourself? Some experts recommend using common sense. Don't push yourself to the point where you can't carry on a normal conversation while exercising. Your intensity level should leave you feeling that this exercise is something you could continue for an extended period of time. If you want to increase your exercise intensity, such as walking up a steep hill, you can do so for a brief period, provided your physician has given you permission to do so. Your goal is level five, which means walking one hour each day for at least five days a week at a brisk pace (4 to 4.5 miles per hour). Remember, start off slowly and gradually increase your distance and speed over the course of ten weeks. Walk with a friend, relative, or spouse. Use indoor shopping malls during inclement weather. Wear a pair of shoes designed for walking, jogging, or cross training.

A TEN-WEEK EXERCISE PLAN FOR BEGINNERS

Week 1:	Time	Level
Day 1	15 minutes	1
Day 2	15 minutes	1
Day 3	15 minutes	1
Day 4	20 minutes	1
Day 5	20 minutes	1
Week 2:	Time	Level
Day 1	20 minutes	1
Day 2	20 minutes	1

Day 3	20 minutes	1
Day 4	25 minutes	1
Day 5	25 minutes	1
Week 3:	**Time**	**Level**
Day 1	25 minutes	1
Day 2	25 minutes	1
Day 3	25 minutes	1
Day 4	30 minutes	2
Day 5	30 minutes	2
Week 4:	**Time**	**Level**
Day 1	30 minutes	2
Day 2	30 minutes	2
Day 3	30 minutes	2
Day 4	35 minutes	2
Day 5	35 minutes	2
Week 5:	**Time**	**Level**
Day 1	35 minutes	2
Day 2	35 minutes	2
Day 3	35 minutes	2
Day 4	40 minutes	2+
Day 5	40 minutes	2+
Week 6:	**Time**	**Level**
Day 1	40 minutes	2+
Day 2	40 minutes	2+
Day 3	40 minutes	2+
Day 4	45 minutes	3
Day 5	45 minutes	3

Week 7:	Time	Level
Day 1	45 minutes	3
Day 2	45 minutes	3
Day 3	45 minutes	3
Day 4	50 minutes	3+
Day 5	50 minutes	3+
Week 8:	Time	Level
Day 1	50 minutes	3+
Day 2	50 minutes	3+
Day 3	50 minutes	4
Day 4	55 minutes	4
Day 5	55 minutes	4
Week 9:	Time	Level
Day 1	55 minutes	4
Day 2	55 minutes	4
Day 3	55 minutes	4
Day 4	60 minutes	4+
Day 5	60 minutes	moderate 4+
Week 10:	Time	Level
Day 1	60 minutes	4+
Day 2	60 minutes	4+
Day 3	60 minutes	brisk 4+
Day 4	60 minutes	4+
Day 5	60 minutes	4+

To get to level five, increase walking speed to brisk (4 to 4.5 miles per hour) with permission from a physician. Always consult with a physician before beginning this or any other exercise program.

Section II

Eat to Win Recipes

ere are some suggestions to make meal preparation and shopping more convenient and enjoyable. If you have trouble finding any of the products in the recipe ingredients lists, on p. 000 or ask your supermarket manager to order them. I've suggested some of the food items by brand name in the recipes because they provide the best results. Reasonable substitutions may work as well.

CONCERNING EAT TO WIN POWER SHAKES AND SMOOTHIES

- Have at least two ice cube trays with standard-size square holes. You will find that cubes of juice and soy milk impart a richer texture to the finished drink. (Two frozen cubes of beverage equal ⅓ cup of liquid.) Once you settle on your favorite functional drink, you will know what cubes to keep ready.

- Always make new frozen cubes as you use them so you won't be disappointed when you go to the freezer with a craving for your favorite drink. It's easier to make blender drinks in the morning if you start them the night before. I find that it's easier to measure all the ingredients except the frozen ones (e.g., soy milk cubes, juice cubes, and frozen fruit) into the blender container, blend briefly, and store covered in the refrigerator overnight. In the morning, pulse the ingredients to remix them and add frozen cubes and/or fruit, then process until smooth. This way you are not forced to "think" before you've had one of these eye-opening smart drinks!

• Purchase a tall thermos cup like the ones for sale at coffeehouses and kitchen stores. They will keep the shakes frosty cold for hours. Bring yours with you to work in the morning and sip it at your leisure.

ABOUT YOUR NEW FOODS

Many of the Eat to Win Power Meal recipes are based on some of the most popular foods and fast foods in America. You can make most of them in minutes. Some take a little longer but can be prepared in stages. For example, you can prepare some Power Meal recipes several days ahead of time. They'll heat up in the microwave in seconds and taste freshly made.

Whenever possible, serve a fresh vegetable along with lunch and dinner to complete your Eat to Win Power Meal. Lightly steam or microwave your vegetable of choice and flavor with lemon juice if desired.

I know you will benefit from my Eat to Win Power Meal recipes. They have a rich history of helping my athletic champion clients eat to win. Now, they will do the same for you. Bon appetit!

Eat to Win Power Meals Recipes

INDEX

Italian-style Zucchini
Leftover Turkey-stuffed Potatoes
Louisiana Fruit Salad
Lyonnaise Potatoes
Mahi-mahi with Spicy Corn Salsa
Marathon Snapper
Mediterranean Broiled Sole
MediterrAsian Chicken Salad
MediterrAsian Hummus
Mississippi Caviar
Moroccan Salad
Power "Franks" and Beans
Power-packed Tuna Salad
Ratatouille
Rigatoni Romana
Rock Shrimp Salad
Salmon and Pasta Skillet Dinner
Shrimp Creole
Shrimp de Jacques
Smart Fries
Smoked Salmon Scramble
Spicy Black-bean Quiche
Spinach Noodle Casserole
Strawberry Power Smoothie
Super Chicken Stir-fry
Super Power Smoothie
Tasty Oatmeal
Thai Noodle Medley
Thick 'n' Frosty Malted
Tuna Fagiole Salad
Ultimate Chicken Salad
Whey Cool Vanilla Malted
Winner's Circle Salad
Ziti Bolognese

Albacore Tuna Skillet Dinner

Serves 4

2 tablespoons light whipped butter (like Land O Lakes)
2 tablespoons lemon juice
1 tablespoon tamari soy sauce
2 tablespoons water
1 teaspoon dried minced garlic
¼ cup chopped celery
¼ cup finely chopped fresh parsley
2 cups cooked brown rice
6½-ounce can solid white albacore tuna packed in springwater
½ cup chopped scallion (green part only)
⅛ teaspoon pepper
1 tablespoon grated Parmesan cheese (or soy substitute)

Coat a nonstick frying pan with olive oil cooking spray. Cook the butter, lemon juice, soy sauce, and water at medium-high heat. Add the garlic, celery, and parsley. Sauté until the celery is just tender. Add the brown rice, stirring constantly to coat it with the mixture. Blend in the tuna, onions, pepper, and Parmesan cheese. Cook until heated through.

Nutrition Totals Per Serving

KCal Breakdown: 28.3% Protein; 56.1% Carbohydrate; 15.6% Fat

Calories: 212
Protein: 16.1 (g)
Carbohydrate: 31.9 (g)

Fat: 3.9 (g)
Sodium: 710 (mg)
Cholesterol: 25 (mg)

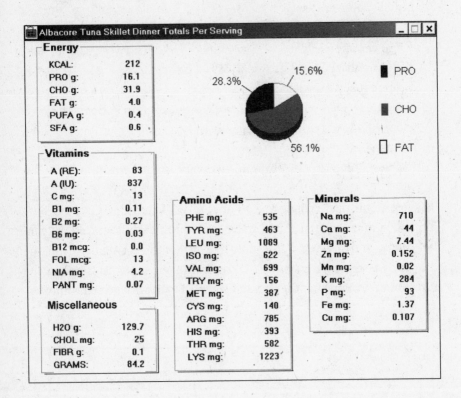

Albacore Tuna Skillet Dinner Totals Per Serving		_ □ X

Energy

KCAL:	212
PRO g:	16.1
CHO g:	31.9
FAT g:	4.0
PUFA g:	0.4
SFA g:	0.6

28.3%   15.6%   ■ PRO

■ CHO

56.1%   □ FAT

Vitamins

A (RE):	83
A (IU):	837
C mg:	13
B1 mg:	0.11
B2 mg:	0.27
B6 mg:	0.03
B12 mcg:	0.0
FOL mcg:	13
NIA mg:	4.2
PANT mg:	0.07

Amino Acids

PHE mg:	535
TYR mg:	463
LEU mg:	1089
ISO mg:	622
VAL mg:	699
TRY mg:	156
MET mg:	387
CYS mg:	140
ARG mg:	785
HIS mg:	393
THR mg:	582
LYS mg:	1223

Minerals

Na mg:	710
Ca mg:	44
Mg mg:	7.44
Zn mg:	0.152
Mn mg:	0.02
K mg:	284
P mg:	93
Fe mg:	1.37
Cu mg:	0.107

Miscellaneous

H2O g:	129.7
CHOL mg:	25
FIBR g:	0.1
GRAMS:	84.2

Strawberry Power Smoothie

Serves 1

⅔ cup reduced-fat soy milk (like Westsoy 1% Lite Soy Beverage)
1 packet whey protein powder (natural or vanilla flavor)
3 tablespoons Eagle Brand Fat Free Sweetened Condensed Milk

1 heaping cup frozen strawberries (unsweetened)
4 cubes frozen reduced-fat soy milk

In a blender combine the liquid soy milk, whey powder, and chocolate syrup. Pulse to blend. Add the frozen cubes and process till smooth. Serve immediately.

Nutrition Totals Per Serving

KCAL Breakdown: 17.0% Protein; 76.3% Carbohydrate; 6.6% Fat

Calories: 345
Protein: 14.4 (g)
Carbohydrate 64.6 (g)

Fat: 2.5 (g)
Sodium: 283 (mg)
Cholesterol: 5 (mg)

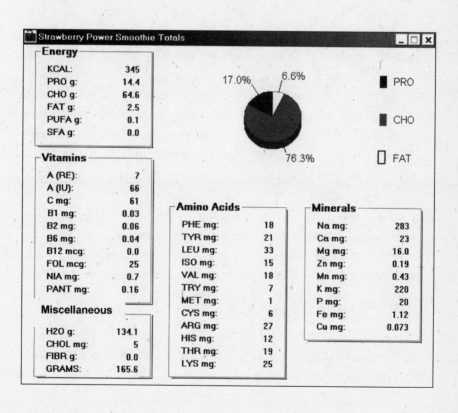

Strawberry Power Smoothie Totals

Energy

KCAL:	345
PRO g:	14.4
CHO g:	64.6
FAT g:	2.5
PUFA g:	0.1
SFA g:	0.0

17.0%   6.6%   76.3%

PRO
CHO
FAT

Vitamins

A (RE):	7
A (IU):	66
C mg:	61
B1 mg:	0.03
B2 mg:	0.06
B6 mg:	0.04
B12 mcg:	0.0
FOL mcg:	25
NIA mg:	0.7
PANT mg:	0.16

Miscellaneous

H2O g:	134.1
CHOL mg:	5
FIBR g:	0.0
GRAMS:	165.6

Amino Acids

PHE mg:	18
TYR mg:	21
LEU mg:	33
ISO mg:	15
VAL mg:	18
TRY mg:	7
MET mg:	1
CYS mg:	6
ARG mg:	27
HIS mg:	12
THR mg:	19
LYS mg:	25

Minerals

Na mg:	283
Ca mg:	23
Mg mg:	16.0
Zn mg:	0.19
Mn mg:	0.43
K mg:	220
P mg:	20
Fe mg:	1.12
Cu mg:	0.073

Angry Salmon

Serves 4

1 tablespoon extra-virgin olive oil
1 pound fresh wild Norwegian salmon fillet
½ cup prepared horseradish
4 minced garlic cloves
Salt
Freshly ground black pepper

Rub the entire top surface of the fillet with 1 teaspoon of the oil, and remove any bones. Salt and pepper the fish, cover loosely with plastic wrap, and refrigerate for 15 to 20 minutes.

Adjust oven racks to the middle and broil positions. Preheat oven to 400 degrees.

In a small bowl mix the horseradish, garlic, the remaining 2 teaspoons of oil, and a dash of salt and pepper till blended. Remove fish from the refrigerator and take plastic off. Spoon dollops of the horseradish mixture over the fillet, creating a ¼-inch-thick coating. Pat it firmly with the back of a spoon and make sure that no pink shows through except along the vertical sides. Cover a roasting pan or deep-dish pie pan with foil and gently place the salmon into the center. Cover loosely with more foil (balance on the edges of the pan) and bake for 15 minutes. Remove foil cover and bake for another 10 to 15 minutes or until cooked through. Time will depend on thickness of the fillet. Remove pan from the oven and increase the heat to broil.

Carefully fold the edges of the foil away from the sides of the pan toward the fish so that the pan juices are completely covered and all you see is the coated salmon. (This is necessary to keep the juices from burning while the horseradish browns.) Broil 2 to 3 minutes on low or until you see the first signs of browning. (The coating is still damp, so most of it won't actually char.) Remove and let sit for 5 to 10 minutes. Divide into four servings. May be served hot or chilled.

Nutrition Totals Per Serving

KCal Breakdown: 47.8% Protein; 2.1% Carbohydrate; 50.1% Fat

Calories: 195   Fat: 10.6 (g)
Protein: 22.7 (g)   Sodium: 170 (mg)
Carbohydrate: 1.0 (g) Cholesterol: 63 (mg)

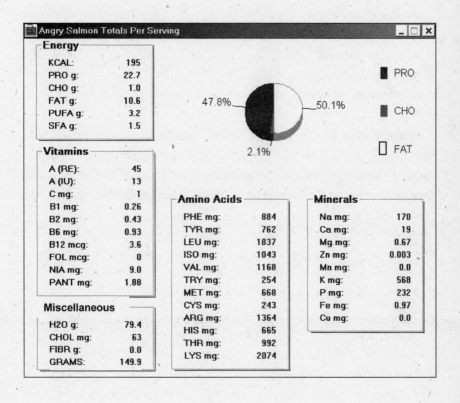

Angry Salmon Totals Per Serving

Energy

KCAL:	195
PRO g:	22.7
CHO g:	1.0
FAT g:	10.6
PUFA g:	3.2
SFA g:	1.5

47.8%   50.1%   2.1%

■ PRO
■ CHO
☐ FAT

Vitamins

A (RE):	45
A (IU):	13
C mg:	1
B1 mg:	0.26
B2 mg:	0.43
B6 mg:	0.93
B12 mcg:	3.6
FOL mcg:	0
NIA mg:	9.0
PANT mg:	1.88

Amino Acids

PHE mg:	884
TYR mg:	762
LEU mg:	1837
ISO mg:	1043
VAL mg:	1168
TRY mg:	254
MET mg:	668
CYS mg:	243
ARG mg:	1364
HIS mg:	665
THR mg:	992
LYS mg:	2074

Minerals

Na mg:	170
Ca mg:	19
Mg mg:	0.67
Zn mg:	0.003
Mn mg:	0.0
K mg:	568
P mg:	232
Fe mg:	0.97
Cu mg:	0.0

Miscellaneous

H2O g:	79.4
CHOL mg:	63
FIBR g:	0.0
GRAMS:	149.9

Apple Crisp

Serves 6

6 medium Rome apples, peeled, cored, and sliced
2 tablespoons lemon juice
1 tablespoon water
1 tablespoon sugar
¾ cup brown sugar
½ cup unbleached wheat flour
½ cup rolled oats
½ teaspoon cinnamon
½ cup light whipped butter

Preheat oven to 375 degrees. Arrange apples in an 8-by-8 inch baking pan. Sprinkle with the lemon juice, water, and 1 teaspoon of the sugar. Combine the rest of the ingredients in a small bowl. Mix with a fork until the mixture is crumbly. Sprinkle the mixture evenly over the apples. Bake 40 to 45 minutes or until the apples are tender.

Nutrition Totals Per Serving

KCal Breakdown: 2.1% Protein; 81.6% Carbohydrate; 16.3% Fat

Calories: 241
Protein: 1.6 (g)
Carbohydrate: 61.3 (g)

Fat: 5.4 (g)
Sodium: 67 (mg)
Cholesterol: 13 (mg)

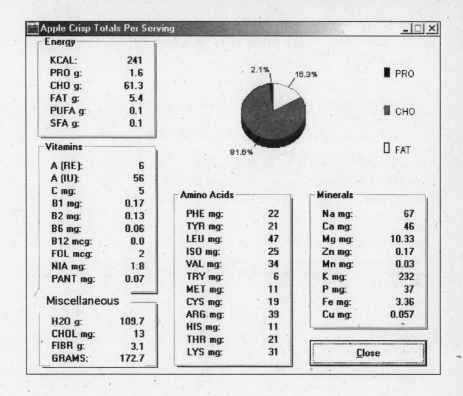

Apple Crisp Totals Per Serving

Energy

KCAL:	241
PRO g:	1.6
CHO g:	61.3
FAT g:	5.4
PUFA g:	0.1
SFA g:	0.1

Vitamins

A (RE):	6
A (IU):	56
C mg:	5
B1 mg:	0.17
B2 mg:	0.13
B6 mg:	0.06
B12 mcg:	0.0
FOL mcg:	2
NIA mg:	1.8
PANT mg:	0.07

Miscellaneous

H2O g:	109.7
CHOL mg:	13
FIBR g:	3.1
GRAMS:	172.7

Amino Acids

PHE mg:	22
TYR mg:	21
LEU mg:	47
ISO mg:	25
VAL mg:	34
TRY mg:	6
MET mg:	11
CYS mg:	19
ARG mg:	39
HIS mg:	11
THR mg:	21
LYS mg:	31

Minerals

Na mg:	67
Ca mg:	46
Mg mg:	10.33
Zn mg:	0.17
Mn mg:	0.03
K mg:	232
P mg:	37
Fe mg:	3.36
Cu mg:	0.057

2.1% 16.3% 81.6%

PRO CHO FAT

Close

Asian Grilled Halibut

Serves 4

¼ cup canola oil
2 tablespoons lemon juice
1 teaspoon tarragon
⅛ teaspoon pepper
2 teaspoons tamari soy sauce
1 pound halibut steaks

Preheat the broiler. Coat the broiling pan with olive oil cooking spray. Place the first five ingredients in a small bowl. Whisk together to mix. Place the fish on the broil pan and spoon half the mixture over it. Broil 5 to 6 minutes on one side. Turn the fish and spoon the rest of the mixture over the other sides. Broil 5 to 6 more minutes, or until the fish is flaky when touched with a fork. Cut into four equal portions. Serve with jasmine rice if desired.

Nutrition Totals Per Serving

KCal Breakdown: 38.3% Protein; 1.7% Carbohydrate; 60.0% Fat

Calories: 249   Fat: 16.7 (g)
Protein: 24.0 (g)   Sodium: 197 (mg)
Carbohydrates: 1.0 (g)   Cholesterol: 36 (mg)

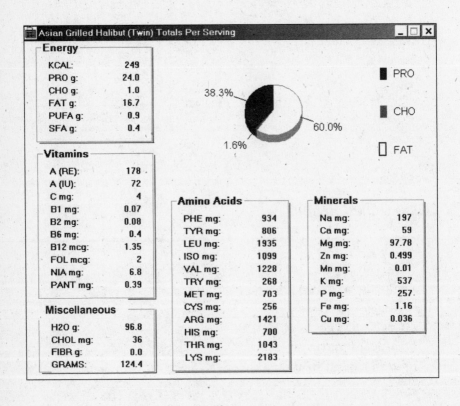

Asian Grilled Halibut (Twin) Totals Per Serving

Energy

KCAL:	249
PRO g:	24.0
CHO g:	1.0
FAT g:	16.7
PUFA g:	0.9
SFA g:	0.4

38.3%   1.6%   60.0%

PRO
CHO
FAT

Vitamins

A (RE):	178
A (IU):	72
C mg:	4
B1 mg:	0.07
B2 mg:	0.08
B6 mg:	0.4
B12 mcg:	1.35
FOL mcg:	2
NIA mg:	6.8
PANT mg:	0.39

Miscellaneous

H2O g:	96.8
CHOL mg:	36
FIBR g:	0.0
GRAMS:	124.4

Amino Acids

PHE mg:	934
TYR mg:	806
LEU mg:	1935
ISO mg:	1099
VAL mg:	1228
TRY mg:	268
MET mg:	703
CYS mg:	256
ARG mg:	1421
HIS mg:	700
THR mg:	1043
LYS mg:	2183

Minerals

Na mg:	197
Ca mg:	59
Mg mg:	97.78
Zn mg:	0.499
Mn mg:	0.01
K mg:	537
P mg:	257
Fe mg:	1.16
Cu mg:	0.036

Athenian Chicken Salad

Serves 4

2 cups macaroni shells cooked according to package directions
Cooked chicken breast cut in strips to make 2 cups
1½ cups seedless green grapes
½ cup chopped celery
1 cup low-fat buttermilk
¼ teaspoon dried dill weed
Pinch of onion powder
Pinch of garlic powder
½ teaspoon tamari soy sauce

Combine first four ingredients in a mixing bowl. Toss to mix. In another bowl mix remaining ingredients. Pour over chicken mixture. Toss to coat.

Nutrition Totals Per Serving

KCal Breakdown: 44.6% Protein; 43.4% Carbohydrate; 12.0% Fat

Calories: 376
Protein: 41.0 (g)
Carbohydrate: 40.0 (g)

Fat: 4.9 (g)
Cholesterol: 94 (mg)
Sodium: 178 (mg)

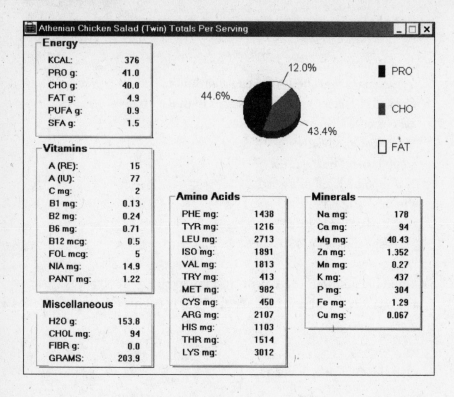

Athenian Chicken Salad (Twin) Totals Per Serving

Energy

KCAL:	376
PRO g:	41.0
CHO g:	40.0
FAT g:	4.9
PUFA g:	0.9
SFA g:	1.5

12.0% PRO
44.6%
43.4%
CHO
FAT

Vitamins

A (RE):	15
A (IU):	77
C mg:	2
B1 mg:	0.13
B2 mg:	0.24
B6 mg:	0.71
B12 mcg:	0.5
FOL mcg:	5
NIA mg:	14.9
PANT mg:	1.22

Amino Acids

PHE mg:	1438
TYR mg:	1216
LEU mg:	2713
ISO mg:	1891
VAL mg:	1813
TRY mg:	413
MET mg:	982
CYS mg:	450
ARG mg:	2107
HIS mg:	1103
THR mg:	1514
LYS mg:	3012

Minerals

Na mg:	178
Ca mg:	94
Mg mg:	40.43
Zn mg:	1.352
Mn mg:	0.27
K mg:	437
P mg:	304
Fe mg:	1.29
Cu mg:	0.067

Miscellaneous

H2O g:	153.8
CHOL mg:	94
FIBR g:	0.0
GRAMS:	203.9

Baked Sicilian Omelet

Serves 2

8 egg whites
1 cup evaporated skim milk
½ cup low-fat cottage cheese
½ cup grated Parmesan cheese
⅛ teaspoon pepper
1 tablespoon Italian parsley (optional)

Preheat oven to 350 degrees. Coat a 9-inch cake pan with olive oil cooking spray. Place all the ingredients in a food processor or blender. Mix till smooth. Pour into the prepared pan and bake for 30 to 35 minutes or until mixture is set. Sprinkle with parsley. Serve warm.

Nutrition Totals Per Serving

KCal Breakdown: 55.2% Protein; 24.2% Carbohydrate; 20.5% Fat

Calories: 339

Protein: 45.7 (g)

Carbohydrate: 20.1 (g)

Fat: 7.6 (g)

Sodium: 1180 (mg)

Cholesterol: 25 (mg)

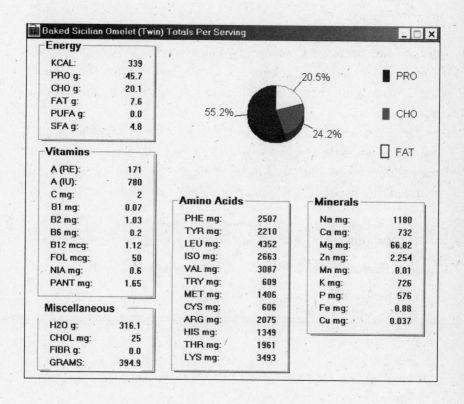

Baked Sicilian Omelet (Twin) Totals Per Serving

Energy

KCAL:	339
PRO g:	45.7
CHO g:	20.1
FAT g:	7.6
PUFA g:	0.0
SFA g:	4.8

20.5%

55.2%

24.2%

■ PRO

■ CHO

☐ FAT

Vitamins

A (RE):	171
A (IU):	780
C mg:	2
B1 mg:	0.07
B2 mg:	1.03
B6 mg:	0.2
B12 mcg:	1.12
FOL mcg:	50
NIA mg:	0.6
PANT mg:	1.65

Amino Acids

PHE mg:	2507
TYR mg:	2210
LEU mg:	4352
ISO mg:	2663
VAL mg:	3087
TRY mg:	609
MET mg:	1406
CYS mg:	606
ARG mg:	2075
HIS mg:	1349
THR mg:	1961
LYS mg:	3493

Minerals

Na mg:	1180
Ca mg:	732
Mg mg:	66.82
Zn mg:	2.254
Mn mg:	0.01
K mg:	726
P mg:	576
Fe mg:	0.88
Cu mg:	0.037

Miscellaneous

H2O g:	316.1
CHOL mg:	25
FIBR g:	0.0
GRAMS:	394.9

Black Forest Pudding

Serves 4

12 reduced-fat vanilla wafers
1 3-ounce package Jell-O chocolate Cook & Serve Pudding
2 cups soy milk (like Edensoy Original Soy Beverage)
8 teaspoons raspberry preserves

Arrange four dessert dishes with three vanilla wafers in the bottom of each one. Set aside. Cook the pudding according to package instructions, substituting the soy beverage for the milk. When the pudding starts to boil, remove from heat and pour an even amount into each dish (approx. ½ cup).

Drop 2 teaspoons of preserves into the center of each pudding. If the wafers rise to the top, gently push them back down with a spoon. Let the pudding cool slightly and then refrigerate, or serve warm. Garnish with Reddi-wip Fat Free Whipped Topping, if desired.

Nutrition Totals Per Serving

KCAL Breakdown: 10.8% Protein; 73.2% Carbohydrate; 16.1% Fat

Calories: 231
Protein: 5.8 (g)
Carbohydrate: 39.1 (g)

Fat: 3.8 (g)
Sodium: 240 (mg)
Cholesterol: 0 (mg)

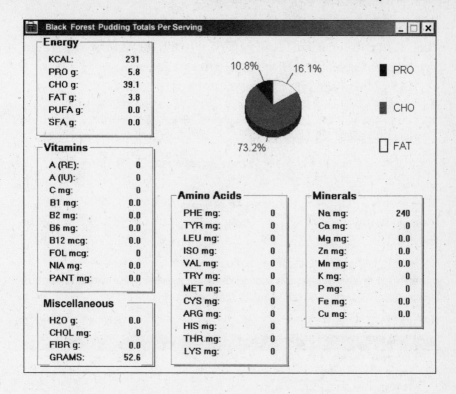

Black Forest Pudding Totals Per Serving

Energy
KCAL:	231
PRO g:	5.8
CHO g:	39.1
FAT g:	3.8
PUFA g:	0.0
SFA g:	0.0

10.8% 16.1% 73.2%

PRO
CHO
FAT

Vitamins
A (RE):	0
A (IU):	0
C mg:	0
B1 mg:	0.0
B2 mg:	0.0
B6 mg:	0.0
B12 mcg:	0.0
FOL mcg:	0
NIA mg:	0.0
PANT mg:	0.0

Amino Acids
PHE mg:	0
TYR mg:	0
LEU mg:	0
ISO mg:	0
VAL mg:	0
TRY mg:	0
MET mg:	0
CYS mg:	0
ARG mg:	0
HIS mg:	0
THR mg:	0
LYS mg:	0

Minerals
Na mg:	240
Ca mg:	0
Mg mg:	0.0
Zn mg:	0.0
Mn mg:	0.0
K mg:	0
P mg:	0
Fe mg:	0.0
Cu mg:	0.0

Miscellaneous
H2O g:	0.0
CHOL mg:	0
FIBR g:	0.0
GRAMS:	52.6

Bow-tie Pesto Pasta

Serves 4

1½ cups basil leaves, rinsed and stems removed

½ cup chopped fresh parsley

¼ cup pine nuts

2½ teaspoons dried minced garlic

1½ cups plus 2 tablespoons Parmesan cheese

½ cup no-oil Italian dressing

1 tablespoon extra-virgin olive oil

16-ounce package bow-tie pasta, cooked according to package
directions

Combine the basil, pine nuts, and garlic in a food processor. Finely chop. Add Parmesan and blend well. Slowly add the olive oil and Italian dressing while blending. Blend until a fine paste forms.

Pour pesto over hot bow-tie pasta and toss to coat.

Nutrition Totals Per Serving

KCal Breakdown: 15.8% Protein; 59.0% Carbohydrate; 25.3% Fat

Calories: 576
Protein: 23.1 (g)
Carbohydrate: 86.2 (g)

Fat: 16.4 (g)
Sodium: 481 (mg)
Cholesterol: 10 (mg)

NOTE: To further reduce the fat and calories of this recipe as well as add valuable soy protein, replace some or all of the Parmesan cheese with a grated soy-based substitute found in health-food stores.

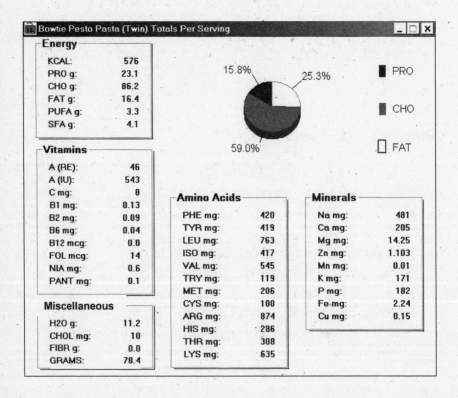

Bowtie Pesto Pasta (Twin) Totals Per Serving

Energy

KCAL:	576
PRO g:	23.1
CHO g:	86.2
FAT g:	16.4
PUFA g:	3.3
SFA g:	4.1

15.8% 25.3% ■ PRO

59.0% ■ CHO □ FAT

Vitamins

A (RE):	46
A (IU):	543
C mg:	8
B1 mg:	0.13
B2 mg:	0.09
B6 mg:	0.04
B12 mcg:	0.0
FOL mcg:	14
NIA mg:	0.6
PANT mg:	0.1

Miscellaneous

H2O g:	11.2
CHOL mg:	10
FIBR g:	0.0
GRAMS:	78.4

Amino Acids

PHE mg:	420
TYR mg:	419
LEU mg:	763
ISO mg:	417
VAL mg:	545
TRY mg:	119
MET mg:	206
CYS mg:	100
ARG mg:	874
HIS mg:	286
THR mg:	308
LYS mg:	635

Minerals

Na mg:	481
Ca mg:	205
Mg mg:	14.25
Zn mg:	1.103
Mn mg:	0.01
K mg:	171
P mg:	182
Fe mg:	2.24
Cu mg:	0.15

Brown Rice Porridge

Serves 4

4 cups cooked brown rice
2 cups skim milk
1 teaspoon cinnamon
4 tablespoons raisins
Sugar substitute of choice (to taste)

Place all ingredients except sugar substitute in a sauce pan. Bring to a boil. Reduce heat. Simmer 1 minute, stirring constantly. Remove from heat and pour into bowls. Sprinkle with sweetener.

Nutrition Totals Per Serving

KCal Breakdown: 12.4% Protein; 83.3% Carbohydrate; 4.3% Fat

Calories: 305
Protein: 9.4 (g)
Carbohydrate: 63.5 (g)

Fat: 1.5 (g)
Cholesterol: 2 (mg)
Sodium: 614 (mg)

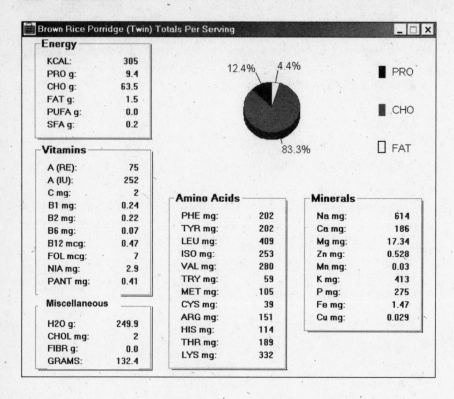

Brown Rice Porridge (Twin) Totals Per Serving

Energy

KCAL:	305
PRO g:	9.4
CHO g:	63.5
FAT g:	1.5
PUFA g:	0.0
SFA g:	0.2

12.4%   4.4%

83.3%

■ PRO

■ CHO

☐ FAT

Vitamins

A (RE):	75
A (IU):	252
C mg:	2
B1 mg:	0.24
B2 mg:	0.22
B6 mg:	0.07
B12 mcg:	0.47
FOL mcg:	7
NIA mg:	2.9
PANT mg:	0.41

Amino Acids

PHE mg:	202
TYR mg:	202
LEU mg:	409
ISO mg:	253
VAL mg:	280
TRY mg:	59
MET mg:	105
CYS mg:	39
ARG mg:	151
HIS mg:	114
THR mg:	189
LYS mg:	332

Minerals

Na mg:	614
Ca mg:	186
Mg mg:	17.34
Zn mg:	0.528
Mn mg:	0.03
K mg:	413
P mg:	275
Fe mg:	1.47
Cu mg:	0.029

Miscellaneous

H2O g:	249.9
CHOL mg:	2
FIBR g:	0.0
GRAMS:	132.4

Candy Apple Oatmeal

Serves 1

¾ cup pure apple juice
¼ cup soy milk (like Edensoy Original Soy Beverage)
⅛ teaspoon ground cinnamon (optional)
½ cup Quaker Old Fashioned Oats
2 tablespoons golden raisins or dried apple pieces (optional)

In a saucepan combine juice, soy beverage, and cinnamon (if using). Add the oats and bring mixture back to a boil. Cook for 5 minutes stirring constantly and gradually reducing heat. Stir in raisins or apple pieces (if using), and sweeten with sugar substitute if needed. For thicker oatmeal use a heaping ½ cup of oats.

In a hurry? Instant oatmeal can be improved as well, by mixing in one part soy milk to one part apple juice, instead of water. Microwave as per directions on label. Garnish as above.

Nutrition Totals Per Serving

KCal Breakdown: 7.5% Protein; 84.3% Carbohydrate; 8.2% Fat

Calories: 261

Protein: 4.9 (g)

Carbohydrate: 55.4 (g)

Fat: 2.4 (g)

Sodium: 45 (mg)

Cholesterol: 0 (mg)

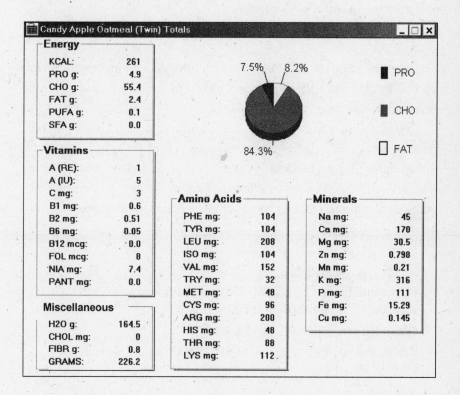

Chicken à la Papa Milano

Serves 4

4 skinned chicken breast halves (2 pounds total)
Pepper to taste
1 medium-size onion, sliced into ½-inch rings
1 teaspoon dried minced garlic (or 2 fresh cloves minced)
1 28-ounce can tomatoes, drained and chopped
1 14½-ounce can tomato sauce
½ teaspoon dried basil
½ teaspoon dried oregano
1 teaspoon tamari soy sauce
1 pound linguine, cooked according to package instructions

Coat a large nonstick frying pan with olive oil cooking spray. Sprinkle chicken breasts with pepper and brown in frying pan over medium heat. Remove from pan and set aside.

Recoat the pan with cooking spray. Add onion and garlic and cook until browned. Add remaining ingredients except linguine. Cook for 5 to 7 minutes. Return chicken to the pan, cover, and simmer for 20 to 30 minutes or until chicken is no longer pink in the center. Arrange linguine on a serving platter. Spoon chicken breasts and sauce over linguine.

Nutrition Totals Per Serving

KCal Breakdown: 30.6% Protein; 63.0 Carbohydrate; 6.4% Fat

Calories: 637
Protein: 45.3 (g)
Carbohydrate: 93.2 (g)
Fat: 4.2 (g)
Sodium: 1054 (mg)
Cholesterol: 73 (mg)

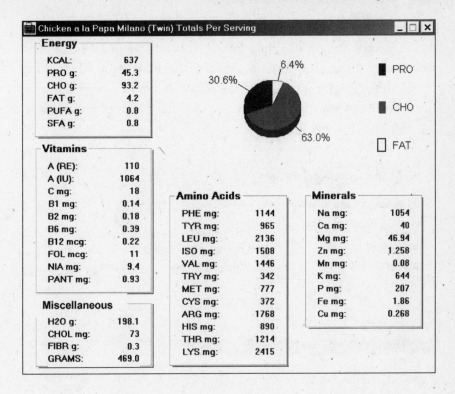

Chicken a la Papa Milano (Twin) Totals Per Serving

Energy

KCAL:	637
PRO g:	45.3
CHO g:	93.2
FAT g:	4.2
PUFA g:	0.8
SFA g:	0.8

6.4%
30.6%
63.0%

■ PRO
■ CHO
□ FAT

Vitamins

A (RE):	110
A (IU):	1064
C mg:	18
B1 mg:	0.14
B2 mg:	0.18
B6 mg:	0.39
B12 mcg:	0.22
FOL mcg:	11
NIA mg:	9.4
PANT mg:	0.93

Amino Acids

PHE mg:	1144
TYR mg:	965
LEU mg:	2136
ISO mg:	1508
VAL mg:	1446
TRY mg:	342
MET mg:	777
CYS mg:	372
ARG mg:	1768
HIS mg:	890
THR mg:	1214
LYS mg:	2415

Minerals

Na mg:	1054
Ca mg:	40
Mg mg:	46.94
Zn mg:	1.258
Mn mg:	0.08
K mg:	644
P mg:	207
Fe mg:	1.86
Cu mg:	0.268

Miscellaneous

H2O g:	198.1
CHOL mg:	73
FIBR g:	0.3
GRAMS:	469.0

Chicken-stuffed Tomatoes

Serves 4

4 medium-size firm tomatoes
1¼ cups chicken breast, cubed, cooked, skin removed
½ cup low-fat mayonnaise
2 tablespoons chopped green onion, including some of the green
    part
½ teaspoon dried dill weed
⅛ teaspoon garlic powder
⅛ teaspoon pepper
⅛ teaspoon paprika

Cut off the tops of the tomatoes and scoop out the flesh. Remove
the seeds and chop the pulp to equal 1 cup. Set aside. Place the toma-

toes upside down to drain the excess liquid. Place the rest of the ingre-dients, except the paprika, in a bowl. Add the chopped tomato. Mix well. Spoon the mixture into the tomatoes. Sprinkle tops with paprika.

(If you are not going to serve the tomatoes immediately, do not fill the tomatoes, but refrigerate the filling and the tomatoes upside down separately until ready to serve.)

Nutrition Totals Per Serving

KCal Breakdown: 38.6% Protein; 23.4% Carbohydrate; 38.0% Fat

Calories: 117

Protein: 11.6 (g)

Carbohydrate: 7.0 (g)

Fat: 5.1 (g)

Cholesterol: 27 (mg)

Sodium: 68 (mg)

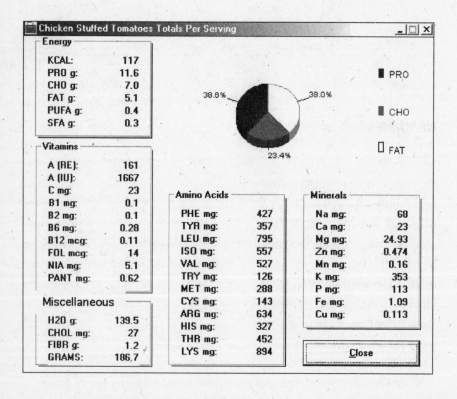

Chicken Stuffed Tomatoes Totals Per Serving

Energy

KCAL:	117
PRO g:	11.6
CHO g:	7.0
FAT g:	5.1
PUFA g:	0.4
SFA g:	0.3

Vitamins

A (RE):	161
A (IU):	1667
C mg:	23
B1 mg:	0.1
B2 mg:	0.1
B6 mg:	0.28
B12 mcg:	0.11
FOL mcg:	14
NIA mg:	5.1
PANT mg:	0.62

Miscellaneous

H2O g:	139.5
CHOL mg:	27
FIBR g:	1.2
GRAMS:	186.7

Amino Acids

PHE mg:	427
TYR mg:	357
LEU mg:	795
ISO mg:	557
VAL mg:	527
TRY mg:	126
MET mg:	288
CYS mg:	143
ARG mg:	634
HIS mg:	327
THR mg:	452
LYS mg:	894

Minerals

Na mg:	68
Ca mg:	23
Mg mg:	24.93
Zn mg:	0.474
Mn mg:	0.16
K mg:	353
P mg:	113
Fe mg:	1.09
Cu mg:	0.113

38.6%   38.0%

23.4%

■ PRO

■ CHO

☐ FAT

Close

Chicken Tetrazzini da Nello

Serves 6

One 16-ounce package spaghetti, cooked according to package
    directions
2 pounds chicken breast fillets, cubed
2 small onions, chopped
2 tablespoons tamari soy sauce
Water
¼ teaspoon pepper
½ pound mushrooms, sliced
1 tablespoon lemon juice
½ cup flour
Pinch of nutmeg
½ teaspoon paprika
¼ cup dry sherry
1 cup skim milk
4 tablespoons grated Parmesan cheese, or soy substitute

Place chicken, onions, and tamari in a large nonstick frying pan.
Pour enough water in pan to cover chicken. Cook over medium-high
heat for 15 to 20 minutes. Meanwhile, prepare spaghetti according to
package directions. Coat a 13-by-9-inch baking pan with olive oil cooking spray. Spread cooked spaghetti evenly in the dish. Remove chicken
and onion from pan with a slotted spoon. Add 1 cup water, pepper,
mushrooms, and lemon juice to remaining liquid. Cook five minutes
over high heat. Set aside. Preheat oven to 350 degrees. Place flour, nutmeg, paprika, sherry, 2½ cups water, and skim milk in a food processor
or blender. Process until smooth. Pour into a 4-quart saucepan. Heat
mixture on medium high, stirring constantly, until sauce thickens. Add
chicken, onions, and mushroom mixture. Cook until heated through.
Spoon over spaghetti. Sprinkle top with Parmesan. Bake 30 minutes or
until bubbly and top is golden brown.

Nutrition Totals Per Serving

KCal Breakdown: 29.6% Protein; 61.9% Carbohydrate; 8.5% Fat

Calories: 342	Fat: 3.1 (g)
Protein: 24.2 (g)	Sodium: 297 (mg)
Carbohydrate: 50.6 (g)	Cholesterol: 39 (mg)

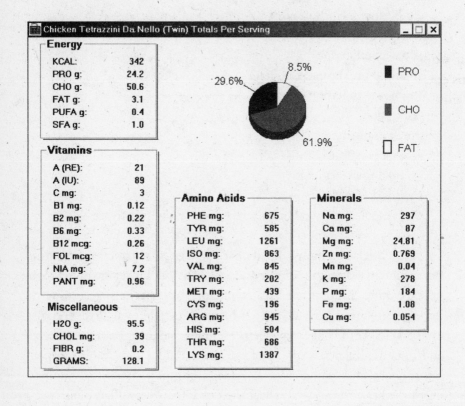

Chicken Tetrazzini Da Nello (Twin) Totals Per Serving

Energy

KCAL:	342
PRO g:	24.2
CHO g:	50.6
FAT g:	3.1
PUFA g:	0.4
SFA g:	1.0

8.5%
29.6%
61.9%

■ PRO
■ CHO
☐ FAT

Vitamins

A (RE):	21
A (IU):	89
C mg:	3
B1 mg:	0.12
B2 mg:	0.22
B6 mg:	0.33
B12 mcg:	0.26
FOL mcg:	12
NIA mg:	7.2
PANT mg:	0.96

Amino Acids

PHE mg:	675
TYR mg:	585
LEU mg:	1261
ISO mg:	863
VAL mg:	845
TRY mg:	202
MET mg:	439
CYS mg:	196
ARG mg:	945
HIS mg:	504
THR mg:	686
LYS mg:	1387

Minerals

Na mg:	297
Ca mg:	87
Mg mg:	24.81
Zn mg:	0.769
Mn mg:	0.04
K mg:	278
P mg:	184
Fe mg:	1.08
Cu mg:	0.054

Miscellaneous

H2O g:	95.5
CHOL mg:	39
FIBR g:	0.2
GRAMS:	128.1

Citrus Baked Chicken

Serves 4

4 skinned chicken breast halves
1½-ounce package Butter Buds or 3 tablespoons similar powdered
  butter substitute
¾ cup frozen orange juice concentrate
¼ teaspoon dried orange peel
¼ cup water
1 teaspoon ground ginger
½ teaspoon ground allspice

Preheat oven to 350 degrees. Coat a 12-by-8-inch baking dish with olive oil cooking spray. Arrange chicken in baking dish. Whisk together remaining ingredients until powdered butter is dissolved. Pour over chicken. Bake for 50 to 60 minutes or until chicken is no longer pink in the middle, basting often with the orange sauce in the baking dish.

Nutrition Totals Per Serving

KCal Breakdown: 53.4% Protein; 32.7% Carbohydrate; 13.9% Fat

Calories: 212
Protein: 27.6 (g)
Carbohydrate: 16.9 (g)

Fat: 3.2 (g)
Sodium: 315 (mg)
Cholesterol: 73 (mg)

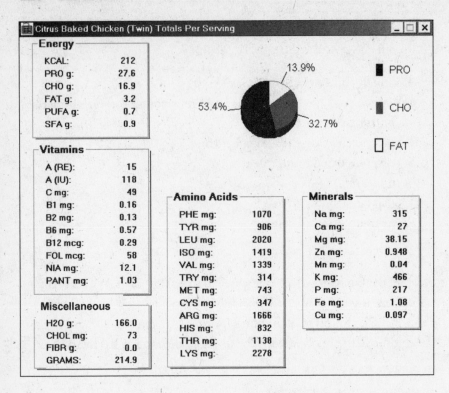

Citrus Baked Chicken (Twin) Totals Per Serving			_ □ ×

Energy

KCAL:	212
PRO g:	27.6
CHO g:	16.9
FAT g:	3.2
PUFA g:	0.7
SFA g:	0.9

13.9%
53.4%
32.7%

■ PRO
■ CHO
□ FAT

Vitamins

A (RE):	15
A (IU):	118
C mg:	49
B1 mg:	0.16
B2 mg:	0.13
B6 mg:	0.57
B12 mcg:	0.29
FOL mcg:	58
NIA mg:	12.1
PANT mg:	1.03

Amino Acids

PHE mg:	1070
TYR mg:	906
LEU mg:	2020
ISO mg:	1419
VAL mg:	1339
TRY mg:	314
MET mg:	743
CYS mg:	347
ARG mg:	1666
HIS mg:	832
THR mg:	1138
LYS mg:	2278

Minerals

Na mg:	315
Ca mg:	27
Mg mg:	38.15
Zn mg:	0.948
Mn mg:	0.04
K mg:	466
P mg:	217
Fe mg:	1.08
Cu mg:	0.097

Miscellaneous

H2O g:	166.0
CHOL mg:	73
FIBR g:	0.0
GRAMS:	214.9

Country Vegetable Soup

Serves 8

½ cup sliced carrots

½ cup sliced celery

½ cup chopped onions

10-ounce package frozen peas

14½-ounce can defatted chicken broth

1½ cups water

1 teaspoon dried parsley

1 teaspoon tamari soy sauce

⅛ teaspoon pepper

¾ teaspoon garlic powder

28-ounce can chopped tomatoes, drained

8-ounce can tomato sauce
16-ounce can red kidney beans, drained
Grated Parmesan cheese (or soy substitute) to sprinkle on
    individual servings (1 to 2 teaspoons)

Coat a large pot with olive oil cooking spray. Place the carrots, celery, and onions in the pot. Cook over medium-high heat until tender. Add a little of the water, if needed, while cooking.

Add the rest of the ingredients. Bring to a boil. Reduce the heat and simmer, uncovered, 15 to 20 minutes. Serve with crusty bread if desired.

Nutrition Totals Per Serving

KCal Breakdown: 27.9% Protein; 66.3% Carbohydrate; 5.8% Fat

Calories: 119   Fat: 0.7 (g)
Protein: 7.2 (g)   Sodium: 785 (mg)
Carbohydrate: 17.2 (g)   Cholesterol: 0 (mg)

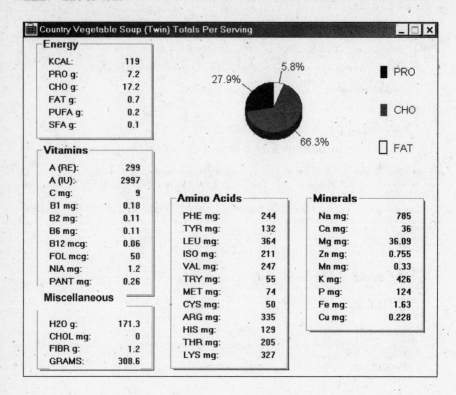

Country Vegetable Soup (Twin) Totals Per Serving	_ □ X

Energy

KCAL:	119
PRO g:	7.2
CHO g:	17.2
FAT g:	0.7
PUFA g:	0.2
SFA g:	0.1

5.8%
27.9%
66.3%

■ PRO
■ CHO
□ FAT

Vitamins

A (RE):	299
A (IU):	2997
C mg:	9
B1 mg:	0.18
B2 mg:	0.11
B6 mg:	0.11
B12 mcg:	0.06
FOL mcg:	50
NIA mg:	1.2
PANT mg:	0.26

Amino Acids

PHE mg:	244
TYR mg:	132
LEU mg:	364
ISO mg:	211
VAL mg:	247
TRY mg:	55
MET mg:	74
CYS mg:	50
ARG mg:	335
HIS mg:	129
THR mg:	205
LYS mg:	327

Minerals

Na mg:	785
Ca mg:	36
Mg mg:	36.09
Zn mg:	0.755
Mn mg:	0.33
K mg:	426
P mg:	124
Fe mg:	1.63
Cu mg:	0.228

Miscellaneous

H2O g:	171.3
CHOL mg:	0
FIBR g:	1.2
GRAMS:	308.6

Crabmeat Salad

Serves 2

8 ounces shredded crabmeat (cooked or canned)
½ cup Nasoya Nayonaise (soy-based mayonnaise)
1 cup chopped celery
¼ cup finely chopped green onion, including the green part
1 teaspoon lemon juice
Pinch of pepper

Combine all the ingredients in a bowl. Mix well. Chill. Serve as a sandwich with whole-wheat pita bread, or on a bed of lettuce garnished with whole-grain rice crackers.

Nutrition Totals Per Serving

KCal Breakdown: 37.4% Protein; 10.6% Carbohydrate; 51.9% Fat

Calories: 260
Protein: 22.6 (g)
Carbohydrate: 6.4 (g)

Fat: 13.9 (g)
Sodium: 1670 (mg)
Cholesterol: 60 (mg)

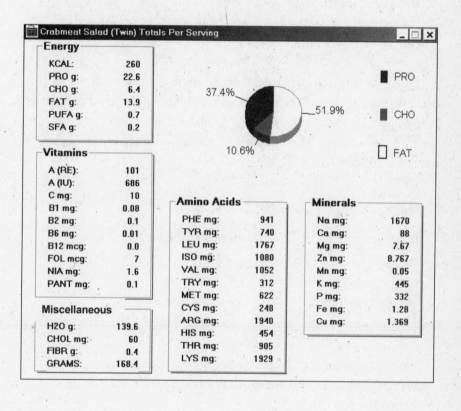

Crabmeat Salad (Twin) Totals Per Serving

Energy

KCAL:	260
PRO g:	22.6
CHO g:	6.4
FAT g:	13.9
PUFA g:	0.7
SFA g:	0.2

Vitamins

A (RE):	101
A (IU):	686
C mg:	10
B1 mg:	0.08
B2 mg:	0.1
B6 mg:	0.01
B12 mcg:	0.0
FOL mcg:	7
NIA mg:	1.6
PANT mg:	0.1

Miscellaneous

H2O g:	139.6
CHOL mg:	60
FIBR g:	0.4
GRAMS:	168.4

Amino Acids

PHE mg:	941
TYR mg:	740
LEU mg:	1767
ISO mg:	1080
VAL mg:	1052
TRY mg:	312
MET mg:	622
CYS mg:	248
ARG mg:	1940
HIS mg:	454
THR mg:	905
LYS mg:	1929

Minerals

Na mg:	1670
Ca mg:	88
Mg mg:	7.67
Zn mg:	8.767
Mn mg:	0.05
K mg:	445
P mg:	332
Fe mg:	1.28
Cu mg:	1.369

37.4%   51.9%   10.6%

■ PRO
■ CHO
☐ FAT

Eat to Win Penne Bolognese

1 serving

1 cup textured soy protein (like Yves Veggie Ground Round, Boca
   Burger Recipe Basics, or Morningstar Farms Grillers Burger
   Style Recipe Crumbles)
½ cup low-fat spaghetti sauce (tomato and olive oil based)
⅓ cup (dry) penne pasta (whole-wheat or multigrain if available)
Hot sauce (optional; Crystal brand recommended)

Heat the textured soy protein along with the pasta sauce in a pan
over medium heat until heated through. At the same time, in another
pan, cook the penne to the al dente stage. Drain the pasta and add it to
the Bolognese sauce. Mix to combine. Add several dashes of hot sauce
to taste if desired.

Nutrition Totals Per Serving

KCal Breakdown: Protein: 32.1%; Carbohydrate: 62.3%; Fat: 5.7%

Calories: 396
Protein: 31.7(g)
Carbohydrate: 61.6 (g)

Fat: 2.5 (g)
Cholesterol: 0 (mg)
Sodium: 951 (mg)

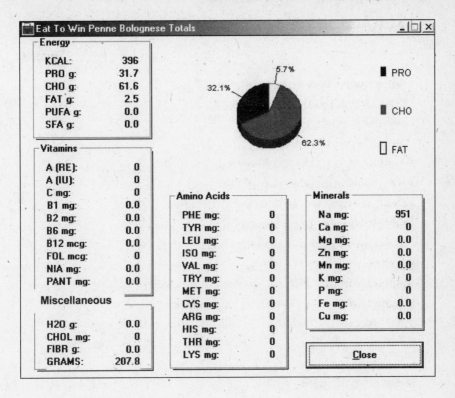

Eat To Win Penne Bolognese Totals

Energy

KCAL:	396
PRO g:	31.7
CHO g:	61.6
FAT g:	2.5
PUFA g:	0.0
SFA g:	0.0

Pie chart: 5.7% PRO, 32.1%, 62.3%, CHO, FAT

Vitamins

A (RE):	0
A (IU):	0
C mg:	0
B1 mg:	0.0
B2 mg:	0.0
B6 mg:	0.0
B12 mcg:	0.0
FOL mcg:	0
NIA mg:	0.0
PANT mg:	0.0

Miscellaneous

H2O g:	0.0
CHOL mg:	0
FIBR g:	0.0
GRAMS:	207.8

Amino Acids

PHE mg:	0
TYR mg:	0
LEU mg:	0
ISO mg:	0
VAL mg:	0
TRY mg:	0
MET mg:	0
CYS mg:	0
ARG mg:	0
HIS mg:	0
THR mg:	0
LYS mg:	0

Minerals

Na mg:	951
Ca mg:	0
Mg mg:	0.0
Zn mg:	0.0
Mn mg:	0.0
K mg:	0
P mg:	0
Fe mg:	0.0
Cu mg:	0.0

Close

Eat to Win Power Chili

Serves 10

1 tablespoon extra-virgin olive oil

2 cups chopped onion

1 cup chopped green pepper

½ pound ground turkey

½ pound turkey sausage, chopped

3 teaspoons minced garlic

2 28-ounce cans whole tomatoes with juice

3 tablespoons chopped green chilies

2 tablespoons plus 2 teaspoons chili powder

½ teaspoons pepper

30-ounce can pinto beans, drained and rinsed

15-ounce can kidney beans, drained and rinsed

3 tablespoons imitation bacon bits

½ teaspoon paprika

½ teaspoon garlic powder

⅛ teaspoon allspice

Place the first six ingredients in a large pot. Cook at medium heat until turkey is browned. Add the rest of the ingredients. Simmer 45 minutes to 1 hour, stirring frequently with a wooden spoon. Mash the tomatoes with the spoon while cooking.

Nutrition Totals Per Serving

KCal Breakdown: 25.1% Protein; 49.4% Carbohydrate; 25.5% Fat

Calories: 313	Fat: 9.4 (g)
Protein: 20.9 (g)	Sodium: 1634 (mg)
Carbohydrate: 41.2 (g)	Cholesterol: 28 (mg)

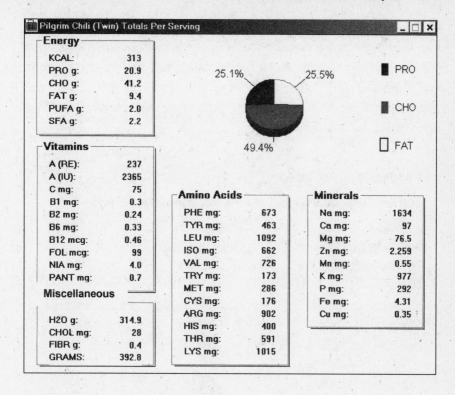

Pilgrim Chili (Twin) Totals Per Serving				_ □ ×

Energy

KCAL:	313
PRO g:	20.9
CHO g:	41.2
FAT g:	9.4
PUFA g:	2.0
SFA g:	2.2

25.1%   25.5%   ■ PRO

49.4%   ■ CHO

□ FAT

Vitamins

A (RE):	237
A (IU):	2365
C mg:	75
B1 mg:	0.3
B2 mg:	0.24
B6 mg:	0.33
B12 mcg:	0.46
FOL mcg:	99
NIA mg:	4.0
PANT mg:	0.7

Miscellaneous

H2O g:	314.9
CHOL mg:	28
FIBR g:	0.4
GRAMS:	392.8

Amino Acids

PHE mg:	673
TYR mg:	463
LEU mg:	1092
ISO mg:	662
VAL mg:	726
TRY mg:	173
MET mg:	286
CYS mg:	176
ARG mg:	902
HIS mg:	400
THR mg:	591
LYS mg:	1015

Minerals

Na mg:	1634
Ca mg:	97
Mg mg:	76.5
Zn mg:	2.259
Mn mg:	0.55
K mg:	977
P mg:	292
Fe mg:	4.31
Cu mg:	0.35

Eggplant Lasagna

8 servings

1 large (about 1 pound) eggplant peeled and cut into ½-inch slices
26-ounce jar low-fat, olive oil–based spaghetti sauce
1 pound lasagna noodles
1 pound low-fat cottage cheese
8 ounces reduced-fat shredded mozzarella cheese
¼ cup grated Parmesan cheese (or soy substitute)

Preheat oven to 375 degrees. Coat a 13-by-9-inch baking dish with
olive oil cooking spray. Over medium-high heat, cook eggplant slices in
a small amount of water in a nonstick frying pan until slices are
browned and tender. Add water as needed (it will evaporate quickly).

Spread a small amount of sauce on the bottom of the prepared baking dish. Arrange uncooked noodles in the bottom of the pan, spread one-third of the cottage cheese over noodles, followed by one-third of the mozzarella and Parmesan cheeses, and top with a few of the eggplant slices. Repeat layers ending with noodles, sauce, and a sprinkling of the mozzarella and Parmesan.

Nutrition Totals Per Serving

KCal Breakdown: 32.2% Protein; 51.6% Carbohydrate; 16.2% Fat

Calories: 429
Protein: 33.8 (g)
Carbohydrate: 54.1 (g)

Fat: 7.5 (g)
Sodium: 1039 (mg)
Cholesterol: 15 (mg)

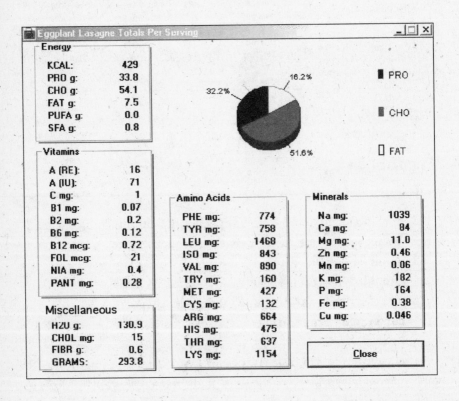

Hearty Lentil Soup

Serves 8

1 cup lentils (rinsed)
1 cup barley
1 16-ounce can chopped tomatoes
1 cup chopped onion
1 cup sliced celery
¾ cup sliced carrot
2 tablespoons tamari soy sauce
½ teaspoon pepper
1 teaspoon dried dill weed
1 teaspoon garlic powder
10 cups defatted chicken broth

Place all ingredients in a large saucepan. Bring to a boil. Cover and reduce heat to a simmer. Cook 50 minutes, stirring occasionally. Add water if soup becomes too thick.

Nutrition Totals Per Serving

KCal Breakdown: 26.6% Protein; 68.6% Carbohydrate; 4.8% Fat

Calories: 138
Protein: 8.8 (g)
Carbohydrate: 22.5 (g)

Fat: 0.7 (g)
Sodium: 402 (mg)
Cholesterol: 0 (mg)

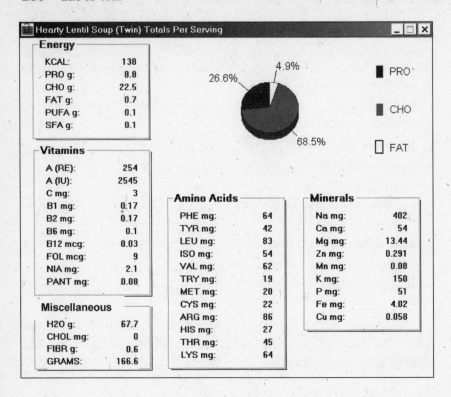

Hearty Lentil Soup (Twin) Totals Per Serving

Energy

KCAL:	138
PRO g:	8.8
CHO g:	22.5
FAT g:	0.7
PUFA g:	0.1
SFA g:	0.1

Pie chart: PRO 4.9%, CHO 68.5%, FAT 26.6%
■ PRO   ■ CHO   □ FAT

Vitamins

A (RE):	254
A (IU):	2545
C mg:	3
B1 mg:	0.17
B2 mg:	0.17
B6 mg:	0.1
B12 mcg:	0.03
FOL mcg:	9
NIA mg:	2.1
PANT mg:	0.08

Amino Acids

PHE mg:	64
TYR mg:	42
LEU mg:	83
ISO mg:	54
VAL mg:	62
TRY mg:	19
MET mg:	20
CYS mg:	22
ARG mg:	86
HIS mg:	27
THR mg:	45
LYS mg:	64

Minerals

Na mg:	402
Ca mg:	54
Mg mg:	13.44
Zn mg:	0.291
Mn mg:	0.08
K mg:	150
P mg:	51
Fe mg:	4.02
Cu mg:	0.058

Miscellaneous

H2O g:	67.7
CHOL mg:	0
FIBR g:	0.6
GRAMS:	166.6

Hiro Chicken Kebabs

Serves 4

1 cup dry sherry

½ cup tamari soy sauce

½ cup filtered water

2 teaspoons ground ginger

½ teaspoon garlic powder

2 teaspoons dry mustard

2 pounds boned and skinned chicken breast, cut into 1-inch cubes

1 medium-sized onion, peeled quartered and separated into
    sections

Place first six ingredients into a bowl. Mix until blended. Using four pieces of chicken and four pieces of onion for each skewer, alternate chicken and onion on eight wooden skewers. Arrange skewers in baking dish.

Pour marinade over skewers, turning to coat. Marinate for at least 2 hours in the refrigerator.

Broil for 10 to 15 minutes, turning skewers every 5 minutes and basting with marinade. Serve with steamed brown rice.

Nutrition Totals Per Serving

KCal Breakdown: 72.6% Protein; 9.3% Carbohydrate; 18.1% Fat

Calories: 246   Fat: 3.4 (g)
Protein: 30.2 (g)   Sodium: 1716 (mg)
Carbohydrate: 3.9 (g)   Cholesterol: 73 (mg)

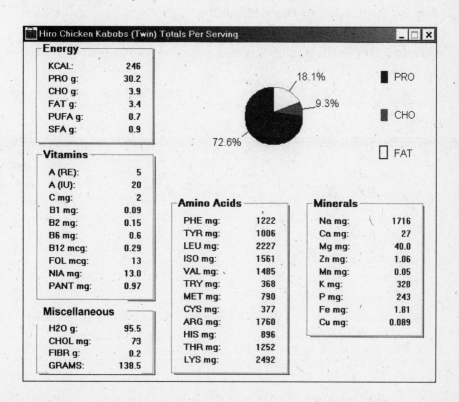

Hiro Chicken Kabobs (Twin) Totals Per Serving

Energy

KCAL:	246
PRO g:	30.2
CHO g:	3.9
FAT g:	3.4
PUFA g:	0.7
SFA g:	0.9

18.1% — PRO
9.3% — CHO
72.6% — FAT

Vitamins

A (RE):	5
A (IU):	20
C mg:	2
B1 mg:	0.09
B2 mg:	0.15
B6 mg:	0.6
B12 mcg:	0.29
FOL mcg:	13
NIA mg:	13.0
PANT mg:	0.97

Amino Acids

PHE mg:	1222
TYR mg:	1006
LEU mg:	2227
ISO mg:	1561
VAL mg:	1485
TRY mg:	368
MET mg:	790
CYS mg:	377
ARG mg:	1760
HIS mg:	896
THR mg:	1252
LYS mg:	2492

Minerals

Na mg:	1716
Ca mg:	27
Mg mg:	40.0
Zn mg:	1.06
Mn mg:	0.05
K mg:	328
P mg:	243
Fe mg:	1.81
Cu mg:	0.089

Miscellaneous

H2O g:	95.5
CHOL mg:	73
FIBR g:	0.2
GRAMS:	138.5

Italian-style Zucchini

Serves 6

4 cups sliced (¼-inch thick) zucchini
2 teaspoons dried minced garlic
1 28-ounce can tomatoes, drained and chopped
¾ cup low-sodium tomato sauce
¼ teaspoon pepper
1 teaspoon dried oregano
2 tablespoons finely chopped fresh parsley
3 tablespoons grated Parmesan cheese (or soy substitute)

Preheat oven to 350 degrees. Coat a 13-by-9-inch baking dish with olive oil cooking spray. Arrange zucchini in dish.

Coat a nonstick frying pan with olive oil cooking spray. Place remaining ingredients except Parmesan in pan. Cook over medium-high heat for 20 minutes, stirring occasionally.

Pour sauce over zucchini. Sprinkle with Parmesan cheese. Bake for 30 minutes or until zucchini is tender.

Nutrition Totals Per Serving

KCal Breakdown: 33.9% Protein; 47.0% Carbohydrate; 19.1% Fat

Calories: 64	Fat: 0.9 (g)
Protein: 3.8 (g)	Sodium: 421 (mg)
Carbohydrate: 5.3 (g)	Cholesterol: 2 (mg)

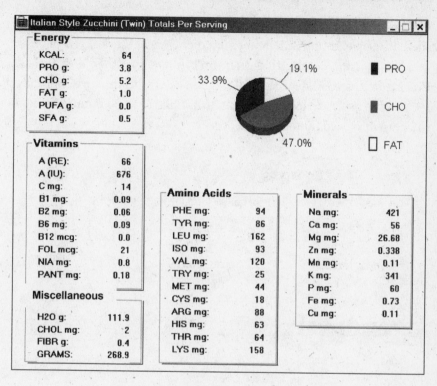

Italian Style Zucchini (Twin) Totals Per Serving

Energy
KCAL:	64
PRO g:	3.8
CHO g:	5.2
FAT g:	1.0
PUFA g:	0.0
SFA g:	0.5

19.1% PRO
33.9%
47.0% CHO
FAT

Vitamins
A (RE):	66
A (IU):	676
C mg:	14
B1 mg:	0.09
B2 mg:	0.06
B6 mg:	0.09
B12 mcg:	0.0
FOL mcg:	21
NIA mg:	0.8
PANT mg:	0.18

Amino Acids
PHE mg:	94
TYR mg:	86
LEU mg:	162
ISO mg:	93
VAL mg:	120
TRY mg:	25
MET mg:	44
CYS mg:	18
ARG mg:	88
HIS mg:	63
THR mg:	64
LYS mg:	158

Minerals
Na mg:	421
Ca mg:	56
Mg mg:	26.68
Zn mg:	0.338
Mn mg:	0.11
K mg:	341
P mg:	60
Fe mg:	0.73
Cu mg:	0.11

Miscellaneous
H2O g:	111.9
CHOL mg:	2
FIBR g:	0.4
GRAMS:	268.9

Leftover Turkey-stuffed Potatoes

Serves 4

2 large baking potatoes, baked and cooled
⅔ cup plain low-fat yogurt
⅔ cup low-fat cottage cheese
½ cup grated Parmesan cheese
½ cup finely chopped onion
¼ teaspoon pepper
1 teaspoon tamari soy sauce
½ teaspoon dried dill weed
2 cups cubed cooked turkey breast
Paprika

Cut each potato in half and scoop out centers, leaving a ¼-inch shell. Place potato and remaining ingredients except turkey and paprika in a bowl. Using an electric beater, mix until smooth. Fold in turkey. Preheat oven to 350 degrees. Fill potato shells with mixture. Sprinkle tops with paprika. Place in a baking dish. Bake 25 to 30 minutes or until lightly browned on top.

Nutrition Totals Per Serving

KCal Breakdown: 24.0% Protein; 65.4% Carbohydrate; 10.6% Fat

Calories: 406
Protein: 24.6 (g)
Carbohydrate: 66.9 (g)

Fat: 4.8 (g)
Sodium: 905 (mg)
Cholesterol: 26 (mg)

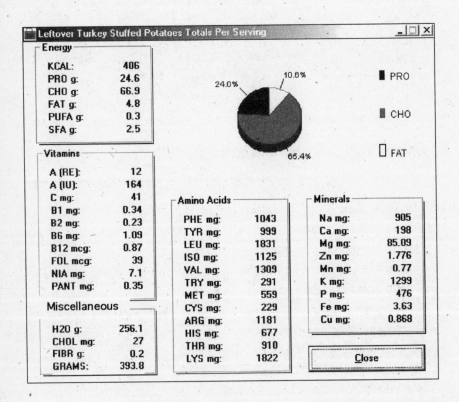

Louisiana Fruit Salad

Serves 5

3 cups cooked, peeled, and cubed sweet potatoes
2 cups chopped Red Delicious apples
2 cups seedless green grapes
2 cups sliced bananas
¾ cup plain low-fat yogurt
1 tablespoon lemon juice
3 packets sugar substitute
¼ teaspoon dried orange peel

Place the first four ingredients in a large bowl and mix together. Combine remaining ingredients in a small bowl. Pour over the sweet potatoes and fruit and toss to coat. Chill before serving.

Nutrition Totals Per Serving

KCal Breakdown: 6.8% Protein; 88.6% Carbohydrate; 4.6% Fat

Calories: 349
Protein: 6.2 (g)
Carbohydrate: 81.5 (g)

Fat:1.9 (g)
Sodium: 53 (mg)
Cholesterol: 3 (mg)

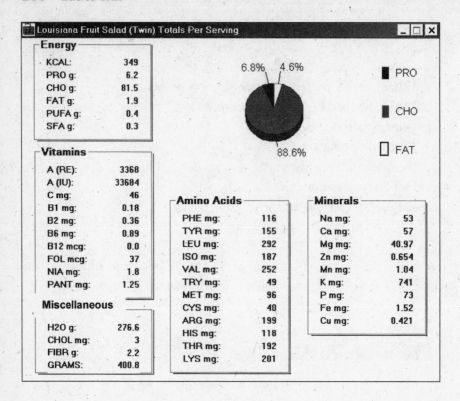

Lyonnaise Potatoes

Serves 4

3 medium or 2 large baking potatoes, peeled and thinly sliced

1 tablespoon extra-virgin olive oil

¼ cup chopped onion

2 tablespoon whole-wheat flour

1 vegetable bouillon cube (choose one that yields 2 cups broth)

1¼ cups reduced-fat soy milk (like Westsoy 1% Lite)

1 tablespoon whipped light butter (like Land O Lakes)

¾ cup nonfat grated mozzarella cheese

¼ teaspoon salt

⅛ teaspoon freshly ground pepper

2 soy substitute bacon strips (like Morningstar Farms Breakfast
   Strips) cooked according to package instructions

Preheat oven to 350 degrees. In a saucepan, sauté the onion in the oil till tender. Gradually stir in flour, bouillon cube, soy milk, butter, cheese, salt, and pepper. Continue stirring mixture till it's smooth and slightly thickened. Remove the saucepan from the heat.

Coat a 1-quart casserole dish with olive oil cooking spray. Place half the potato slices in the bottom and cover with half the sauce. Add the remaining potatoes and the rest of the sauce. Cook the potatoes covered for 35 minutes. Uncover the dish and bake the potatoes 30 minutes more or till they are tender. Crumble soy bacon over potatoes during the last few minutes of baking.

Nutrition Totals Per Serving

KCal Breakdown: 20.7% Protein; 51.6% Carbohydrate; 27.7% Fat

Calories: 156
Protein: 8.2 (g)
Carbohydrate: 20.3 (g)

Fat: 4.8 (g)
Sodium: 436 (mg)
Cholesterol: 5 (mg)

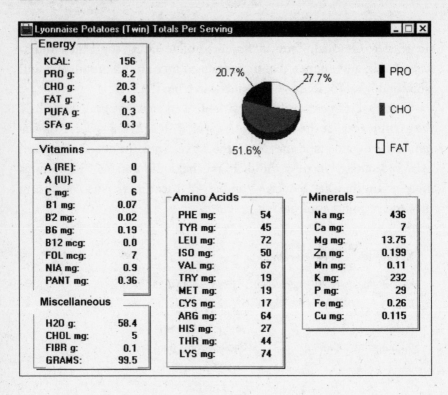

Lyonnaise Potatoes (Twin) Totals Per Serving

Energy

KCAL:	156
PRO g:	8.2
CHO g:	20.3
FAT g:	4.8
PUFA g:	0.3
SFA g:	0.3

PRO 27.7%
CHO 51.6%
FAT 20.7%

Vitamins

A (RE):	0
A (IU):	0
C mg:	6
B1 mg:	0.07
B2 mg:	0.02
B6 mg:	0.19
B12 mcg:	0.0
FOL mcg:	7
NIA mg:	0.9
PANT mg:	0.36

Amino Acids

PHE mg:	54
TYR mg:	45
LEU mg:	72
ISO mg:	50
VAL mg:	67
TRY mg:	19
MET mg:	19
CYS mg:	17
ARG mg:	64
HIS mg:	27
THR mg:	44
LYS mg:	74

Minerals

Na mg:	436
Ca mg:	7
Mg mg:	13.75
Zn mg:	0.199
Mn mg:	0.11
K mg:	232
P mg:	29
Fe mg:	0.26
Cu mg:	0.115

Miscellaneous

H2O g:	58.4
CHOL mg:	5
FIBR g:	0.1
GRAMS:	99.5

Mahi-mahi with Spicy Corn Salsa

Serves 4

1 pound mahi-mahi fillets, ½- to 1-inch thick

1 tablespoon plus 2 teaspoons olive oil

¼ teaspoon paprika

¼ cup chopped onion

¼ cup water

2 teaspoons chili powder

¼ cup chopped red pepper

¼ cup chopped green pepper

10 ounces corn kernels, thawed if frozen

1 teaspoon tamari soy sauce

Preheat the broiler. Coat a broiling pan with olive oil cooking spray. Brush the fillets with 2 teaspoons of the olive oil and sprinkle with paprika. Place the fillets on the prepared broiling pan and broil 4 minutes. Turn and broil 4 to 5 minutes on the other side, or until the fillets are flaky when touched with a fork.

In the meantime, heat the remaining tablespoon of olive oil in a skillet. Add the onion and sauté until tender. Add the water, chili powder, corn, red and green pepper, and tamari and stir. Cook 2 to 3 minutes on high heat, reduce the heat, and simmer until the fillets are done.

Cut the fillets into four equal portions. Spoon the corn salsa over them. Serve immediately.

Nutrition Totals Per Serving

KCal Breakdown: 45.6% Protein; 24.7% Carbohydrate; 29.7% Fat

Calories: 192	Fat: 6.4 (g)
Protein: 22.2 (g)	Sodium: 151 (mg)
Carbohydrate: 12.0 (g)	Cholesterol: 41 (mg)

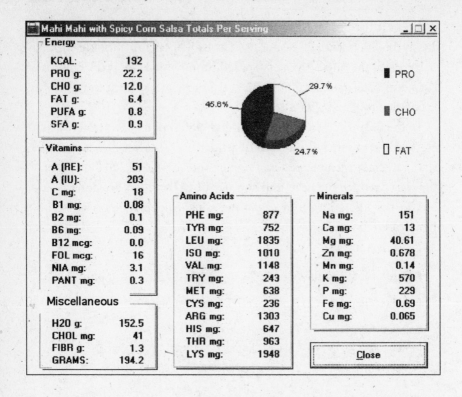

Mahi Mahi with Spicy Corn Salsa Totals Per Serving

Energy

KCAL:	192
PRO g:	22.2
CHO g:	12.0
FAT g:	6.4
PUFA g:	0.8
SFA g:	0.9

- PRO 29.7%
- CHO 24.7%
- FAT 45.6%

Vitamins

A (RE):	51
A (IU):	203
C mg:	18
B1 mg:	0.08
B2 mg:	0.1
B6 mg:	0.09
B12 mcg:	0.0
FOL mcg:	16
NIA mg:	3.1
PANT mg:	0.3

Miscellaneous

H2O g:	152.5
CHOL mg:	41
FIBR g:	1.3
GRAMS:	194.2

Amino Acids

PHE mg:	877
TYR mg:	752
LEU mg:	1835
ISO mg:	1010
VAL mg:	1148
TRY mg:	243
MET mg:	638
CYS mg:	236
ARG mg:	1303
HIS mg:	647
THR mg:	963
LYS mg:	1948

Minerals

Na mg:	151
Ca mg:	13
Mg mg:	40.61
Zn mg:	0.678
Mn mg:	0.14
K mg:	570
P mg:	229
Fe mg:	0.69
Cu mg:	0.065

Close

Marathon Snapper

Serves 4

3 egg whites
1½ teaspoons garlic powder
1 tablespoon grated Parmesan cheese (or soy substitute)
4 snapper fillets
Lemon wedges

Preheat oven to 350 degrees. Coat a 12-by-8-inch baking dish with olive oil cooking spray. Whisk together the first three ingredients. Dip each fillet in the mixture to coat. Arrange the fillets in the baking dish. Bake for 10 minutes. Turn fillets and bake for 20 minutes more. Serve with lemon wedges.

Nutrition Totals Per Serving

KCal Breakdown; 83.4% Protein; 3.5% Carbohydrate; 13.1% Fat

Calories: 135   Fat: 1.9 (g)
Protein: 26.5 (g)   Sodium: 133 (mg)
Carbohydrate: 1.1 (g) Cholesterol: 42 (mg)

Marathon Snapper (Twin) Totals Per Serving

Energy

KCAL:	135
PRO g:	26.5
CHO g:	1.1
FAT g:	1.9
PUFA g:	0.5
SFA g:	0.5

Pie chart: 13.1%, 3.5%, 83.4% — PRO, CHO, FAT

Vitamins

A (RE):	0
A (IU):	9
C mg:	0
B1 mg:	0.06
B2 mg:	0.07
B6 mg:	0.0
B12 mcg:	0.02
FOL mcg:	4
NIA mg:	0.3
PANT mg:	0.07

Amino Acids

PHE mg:	1099
TYR mg:	916
LEU mg:	2169
ISO mg:	1258
VAL mg:	1429
TRY mg:	309
MET mg:	803
CYS mg:	317
ARG mg:	1574
HIS mg:	765
THR mg:	1155
LYS mg:	2343

Minerals

Na mg:	133
Ca mg:	57
Mg mg:	39.75
Zn mg:	0.474
Mn mg:	0.01
K mg:	520
P mg:	243
Fe mg:	0.25
Cu mg:	0.039

Miscellaneous

H2O g:	109.2
CHOL mg:	42
FIBR g:	0.0
GRAMS:	140.5

Mediterranean Broiled Sole

Serves 4

1 pound sole fillets, ¼- to ½-inch thick (4 fillets)
2 egg whites
1 tablespoon lemon juice
⅛ teaspoon pepper
½ teaspoon garlic powder
½ cup Italian bread crumbs
¼ cup grated Parmesan cheese (or soy substitute)

Preheat the broiler. Coat a broiling pan with olive oil cooking spray. Place the egg whites and lemon juice in a small bowl. Beat together with a whisk. Place the rest of the ingredients in another bowl. Mix.

Dip the fillets in the egg mixture and coat well. Then dip them in the bread-crumb mixture and coat them lightly. Place the fillets on the broiling pan. Broil 2 to 3 minutes on one side. Turn the fillets and broil them 2 to 3 minutes on the other side until golden and flaky when touched with a fork.

Nutrition Totals Per Serving:

KCal Breakdown: 57.6% Protein; 26.4% Carbohydrate; 16.0% Fat

Calories: 161
Protein: 22.9 (g)
Carbohydrate: 10.5 (g)

Fat: 2.8 (g)
Sodium: 287 (mg)
Cholesterol: 4 (mg)

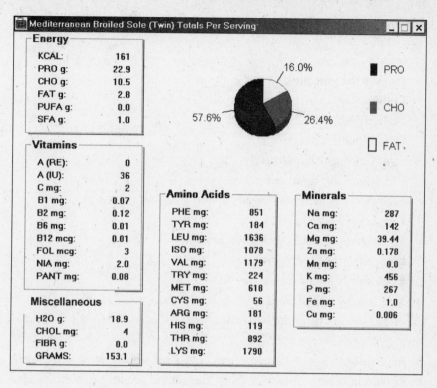

Mediterranean Broiled Sole (Twin) Totals Per Serving

Energy

KCAL:	161
PRO g:	22.9
CHO g:	10.5
FAT g:	2.8
PUFA g:	0.0
SFA g:	1.0

Pie chart: 16.0% PRO, 26.4% CHO, 57.6% FAT

Vitamins

A (RE):	0
A (IU):	36
C mg:	2
B1 mg:	0.07
B2 mg:	0.12
B6 mg:	0.01
B12 mcg:	0.01
FOL mcg:	3
NIA mg:	2.0
PANT mg:	0.08

Miscellaneous

H2O g:	18.9
CHOL mg:	4
FIBR g:	0.0
GRAMS:	153.1

Amino Acids

PHE mg:	851
TYR mg:	184
LEU mg:	1636
ISO mg:	1078
VAL mg:	1179
TRY mg:	224
MET mg:	618
CYS mg:	56
ARG mg:	181
HIS mg:	119
THR mg:	892
LYS mg:	1790

Minerals

Na mg:	287
Ca mg:	142
Mg mg:	39.44
Zn mg:	0.178
Mn mg:	0.0
K mg:	456
P mg:	267
Fe mg:	1.0
Cu mg:	0.006

MediterrAsian Chicken Salad

Serves 4

½ cup wine vinegar
1 tablespoon extra-virgin olive oil
2 tablespoons tamari soy sauce
1 tablespoon water
3 packets sugar substitute
1 teaspoon dry mustard
1 teaspoon gingerroot, freshly ground
1 clove garlic, minced
1½ cups cooked cubed chicken breast
¼ cup chopped green onion
1 cup thinly sliced radishes
5 cups baby field greens
½ cup sliced almonds, toasted

Mix vinegar, oil, soy sauce, water, sugar substitute, mustard, ginger, and garlic in a bowl. Place chicken and onion in vinegar mixture and mix to coat. Marinate 30 to 40 minutes. Meanwhile, toss radishes and field greens. Divide into four bowls. Remove chicken and onion from marinade with slotted spoon. Place equal portions in each bowl. Top with toasted almonds. Drizzle salads with extra marinade as desired.

Nutrition Totals Per Serving

KCal Breakdown: 36.0% Protein; 16.7% Carbohydrate; 47.3% Fat

Calories: 290
Protein: 26.4 (g)
Carbohydrate: 12.2 (g)

Fat: 15.4 (g)
Cholesterol: 55 (mg)
Sodium: 481 (mg)

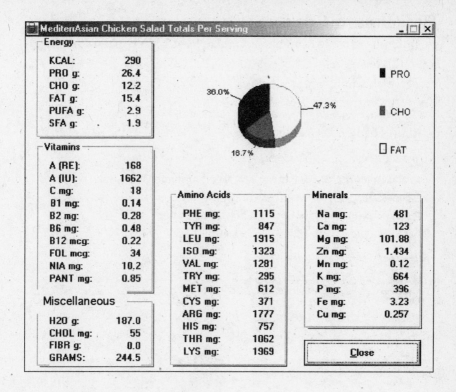

MediterrAsian Chicken Salad Totals Per Serving

Energy

KCAL:	290
PRO g:	26.4
CHO g:	12.2
FAT g:	15.4
PUFA g:	2.9
SFA g:	1.9

47.3% CHO
36.0% PRO
16.7% FAT

Vitamins

A (RE):	168
A (IU):	1662
C mg:	18
B1 mg:	0.14
B2 mg:	0.28
B6 mg:	0.48
B12 mcg:	0.22
FOL mcg:	34
NIA mg:	10.2
PANT mg:	0.85

Amino Acids

PHE mg:	1115
TYR mg:	847
LEU mg:	1915
ISO mg:	1323
VAL mg:	1281
TRY mg:	295
MET mg:	612
CYS mg:	371
ARG mg:	1777
HIS mg:	757
THR mg:	1062
LYS mg:	1969

Minerals

Na mg:	481
Ca mg:	123
Mg mg:	101.88
Zn mg:	1.434
Mn mg:	0.12
K mg:	664
P mg:	396
Fe mg:	3.23
Cu mg:	0.257

Miscellaneous

H2O g:	187.0
CHOL mg:	55
FIBR g:	0.0
GRAMS:	244.5

[Close]

MediterrAsian Hummus

Serves 8

15-ounce can garbanzo beans (chickpeas), drained and rinsed

2 tablespoons fresh lemon juice

1 teaspoon lemon zest

2 teaspoons extra-virgin olive oil

2 teaspoons dark sesame oil

⅓ cup extra-firm tofu

2 cloves garlic (quartered)

¼ teaspoon paprika

¼ teaspoon salt

Combine all the ingredients in a blender or food processor. Transfer the hummus to a bowl and cover. Chill at least 2 hours before serving to attain full flavor.

Serve on whole-wheat pita bread or as a dip for fresh vegetables.

Nutrition Totals Per Serving

KCal Breakdown: 18.3% Protein; 42.4% Carbohydrate; 39.3% Fat

Calories: 81	Fat: 3.9 (g)
Protein: 4.1 (g)	Cholesterol: 0 (mg)
Carbohydrate: 9.5 (g)	Sodium: 231 (mg)

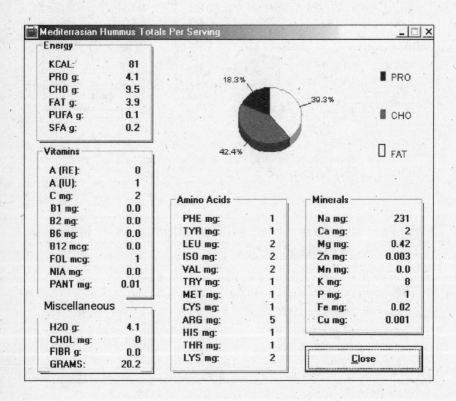

Mediterrasian Hummus Totals Per Serving

Energy

KCAL:	81
PRO g:	4.1
CHO g:	9.5
FAT g:	3.9
PUFA g:	0.1
SFA g:	0.2

18.3%   39.3%   42.4%

■ PRO

■ CHO

☐ FAT

Vitamins

A (RE):	0
A (IU):	1
C mg:	2
B1 mg:	0.0
B2 mg:	0.0
B6 mg:	0.0
B12 mcg:	0.0
FOL mcg:	1
NIA mg:	0.0
PANT mg:	0.01

Amino Acids

PHE mg:	1
TYR mg:	1
LEU mg:	2
ISO mg:	2
VAL mg:	2
TRY mg:	1
MET mg:	1
CYS mg:	1
ARG mg:	5
HIS mg:	1
THR mg:	1
LYS mg:	2

Minerals

Na mg:	231
Ca mg:	2
Mg mg:	0.42
Zn mg:	0.003
Mn mg:	0.0
K mg:	8
P mg:	1
Fe mg:	0.02
Cu mg:	0.001

Miscellaneous

H2O g:	4.1
CHOL mg:	0
FIBR g:	0.0
GRAMS:	20.2

Close

Mississippi Caviar

Serves 8

2 cups frozen black-eyed peas (fresh cooked, frozen, or canned)
1 cup diced red onion
1 cup tomato diced and seeded
2 tablespoons fresh cilantro leaves
1 heaping tablespoon diced jalapeño pepper (seeds and ridges removed)
1 teaspoon ground cumin
1 teaspoon sea salt
¼ cup fresh lemon juice
3 tablespoons balsamic vinegar

Blend all the ingredients except the peas in a blender or food processor (don't liquefy). Pour mixture over the peas in a mixing bowl and stir to coat. For best flavor chill covered overnight and let warm slightly before serving.

Nutrition Totals Per Serving

KCal Breakdown: 21.3% Protein; 73.2% Carbohydrate; 5.5% Fat

Calories: 76	Fat: 0.5 (g)
Protein: 4.2 (g)	Sodium: 294 (mg)
Carbohydrate: 14.6 (g)	Cholesterol: 0 (mg)

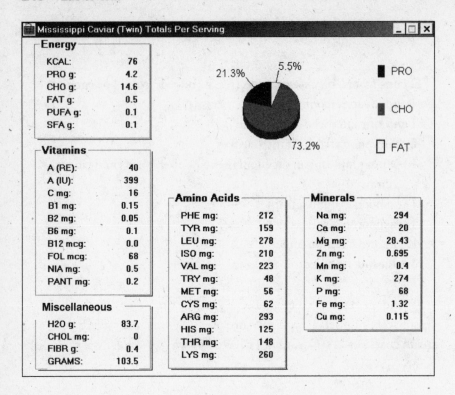

Mississippi Caviar (Twin) Totals Per Serving			

Energy

KCAL:	76
PRO g:	4.2
CHO g:	14.6
FAT g:	0.5
PUFA g:	0.1
SFA g:	0.1

Pie chart: 21.3% PRO, 73.2% CHO, 5.5% FAT

Vitamins

A (RE):	40
A (IU):	399
C mg:	16
B1 mg:	0.15
B2 mg:	0.05
B6 mg:	0.1
B12 mcg:	0.0
FOL mcg:	68
NIA mg:	0.5
PANT mg:	0.2

Amino Acids

PHE mg:	212
TYR mg:	159
LEU mg:	278
ISO mg:	210
VAL mg:	223
TRY mg:	48
MET mg:	56
CYS mg:	62
ARG mg:	293
HIS mg:	125
THR mg:	148
LYS mg:	260

Minerals

Na mg:	294
Ca mg:	20
Mg mg:	28.43
Zn mg:	0.695
Mn mg:	0.4
K mg:	274
P mg:	68
Fe mg:	1.32
Cu mg:	0.115

Miscellaneous

H2O g:	83.7
CHOL mg:	0
FIBR g:	0.4
GRAMS:	103.5

Moroccan Salad

Serves 4

1 cup raw bulgur

1¾ cup defatted chicken stock (or vegetable stock)

¼ cup plus ⅛ cup lemon juice

¼ teaspoon garlic powder

½ cup chopped onion

½ cup chopped green onion

¼ cup chopped fresh parsley

½ cup chopped cucumber

1 cup chopped tomato

1 teaspoon dried mint

¼ cup no-oil vinaigrette
Pepper to taste

Place bulgur, soup stock, ¼ cup lemon juice, and garlic powder in a bowl. Let stand 30 to 45 minutes or until bulgur has softened. Drain well and squeeze out excess liquid. Add remaining ingredients and toss. Chill before serving.

Nutrition Totals Per Serving

KCal Breakdown: 30.0% Protein; 48.7% Carbohydrate; 21.3% Fat

Calories: 147
Protein: 11.3 (g)
Carbohydrate: 44.1 (g)

Fat: 3.6 (g)
Sodium: 357 (mg)
Cholesterol: 0 (mg)

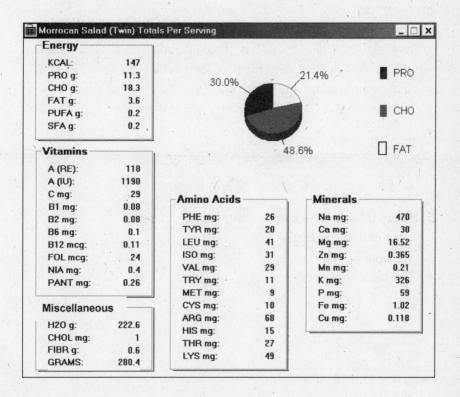

Morrocan Salad (Twin) Totals Per Serving

Energy

KCAL:	147
PRO g:	11.3
CHO g:	18.3
FAT g:	3.6
PUFA g:	0.2
SFA g:	0.2

Pie chart: 30.0%, 21.4%, 48.6% — PRO, CHO, FAT

Vitamins

A (RE):	118
A (IU):	1190
C mg:	29
B1 mg:	0.08
B2 mg:	0.08
B6 mg:	0.1
B12 mcg:	0.11
FOL mcg:	24
NIA mg:	0.4
PANT mg:	0.26

Amino Acids

PHE mg:	26
TYR mg:	20
LEU mg:	41
ISO mg:	31
VAL mg:	29
TRY mg:	11
MET mg:	9
CYS mg:	10
ARG mg:	68
HIS mg:	15
THR mg:	27
LYS mg:	49

Minerals

Na mg:	470
Ca mg:	30
Mg mg:	16.52
Zn mg:	0.365
Mn mg:	0.21
K mg:	326
P mg:	59
Fe mg:	1.02
Cu mg:	0.118

Miscellaneous

H2O g:	222.6
CHOL mg:	1
FIBR g:	0.6
GRAMS:	280.4

Power "Franks" and Beans

Serves 4

2 16-ounce cans Heinz Vegetarian Baked Beans
¼ cup chopped onion (optional)
2 tablespoons prepared yellow mustard
2 tablespoons honey
2 tablespoons Heinz ketchup
4 slices soy-based hot-dog substitute like Yves Tofu Wieners,
     Morningstar Farms Veggie Dogs, or Lightlife Smart Dogs
2 slices soy-based bacon substitute like Morningstar Farms
     Breakfast Strips (at room temperature)

Slice the hot dogs into small circles and dice the "bacon" into small squares. Set them aside. Combine the mustard, honey, and ketchup in a small bowl and mix till uniform in color.

Coat a large skillet with olive oil cooking spray and set over medium-high heat. Add the onion (if using) and sauté in 2 teaspoons of water until the edges start to turn golden in color. Add the beans and the condiment mixture and stir to combine. Add the hot-dog and "bacon" pieces and stir often while bringing all the ingredients up to heat.

Nutrition Totals Per Serving

KCal Breakdown: 23.7% Protein; 70.4% Carbohydrate; 6.0% Fat

Calories: 348
Protein: 20.1 (g)
Carbohydrate: 59.6 (g)

Fat: 2.3 (g)
Sodium: 1183 (mg)
Cholesterol: 0 (mg)

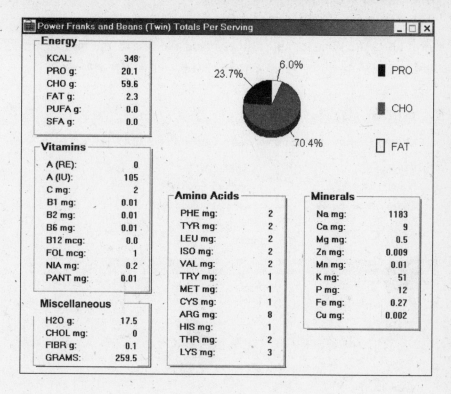

Power Franks and Beans (Twin) Totals Per Serving

Energy

KCAL:	348
PRO g:	20.1
CHO g:	59.6
FAT g:	2.3
PUFA g:	0.0
SFA g:	0.0

23.7%   6.0%   70.4%

■ PRO
■ CHO
□ FAT

Vitamins

A (RE):	0
A (IU):	105
C mg:	2
B1 mg:	0.01
B2 mg:	0.01
B6 mg:	0.01
B12 mcg:	0.0
FOL mcg:	1
NIA mg:	0.2
PANT mg:	0.01

Amino Acids

PHE mg:	2
TYR mg:	2
LEU mg:	2
ISO mg:	2
VAL mg:	2
TRY mg:	1
MET mg:	1
CYS mg:	1
ARG mg:	8
HIS mg:	1
THR mg:	2
LYS mg:	3

Minerals

Na mg:	1183
Ca mg:	9
Mg mg:	0.5
Zn mg:	0.009
Mn mg:	0.01
K mg:	51
P mg:	12
Fe mg:	0.27
Cu mg:	0.002

Miscellaneous

H2O g:	17.5
CHOL mg:	0
FIBR g:	0.1
GRAMS:	259.5

Power-packed Tuna Salad

Serves 4

12-ounce can solid white tuna, packed in springwater
½ cup low-fat yogurt (1½% milkfat)
¼ cup Nasoya Nayonaise
2 tablespoons Dijon mustard
½ cup finely chopped celery
½ cup finely chopped red onion
¼ teaspoon dried dill weed
¼ teaspoon celery seed
1 to 2 tablespoons organic wheat germ (optional)
Pepper to taste

Drain water from tuna and place in a bowl. Mash tuna with a fork until fibers are separate and feathery. Add the rest of the ingredients and mix well. Chill. Serve on a bed of lettuce, or use for sandwiches.

Nutrition Totals Per Serving

KCal Breakdown: 55.2% Protein; 14.4% Carbohydrate; 30.4% Fat

Calories: 197
Protein: 26.0 (g)
Carbohydrate: 6.8 (g)

Fat: 6.4 (g)
Sodium: 564 (mg)
Cholesterol: 38 (mg)

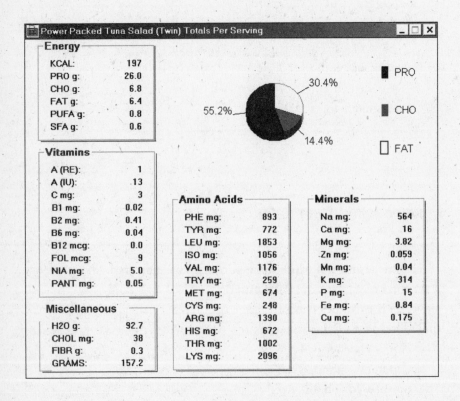

Power Packed Tuna Salad (Twin) Totals Per Serving

Energy

KCAL:	197
PRO g:	26.0
CHO g:	6.8
FAT g:	6.4
PUFA g:	0.8
SFA g:	0.6

55.2% — 30.4% — 14.4%

PRO
CHO
FAT

Vitamins

A (RE):	1
A (IU):	13
C mg:	3
B1 mg:	0.02
B2 mg:	0.41
B6 mg:	0.04
B12 mcg:	0.0
FOL mcg:	9
NIA mg:	5.0
PANT mg:	0.05

Miscellaneous

H2O g:	92.7
CHOL mg:	38
FIBR g:	0.3
GRAMS:	157.2

Amino Acids

PHE mg:	893
TYR mg:	772
LEU mg:	1853
ISO mg:	1056
VAL mg:	1176
TRY mg:	259
MET mg:	674
CYS mg:	248
ARG mg:	1390
HIS mg:	672
THR mg:	1002
LYS mg:	2096

Minerals

Na mg:	564
Ca mg:	16
Mg mg:	3.82
Zn mg:	0.059
Mn mg:	0.04
K mg:	314
P mg:	15
Fe mg:	0.84
Cu mg:	0.175

Ratatouille

Serves 4

1 tablespoon extra-virgin olive oil

⅓ cup diced onion

2 cups zucchini squash (unpeeled) cut in half lengthwise, then into
   ½-inch-wide semicircles

1 cup eggplant, peeled and cubed

1 cup green pepper, seeded, rinsed, and cubed

1 cup red pepper, seeded, rinsed, and cubed

¼ teaspoon sugar

½ teaspoon salt

½ teaspoon freshly ground black pepper

3 sprigs of fresh thyme (or ½ teaspoon dried thyme)

3 fresh chopped basil leaves (or ½ teaspoon dried basil)

14½-ounce can diced tomatoes with roasted garlic

2 tablespoons tomato paste

5 soy sausage links (like Morningstar Farms Breakfast Links)

In a large skillet sauté onions in the oil till tender. Add remaining ingredients except tomatoes, tomato paste, sausages, and basil (if using fresh). Stir well. Reduce heat, cover, and simmer approximately 15 minutes until vegetables soften. Cook sausages according to package instructions. When cool enough to handle, slice sausages into 1-inch pieces on the bias (diagonally), leaving off the ends. Mash the ends into a pulp resembling ground sausage. Add slices and pulp to the skillet along with tomatoes, tomato paste, and fresh basil, if using. Simmer uncovered about 7 minutes. Remove fresh thyme sprigs before serving.

Nutrition Totals Per Serving

KCal Breakdown: 23.3% Protein; 39.4% Carbohydrate; 37.3% Fat

Calories: 120	Fat: 5.3 (g)
Protein: 7.4 (g)	Sodium: 942 (mg)
Carbohydrate: 12.6 (g)	Cholesterol: 0 (mg)

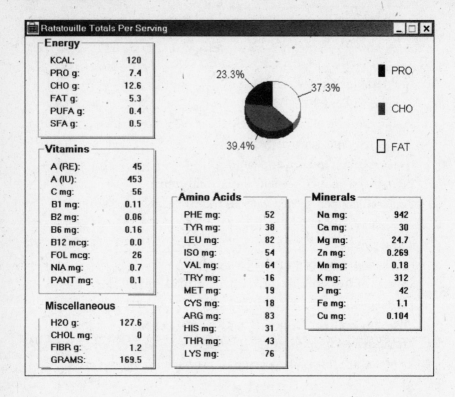

Ratatouille Totals Per Serving		

Energy

KCAL:	120
PRO g:	7.4
CHO g:	12.6
FAT g:	5.3
PUFA g:	0.4
SFA g:	0.5

23.3% 37.3% 39.4%

■ PRO
■ CHO
□ FAT

Vitamins

A (RE):	45
A (IU):	453
C mg:	56
B1 mg:	0.11
B2 mg:	0.06
B6 mg:	0.16
B12 mcg:	0.0
FOL mcg:	26
NIA mg:	0.7
PANT mg:	0.1

Amino Acids

PHE mg:	52
TYR mg:	38
LEU mg:	82
ISO mg:	54
VAL mg:	64
TRY mg:	16
MET mg:	19
CYS mg:	18
ARG mg:	83
HIS mg:	31
THR mg:	43
LYS mg:	76

Minerals

Na mg:	942
Ca mg:	30
Mg mg:	24.7
Zn mg:	0.269
Mn mg:	0.18
K mg:	312
P mg:	42
Fe mg:	1.1
Cu mg:	0.104

Miscellaneous

H2O g:	127.6
CHOL mg:	0
FIBR g:	1.2
GRAMS:	169.5

Rigatoni Romana

Serves 6

16-ounce package rigatoni pasta (preferably imported from Italy)
2 tablespoons Bertolli Extra Light Olive Oil
4 cloves garlic, minced
2 14½-ounce cans Hunt's Choice Cut Tomatoes with Roasted
   Garlic
¼ cup chopped fresh basil leaves

Cook the pasta to the al dente stage and rinse with cold water. Set aside.

In a large pot, heat 1 tablespoon of the oil, along with the tomatoes. When the tomatoes are heated through, add the pasta and toss to distribute evenly. Heat the remaining 2 tablespoons of oil with the garlic in the microwave on high for 30 seconds, or on the stovetop. Pour over the pasta mixture and stir in well. When all the ingredients are sufficiently heated, add the basil and toss a final time to blend. Salt and pepper to taste. Sprinkle with pine nuts or cubed fresh mozzarella, if desired.

Nutrition Totals Per Serving

KCal Breakdown: 11.7% Protein; 68.9% Carbohydrate; 19.4% Fat

Calories: 364   Fat: 7.7 (g)
Protein: 10.6 (g)   Sodium: 596 (mg)
Carbohydrate: 62.0 (g) Cholesterol: 0 (mg)

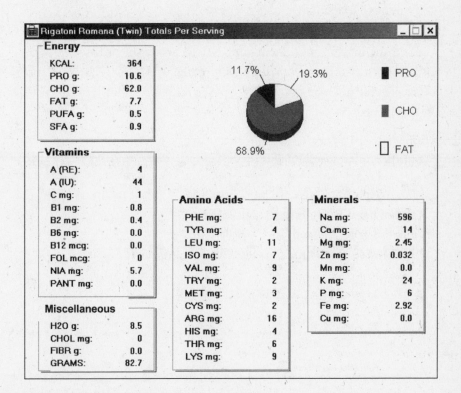

Rigatoni Romana (Twin) Totals Per Serving

Energy
KCAL:	364
PRO g:	10.6
CHO g:	62.0
FAT g:	7.7
PUFA g:	0.5
SFA g:	0.9

11.7%   19.3%   ■ PRO
   ■ CHO
68.9%   □ FAT

Vitamins
A (RE):	4
A (IU):	44
C mg:	1
B1 mg:	0.8
B2 mg:	0.4
B6 mg:	0.0
B12 mcg:	0.0
FOL mcg:	0
NIA mg:	5.7
PANT mg:	0.0

Amino Acids
PHE mg:	7
TYR mg:	4
LEU mg:	11
ISO mg:	7
VAL mg:	9
TRY mg:	2
MET mg:	3
CYS mg:	2
ARG mg:	16
HIS mg:	4
THR mg:	6
LYS mg:	9

Minerals
Na mg:	596
Ca mg:	14
Mg mg:	2.45
Zn mg:	0.032
Mn mg:	0.0
K mg:	24
P mg:	6
Fe mg:	2.92
Cu mg:	0.0

Miscellaneous
H2O g:	8.5
CHOL mg:	0
FIBR g:	0.0
GRAMS:	82.7

Rock Shrimp Salad

Serves 4

1 cup low-fat cottage cheese
½ cup skim milk
3 tablespoons lemon juice
½ teaspoon tamari soy sauce
1 teaspoon prepared mustard
¼ quarter teaspoon pepper
8 ounces elbow macaroni, cooked, rinsed, and drained
1 cup chopped celery
¼ cup chopped onions
½ cup chopped scallions
2 cups cooked, deveined, and coarsely chopped rock shrimp
    (regular shrimp may be substituted if rock shrimp is
    unavailable)

Place the first six ingredients into a food processor or blender. Mix until smooth. Combine remaining ingredients in a large bowl. Pour cottage-cheese mixture over shrimp, pasta, and vegetables. Toss to coat. Chill.

Nutrition Totals Per Serving

KCal Breakdown: 28.6% Protein; 63.7% Carbohydrate; 7.7% Fat

Calories: 295
Protein: 20.9 (g)
Carbohydrate: 46.6 (g)

Fat: 2.5 (g)
Sodium: 352 (mg)
Cholesterol: 47 (mg)

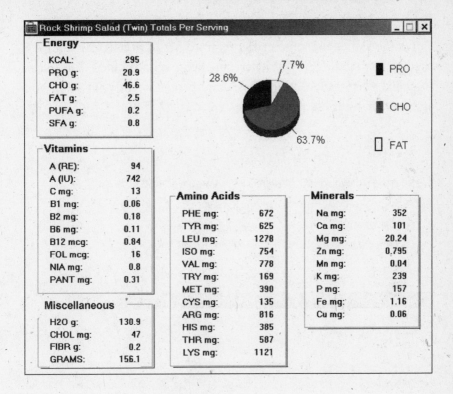

Rock Shrimp Salad (Twin) Totals Per Serving

Energy

KCAL:	295
PRO g:	20.9
CHO g:	46.6
FAT g:	2.5
PUFA g:	0.2
SFA g:	0.8

7.7%
28.6%
63.7%

■ PRO
■ CHO
□ FAT

Vitamins

A (RE):	94
A (IU):	742
C mg:	13
B1 mg:	0.06
B2 mg:	0.18
B6 mg:	0.11
B12 mcg:	0.84
FOL mcg:	16
NIA mg:	0.8
PANT mg:	0.31

Amino Acids

PHE mg:	672
TYR mg:	625
LEU mg:	1278
ISO mg:	754
VAL mg:	778
TRY mg:	169
MET mg:	390
CYS mg:	135
ARG mg:	816
HIS mg:	385
THR mg:	587
LYS mg:	1121

Minerals

Na mg:	352
Ca mg:	101
Mg mg:	20.24
Zn mg:	0.795
Mn mg:	0.04
K mg:	239
P mg:	157
Fe mg:	1.16
Cu mg:	0.06

Miscellaneous

H2O g:	130.9
CHOL mg:	47
FIBR g:	0.2
GRAMS:	156.1

Salmon and Pasta Skillet Dinner

Serves 4

2 cups vegetable broth (can be made with a bouillon cube)

2½ cups rotini or any tube-shaped pasta (dry)

¼ cup whipped cream cheese with chives

½ cup soy milk (like Edensoy Original)

1 tablespoon grated Parmesan cheese (or soy substitute)

1 teaspoon prepared yellow mustard

½ teaspoon dried basil (crushed)

Dash freshly ground black pepper

14½-ounce can red (sockeye) salmon (skin and bones removed and cut into bite-size pieces)

1 cup baby sweet peas (optional)

In a large skillet, bring the vegetable broth to a boil. Add the pasta. Cover the skillet and simmer the mixture for 10 minutes or until the pasta is just tender. Stir in the cream cheese till combined. Stir in the soy milk, Parmesan, mustard, basil, and pepper. Gently stir in salmon and peas (if using) and cook till heated.

Nutrition Totals Per Serving

KCal Breakdown: 27.4% Protein; 51.6% Carbohydrate; 21.0% Fat

Calories: 432

Protein: 28.9 (g)

Carbohydrate: 54.4 (g)

Fat: 9.9 (g)

Sodium: 818 (mg)

Cholesterol: 43 (mg)

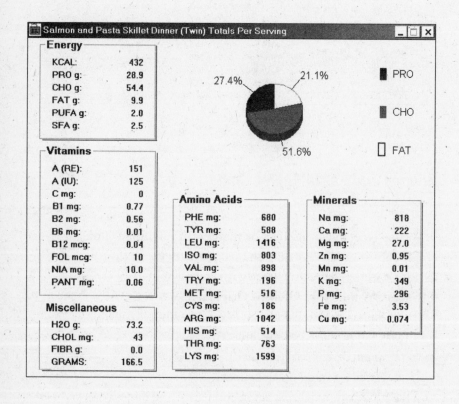

Salmon and Pasta Skillet Dinner (Twin) Totals Per Serving

Energy

KCAL:	432
PRO g:	28.9
CHO g:	54.4
FAT g:	9.9
PUFA g:	2.0
SFA g:	2.5

27.4%   21.1%   51.6%

PRO CHO FAT

Vitamins

A (RE):	151
A (IU):	125
C mg:	0
B1 mg:	0.77
B2 mg:	0.56
B6 mg:	0.01
B12 mcg:	0.04
FOL mcg:	10
NIA mg:	10.0
PANT mg:	0.06

Amino Acids

PHE mg:	680
TYR mg:	588
LEU mg:	1416
ISO mg:	803
VAL mg:	898
TRY mg:	196
MET mg:	516
CYS mg:	186
ARG mg:	1042
HIS mg:	514
THR mg:	763
LYS mg:	1599

Minerals

Na mg:	818
Ca mg:	222
Mg mg:	27.0
Zn mg:	0.95
Mn mg:	0.01
K mg:	349
P mg:	296
Fe mg:	3.53
Cu mg:	0.074

Miscellaneous

H2O g:	73.2
CHOL mg:	43
FIBR g:	0.0
GRAMS:	166.5

Shrimp Creole

Serves 4

1 pound fresh peeled and deveined shrimp, uncooked
½ cup chopped onion
½ cup chopped celery
½ cup chopped green pepper
½ cup sliced okra
2 cloves garlic, minced
1 tablespoon extra-virgin olive oil
14½-ounce can diced tomatoes with garlic
½ cup water
2 tablespoons parsley, chopped
½ teaspoon salt
½ teaspoon paprika
¼ teaspoon ground red pepper
1 bay leaf
3 sprigs fresh thyme
1 tablespoon cornstarch dissolved in 2 tablespoons cold water
2 cups hot cooked rice

Heat the oil in a large skillet. Add onion, celery, green pepper, okra, and garlic. Sauté the mixture until the ingredients start to soften. Stir in undrained tomatoes, ½ cup water, parsley, salt, paprika, red pepper, bay leaf, and thyme. Bring the mixture to a boil, then reduce heat to low. Cover the skillet and simmer the mixture for 15 minutes. Stir together the 2 tablespoons water and the cornstarch. Add the cornstarch mixture to the tomato mixture in the skillet, along with the shrimp. Cook and stir the mixture for several more minutes until the shrimp turn pink. Remove the bay leaf and thyme stalks. Serve over rice.

Nutrition Totals Per Serving

KCal Breakdown: 36.0% Protein; 47.0% Carbohydrate; 17.0% Fat

Calories: 305   Fat: 5.6 (g)
Protein: 27 (g)   Sodium: 1289 (mg)
Carbohydrate: 35.2 (g)   Cholesterol: 173 (mg)

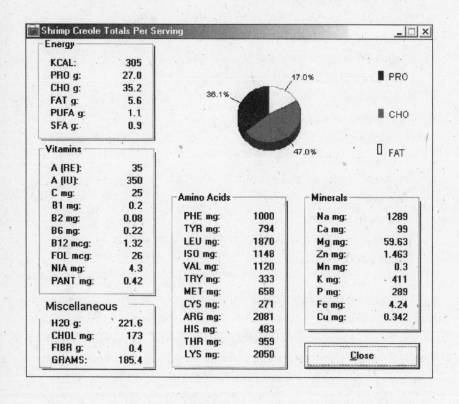

Shrimp Creole Totals Per Serving

Energy

KCAL:	305
PRO g:	27.0
CHO g:	35.2
FAT g:	5.6
PUFA g:	1.1
SFA g:	0.9

Vitamins

A (RE):	35
A (IU):	350
C mg:	25
B1 mg:	0.2
B2 mg:	0.08
B6 mg:	0.22
B12 mcg:	1.32
FOL mcg:	26
NIA mg:	4.3
PANT mg:	0.42

Miscellaneous

H2O g:	221.6
CHOL mg:	173
FIBR g:	0.4
GRAMS:	185.4

Amino Acids

PHE mg:	1000
TYR mg:	794
LEU mg:	1870
ISO mg:	1148
VAL mg:	1120
TRY mg:	333
MET mg:	658
CYS mg:	271
ARG mg:	2081
HIS mg:	483
THR mg:	959
LYS mg:	2050

Minerals

Na mg:	1289
Ca mg:	99
Mg mg:	59.63
Zn mg:	1.463
Mn mg:	0.3
K mg:	411
P mg:	289
Fe mg:	4.24
Cu mg:	0.342

17.0% PRO
36.1% CHO
47.0% FAT

Close

Shrimp de Jacques

Serves 4

¾ cup finely chopped onion
½ cup sliced mushrooms
1½ cups coarsely chopped cooked shrimp
½ teaspoon tarragon vinegar
¼ cup plain low-fat yogurt
¼ teaspoon dry mustard
1 teaspoon tamari soy sauce
¾ teaspoon garlic powder
3 tablespoons grated Parmesan cheese (or soy substitute)
1 egg white
¾ cup whole-wheat bread crumbs
½ teaspoon dried basil
1 tablespoon chopped fresh parsley
⅛ teaspoon dried marjoram
Pinch of pepper
Paprika

Preheat oven broiler. Coat a nonstick frying pan with olive oil cooking spray. Brown onion. Add mushrooms and shrimp. Cook 2 to 3 more minutes. Set aside.

Whisk together vinegar, yogurt, mustard, tamari, ½ teaspoon garlic powder, 1 tablespoon Parmesan, and egg white. Add shrimp, onion, and mushrooms to sauce. Spoon into four ramekins.

Mix bread crumbs, basil, parsley, marjoram, pepper, 2 tablespoons Parmesan, and ¼ teaspoon garlic powder. Sprinkle on top of shrimp equally. Sprinkle with paprika. Place under broiler 3 to 4 minutes or until hot and bubbly.

Nutrition Totals Per Serving

KCal Breakdown: 35.1% Protein; 49.8% Carbohydrate; 15.2% Fat

Calories: 141

Protein: 12.5 (g)

Carbohydrate: 17.7 (g)

Fat: 2.4 (g)

Sodium: 723 (mg)

Cholesterol: 60 (mg)

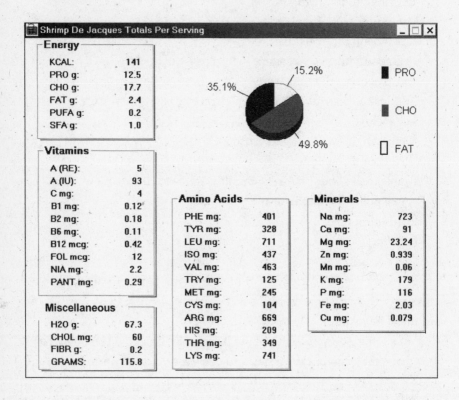

Shrimp De Jacques Totals Per Serving		_ □ x

Energy

KCAL:	141
PRO g:	12.5
CHO g:	17.7
FAT g:	2.4
PUFA g:	0.2
SFA g:	1.0

15.2% 35.1% 49.8%

■ PRO
■ CHO
□ FAT

Vitamins

A (RE):	5
A (IU):	93
C mg:	4
B1 mg:	0.12
B2 mg:	0.18
B6 mg:	0.11
B12 mcg:	0.42
FOL mcg:	12
NIA mg:	2.2
PANT mg:	0.29

Amino Acids

PHE mg:	401
TYR mg:	328
LEU mg:	711
ISO mg:	437
VAL mg:	463
TRY mg:	125
MET mg:	245
CYS mg:	104
ARG mg:	669
HIS mg:	209
THR mg:	349
LYS mg:	741

Minerals

Na mg:	723
Ca mg:	91
Mg mg:	23.24
Zn mg:	0.939
Mn mg:	0.06
K mg:	179
P mg:	116
Fe mg:	2.03
Cu mg:	0.079

Miscellaneous

H2O g:	67.3
CHOL mg:	60
FIBR g:	0.2
GRAMS:	115.8

Smart Fries

Serves 2

1 large potato cut into ½-inch-thick strips

3 egg whites

1½ tablespoons grated Parmesan cheese (or soy substitute)

Pinch of pepper

Preheat oven to 400 degrees. Coat a cookie sheet with olive oil cooking spray. Whisk together egg whites, Parmesan cheese, and pepper.

Dip potato strips in egg-white mixture to coat. Arrange potatoes on prepared cookie sheet and bake them for 15 minutes. Turn and cook them for 15 minutes more or until golden brown. Serve with a side of ketchup.

Nutrition Totals Per Serving

KCal Breakdown: 19.6% Protein; 74.9% Carbohydrate; 5.5% Fat

Calories: 207
Protein: 10.3 (g)
Carbohydrate: 39.0 (g)

Fat: 1.3 (g)
Sodium: 157 (mg)
Cholesterol: 3 (mg)

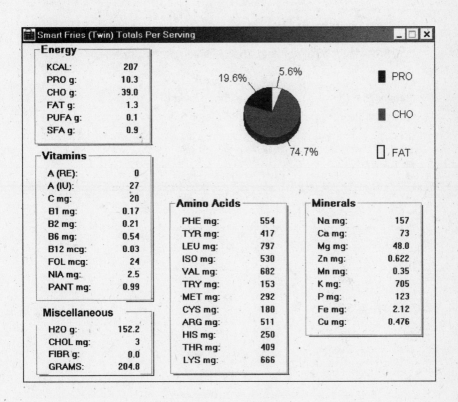

Smart Fries (Twin) Totals Per Serving

Energy

KCAL:	207
PRO g:	10.3
CHO g:	39.0
FAT g:	1.3
PUFA g:	0.1
SFA g:	0.9

19.6% 5.6% 74.7%

■ PRO
■ CHO
□ FAT

Vitamins

A (RE):	0
A (IU):	27
C mg:	20
B1 mg:	0.17
B2 mg:	0.21
B6 mg:	0.54
B12 mcg:	0.03
FOL mcg:	24
NIA mg:	2.5
PANT mg:	0.99

Miscellaneous

H2O g:	152.2
CHOL mg:	3
FIBR g:	0.0
GRAMS:	204.8

Amino Acids

PHE mg:	554
TYR mg:	417
LEU mg:	797
ISO mg:	530
VAL mg:	682
TRY mg:	153
MET mg:	292
CYS mg:	180
ARG mg:	511
HIS mg:	250
THR mg:	409
LYS mg:	666

Minerals

Na mg:	157
Ca mg:	73
Mg mg:	48.0
Zn mg:	0.622
Mn mg:	0.35
K mg:	705
P mg:	123
Fe mg:	2.12
Cu mg:	0.476

Smoked Salmon Scramble

Serves 2

1 small onion, finely diced
2 ounces thinly sliced smoked salmon, diced
8 egg whites
¼ cup skim milk
Dash of pepper

Coat a nonstick skillet with olive oil cooking spray. Lightly brown onion. Add salmon and cook another minute. In the meantime whisk together the egg whites, skim milk, and pepper. Pour over salmon and onion. Cook on medium heat, stirring constantly until eggs are set.

Nutrition Totals Per Serving

KCal Breakdown: 55.5% Protein; 16.3% Carbohydrate; 28.2% Fat

Calories: 154
Protein: 20.6 (g)
Carbohydrate: 6.1 (g)

Fat: 4.6 (g)
Sodium: 562 (mg)
Cholesterol: 6 (mg)

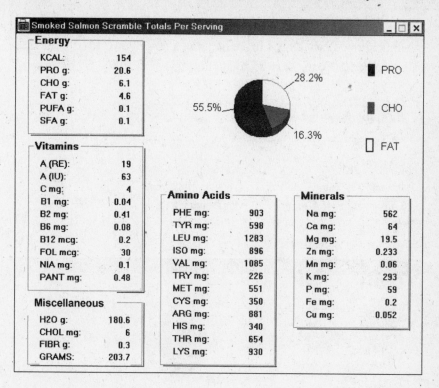

Smoked Salmon Scramble Totals Per Serving

Energy

KCAL:	154
PRO g:	20.6
CHO g:	6.1
FAT g:	4.6
PUFA g:	0.1
SFA g:	0.1

28.2% PRO
55.5% CHO
16.3% FAT

Vitamins

A (RE):	19
A (IU):	63
C mg:	4
B1 mg:	0.04
B2 mg:	0.41
B6 mg:	0.08
B12 mcg:	0.2
FOL mcg:	30
NIA mg:	0.1
PANT mg:	0.48

Amino Acids

PHE mg:	903
TYR mg:	598
LEU mg:	1283
ISO mg:	896
VAL mg:	1085
TRY mg:	226
MET mg:	551
CYS mg:	350
ARG mg:	881
HIS mg:	340
THR mg:	654
LYS mg:	930

Minerals

Na mg:	562
Ca mg:	64
Mg mg:	19.5
Zn mg:	0.233
Mn mg:	0.06
K mg:	293
P mg:	59
Fe mg:	0.2
Cu mg:	0.052

Miscellaneous

H2O g:	180.6
CHOL mg:	6
FIBR g:	0.3
GRAMS:	203.7

Spicy Black-bean Quiche

Serves 4

1 cup chopped onion

½ cup chopped green pepper

2 teaspoons chili powder

½ teaspoon garlic powder

⅛ teaspoon salt

16-ounce can black beans, drained

1½ cups cooked brown rice

¾ cup skim milk

3 egg whites, lightly beaten

1 cup fat-free shredded cheddar cheese

Preheat the oven to 350 degrees. Coat a 9-inch pie pan with olive oil cooking spray. Place all the ingredients in a large bowl. Mix. Pour into the prepared pie pan. Bake 25 to 30 minutes, or until the center is set.

Nutrition Totals Per Serving

KCal Breakdown: 31.3% Protein; 65.8% Carbohydrate; 2.8% Fat

Calories: 281
Protein: 21.7 (g)
Carbohydrate: 45.5 (g)

Fat: 9 (g)
Sodium: 1088 (mg)
Cholesterol: 5 (g)

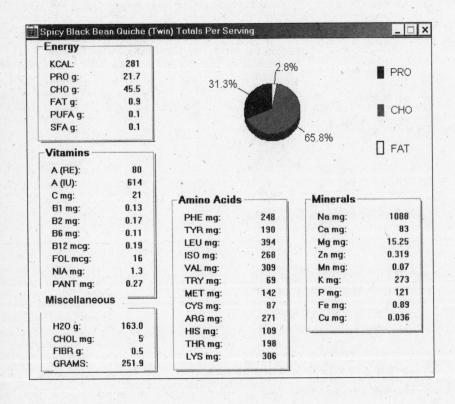

Spicy Black Bean Quiche (Twin) Totals Per Serving

Energy

KCAL:	281
PRO g:	21.7
CHO g:	45.5
FAT g:	0.9
PUFA g:	0.1
SFA g:	0.1

2.8%
31.3%
65.8%

■ PRO
■ CHO
☐ FAT

Vitamins

A (RE):	80
A (IU):	614
C mg:	21
B1 mg:	0.13
B2 mg:	0.17
B6 mg:	0.11
B12 mcg:	0.19
FOL mcg:	16
NIA mg:	1.3
PANT mg:	0.27

Amino Acids

PHE mg:	248
TYR mg:	190
LEU mg:	394
ISO mg:	268
VAL mg:	309
TRY mg:	69
MET mg:	142
CYS mg:	87
ARG mg:	271
HIS mg:	109
THR mg:	198
LYS mg:	306

Minerals

Na mg:	1088
Ca mg:	83
Mg mg:	15.25
Zn mg:	0.319
Mn mg:	0.07
K mg:	273
P mg:	121
Fe mg:	0.89
Cu mg:	0.036

Miscellaneous

H2O g:	163.0
CHOL mg:	5
FIBR g:	0.5
GRAMS:	251.9

Spinach Noodle Casserole

Serves 8

8 ounces no-yolk noodles, cooked according to package directions
2 10-ounce packages frozen chopped spinach, defrosted and
    drained
1 tablespoon light butter, softened at room temperature
1 cup chopped onions
5 egg whites or egg-substitute equivalent, well beaten
1 cup reduced-fat sour cream
1 cup reduced-fat mozzarella cheese, shredded
½ cup reduced-fat cheddar cheese, shredded
⅛ teaspoon pepper

Preheat oven to 350 degrees. Coat a 3- to 4-quart casserole with
olive oil cooking spray. Place the noodles in a large bowl. Add the rest of
the ingredients. Toss to mix. Pour mixture into the prepared casserole.
Bake covered for 30 minutes. Remove the cover and bake 15 more minutes.

Nutrition Totals Per Serving

KCal Breakdown: 26.3% Protein; 47.7% Carbohydrate; 26.0% Fat

Calories: 239
Protein: 16.1 (g)
Carbohydrate: 29.2 (g)

Fat: 7.1 (g)
Sodium: 271 (mg)
Cholesterol: 17 (mg)

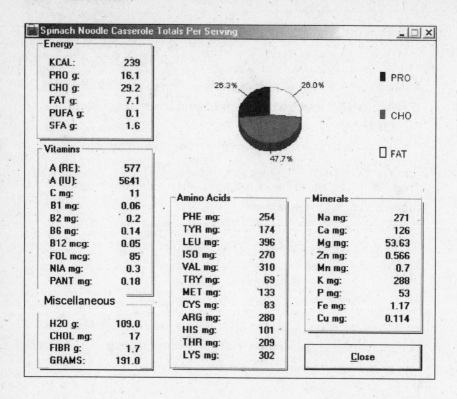

Strawberry Power Smoothie

Serves 1

1 cup soy milk (like Edensoy Original)
1 tablespoon soy protein powder
3 tablespoons Eagle Brand Fat Free Sweetened Condensed Milk
1 heaping cup frozen strawberries (unsweetened)

In a blender combine the soy beverage, soy powder, and condensed milk. Pulse to blend. Add the strawberries and process till smooth.

Nutrition Totals Per Serving

KCal Breakdown: 17.0% Protein; 76.3% Carbohydrate; 6.6% Fat

Calories: 345
Protein: 14.4 (g)
Carbohydrate: 64.6 (g)

Fat: 2.5 (g)
Sodium: 283 (mg)
Cholesterol: 5 (mg)

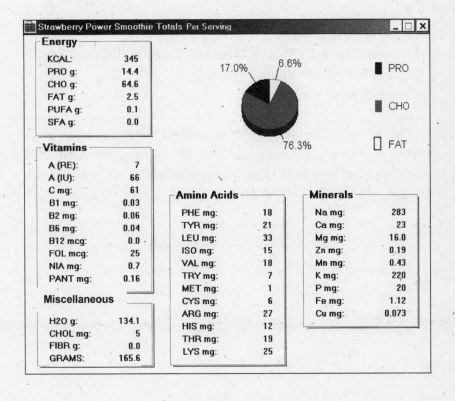

Strawberry Power Smoothie Totals Per Serving

Energy

KCAL:	345
PRO g:	14.4
CHO g:	64.6
FAT g:	2.5
PUFA g:	0.1
SFA g:	0.0

17.0% 6.6%

PRO
CHO
FAT

76.3%

Vitamins

A (RE):	7
A (IU):	66
C mg:	61
B1 mg:	0.03
B2 mg:	0.06
B6 mg:	0.04
B12 mcg:	0.0
FOL mcg:	25
NIA mg:	0.7
PANT mg:	0.16

Amino Acids

PHE mg:	18
TYR mg:	21
LEU mg:	33
ISO mg:	15
VAL mg:	18
TRY mg:	7
MET mg:	1
CYS mg:	6
ARG mg:	27
HIS mg:	12
THR mg:	19
LYS mg:	25

Minerals

Na mg:	283
Ca mg:	23
Mg mg:	16.0
Zn mg:	0.19
Mn mg:	0.43
K mg:	220
P mg:	20
Fe mg:	1.12
Cu mg:	0.073

Miscellaneous

H2O g:	134.1
CHOL mg:	5
FIBR g:	0.0
GRAMS:	165.6

Super Chicken Stir-fry

Serves 2 to 4

½ cup water
4 teaspoons tamari soy sauce
3 cups cooked brown rice
1 cup cubed cooked chicken breast
Pinch of pepper
Pinch of garlic powder
1 10-ounce package broccoli florets (cooked according to package
    instructions and drained well)
Chopped scallions

Coat a nonstick frying pan with olive oil cooking spray. Place water, tamari, and rice in pan. Heat to medium–high, stirring constantly. Add chicken, pepper, and garlic. Heat through. Add broccoli. Stir until hot. Garnish with scallions.

Nutrition Totals Per Serving (based on 4 servings)

KCal Breakdown: 21.7% Protein; 71.1% Carbohydrate; 7.2% Fat

Calories: 228
Protein: 12.4 (g)
Carbohydrate: 40.5 (g)

Fat: 1.8 (g)
Sodium: 703 (mg)
Cholesterol: 18 (mg)

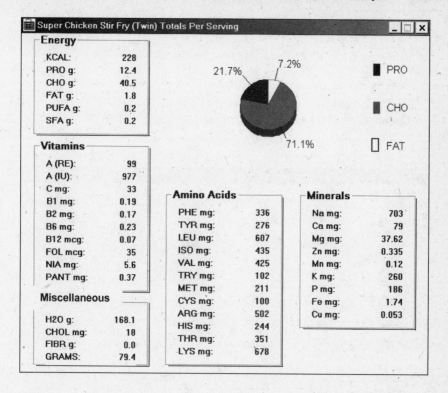

Tasty Oatmeal

Serves 2

¼ cup raisins
2 medium bananas, cut in quarters lengthwise and sliced ½-inch
    thick
⅛ teaspoon cinnamon
1½ cups water
1 cup instant oatmeal

Place the first four ingredients in a saucepan. Bring to a rapid boil. Stir in the oatmeal. Turn off the heat immediately. Stir for 1 minute, leaving the saucepan on the burner. Remove the saucepan from the burner and pour the cereal into two bowls. Serve piping hot. Sprinkle with sweetener and garnish with sliced papaya if desired.

Nutrition Totals Per Serving

KCal Breakdown: 10.9% Protein; 77.8% Carbohydrate; 11.4% Fat

Calories: 261
Protein: 5.8 (g)
Carbohydrate: 41.5 (g)

Fat: 2.7 (g)
Sodium: 83 (mg)
Cholesterol: 0 (mg)

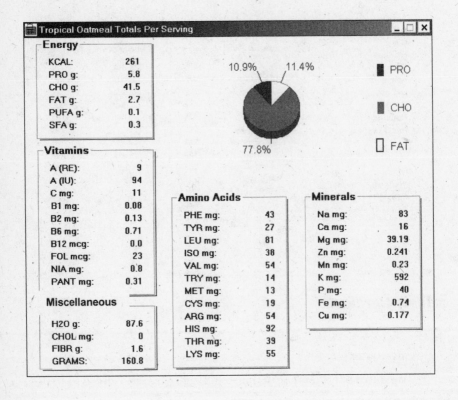

| Tropical Oatmeal Totals Per Serving | | _ □ x |

Energy

KCAL:	261
PRO g:	5.8
CHO g:	41.5
FAT g:	2.7
PUFA g:	0.1
SFA g:	0.3

10.9%   11.4%   ■ PRO
■ CHO
77.8%   □ FAT

Vitamins

A (RE):	9
A (IU):	94
C mg:	11
B1 mg:	0.08
B2 mg:	0.13
B6 mg:	0.71
B12 mcg:	0.0
FOL mcg:	23
NIA mg:	0.8
PANT mg:	0.31

Amino Acids

PHE mg:	43
TYR mg:	27
LEU mg:	81
ISO mg:	38
VAL mg:	54
TRY mg:	14
MET mg:	13
CYS mg:	19
ARG mg:	54
HIS mg:	92
THR mg:	39
LYS mg:	55

Minerals

Na mg:	83
Ca mg:	16
Mg mg:	39.19
Zn mg:	0.241
Mn mg:	0.23
K mg:	592
P mg:	40
Fe mg:	0.74
Cu mg:	0.177

Miscellaneous

H2O g:	87.6
CHOL mg:	0
FIBR g:	1.6
GRAMS:	160.8

Thai Noodle Medley

4 Servings

12-ounce package rice noodles
½ cup carrot (cut into thin strips)
½ cup red bell pepper (cut into thin strips)
½ cup broccoli florets (parboiled and chilled)

FOR SAUCE:
2 chopped scallions, white part only
2-by-1-inch piece of peeled fresh gingerroot, cut into quarters
2 garlic cloves, minced
2 tablespoons smooth natural peanut butter
8 ounces firm tofu cut into 1-inch pieces
1 teaspoon Ka-ME dark sesame oil
¼ cup honey
¼ cup light soy sauce
¼ cup rice wine vinegar
¼ teaspoon ground red pepper

Combine all the ingredients for the sauce together in a food processor or blender till smooth. Pour into a bowl and chill.

Prepare the noodles according to package instructions. Drain and rinse with cold water. Place noodles in a large bowl. Pour chilled Thai sauce over noodles. Toss to coat. Add prepared carrots, red pepper, and broccoli. Toss and serve.

Nutrition Totals Per Serving

KCal Breakdown: 17.8% Protein; 56.3% Carbohydrate; 25.9% Fat

Calories: 291	Fat: 8.7 (g)
Protein: 13.4 (g)	Sodium: 658 (mg)
Carbohydrate: 42.4 (g)	Cholesterol: 5 (mg)

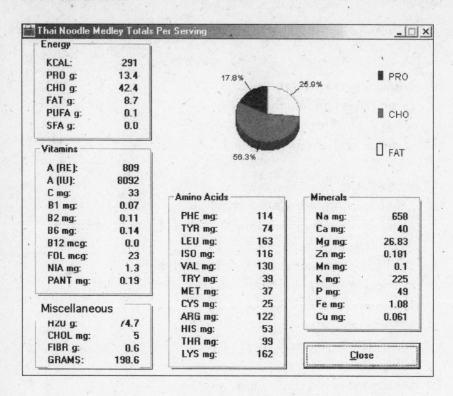

Thai Noodle Medley Totals Per Serving

Energy

KCAL:	291
PRO g:	13.4
CHO g:	42.4
FAT g:	8.7
PUFA g:	0.1
SFA g:	0.0

17.8% / 25.9% / 56.3%

PRO / CHO / FAT

Vitamins

A (RE):	809
A (IU):	8092
C mg:	33
B1 mg:	0.07
B2 mg:	0.11
B6 mg:	0.14
B12 mcg:	0.0
FOL mcg:	23
NIA mg:	1.3
PANT mg:	0.19

Amino Acids

PHE mg:	114
TYR mg:	74
LEU mg:	163
ISO mg:	116
VAL mg:	130
TRY mg:	39
MET mg:	37
CYS mg:	25
ARG mg:	122
HIS mg:	53
THR mg:	99
LYS mg:	162

Minerals

Na mg:	658
Ca mg:	40
Mg mg:	26.83
Zn mg:	0.181
Mn mg:	0.1
K mg:	225
P mg:	49
Fe mg:	1.08
Cu mg:	0.061

Miscellaneous

H2O g:	74.7
CHOL mg:	5
FIBR g:	0.6
GRAMS:	198.6

Close

Thick 'n' Frosty Malted

Serves 1

1 medium-size frozen banana (ripened and peeled before freezing)
¼ cup reduced-calorie chocolate syrup (like Hershey's Lite
    Chocolate Syrup)
¾ cup reduced-fat soy milk (like Westsoy 1%)
1 tablespoon soy or whey protein powder
1 tablespoon malted-milk powder (optional)

Nutrition Totals Per Serving

KCal Breakdown: 12.7% Protein; 79.0% Carbohydrate; 8.2% Fat

Calories: 338
Protein: 10.8 (g)
Carbohydrate: 67 (g)

Fat: 3.1 (g)
Sodium: 289 (mg)
Cholesterol: 2 (g)

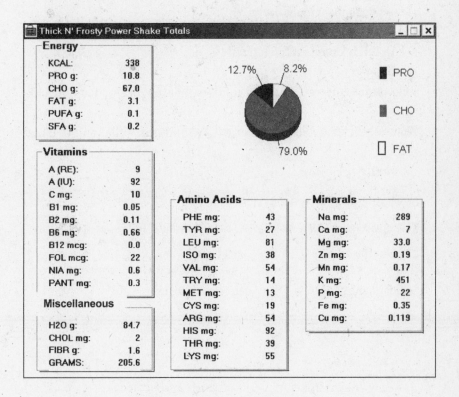

Thick N' Frosty Power Shake Totals

Energy

KCAL:	338
PRO g:	10.8
CHO g:	67.0
FAT g:	3.1
PUFA g:	0.1
SFA g:	0.2

12.7%   8.2%

79.0%

■ PRO
■ CHO
☐ FAT

Vitamins

A (RE):	9
A (IU):	92
C mg:	10
B1 mg:	0.05
B2 mg:	0.11
B6 mg:	0.66
B12 mcg:	0.0
FOL mcg:	22
NIA mg:	0.6
PANT mg:	0.3

Miscellaneous

H2O g:	84.7
CHOL mg:	2
FIBR g:	1.6
GRAMS:	205.6

Amino Acids

PHE mg:	43
TYR mg:	27
LEU mg:	81
ISO mg:	38
VAL mg:	54
TRY mg:	14
MET mg:	13
CYS mg:	19
ARG mg:	54
HIS mg:	92
THR mg:	39
LYS mg:	55

Minerals

Na mg:	289
Ca mg:	7
Mg mg:	33.0
Zn mg:	0.19
Mn mg:	0.17
K mg:	451
P mg:	22
Fe mg:	0.35
Cu mg:	0.119

Tuna Fagiole Salad

Serves 4

1 cup finely chopped onion
½ teaspoon garlic powder
¼ cup no-oil Italian dressing
2 tablespoons lemon juice
1½ tablespoons wine vinegar
1 15-ounce can chickpeas (drained)
¼ cup finely chopped fresh parsley
¼ teaspoon pepper
1 6½-ounce can water-packed solid white tuna, drained and flaked

Place all the ingredients in a large bowl and mix well. Chill to blend flavors.

Nutrition Totals Per Serving

KCal Breakdown: 37.9% Protein; 48.3% Carbohydrate; 13.0% Fat

Calories: 199
Protein: 19.1 (g)
Carbohydrate: 24.3 (g)

Fat: 3.1 (mg)
Sodium: 310 (mg)
Cholesterol: 19 (mg)

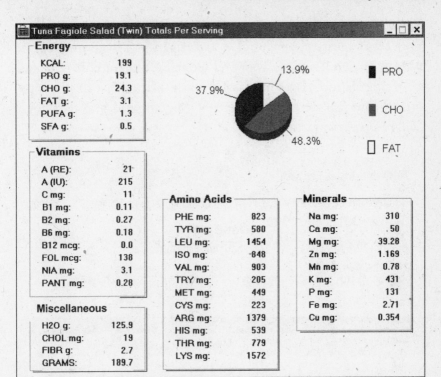

Tuna Fagiole Salad (Twin) Totals Per Serving							

Energy

KCAL:	199
PRO g:	19.1
CHO g:	24.3
FAT g:	3.1
PUFA g:	1.3
SFA g:	0.5

13.9%
37.9%
48.3%

■ PRO
■ CHO
□ FAT

Vitamins

A (RE):	21
A (IU):	215
C mg:	11
B1 mg:	0.11
B2 mg:	0.27
B6 mg:	0.18
B12 mcg:	0.0
FOL mcg:	138
NIA mg:	3.1
PANT mg:	0.28

Amino Acids

PHE mg:	823
TYR mg:	580
LEU mg:	1454
ISO mg:	848
VAL mg:	903
TRY mg:	205
MET mg:	449
CYS mg:	223
ARG mg:	1379
HIS mg:	539
THR mg:	779
LYS mg:	1572

Minerals

Na mg:	310
Ca mg:	.50
Mg mg:	39.28
Zn mg:	1.169
Mn mg:	0.78
K mg:	431
P mg:	131
Fe mg:	2.71
Cu mg:	0.354

Miscellaneous

H2O g:	125.9
CHOL mg:	19
FIBR g:	2.7
GRAMS:	189.7

Ultimate Chicken Salad

Serves 6

2 cups cubed cooked chicken

⅔ cup diced celery

½ cup coarsely chopped pecans

2 cups diced Granny Smith apples

½ cup plain low-fat yogurt

¼ cup low-fat cottage cheese

½ teaspoon prepared mustard

2 teaspoons lemon juice

1 teaspoon tamari soy sauce

12 leaves lettuce

6 slices pineapple (fresh if available)

Combine the first four ingredients in a large bowl. Place yogurt, cottage cheese, mustard, lemon juice, and tamari in a food processor or blender. Mix until smooth. Pour over the chicken mixture. Toss to coat.

Arrange lettuce leaves in six salad bowls. Place a slice of pineapple in each bowl. Spoon equal amounts of chicken salad into each bowl. Chill before serving.

Nutrition Totals Per Serving

KCal Breakdown: 22.6% Protein; 44.3% Carbohydrate; 33.1% Fat

Calories: 212
Protein: 12.6 (g)
Carbohydrate: 24.7 (g)

Fat: 8.2 (g)
Sodium: 130 (mg)
Cholesterol: 27 (mg)

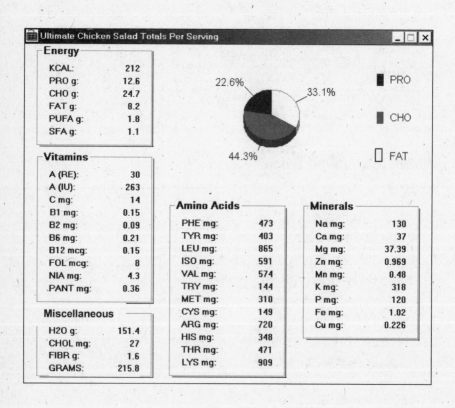

Ultimate Chicken Salad Totals Per Serving

Energy

KCAL:	212
PRO g:	12.6
CHO g:	24.7
FAT g:	8.2
PUFA g:	1.8
SFA g:	1.1

22.6%   33.1%   44.3%

■ PRO
■ CHO
☐ FAT

Vitamins

A (RE):	30
A (IU):	263
C mg:	14
B1 mg:	0.15
B2 mg:	0.09
B6 mg:	0.21
B12 mcg:	0.15
FOL mcg:	8
NIA mg:	4.3
PANT mg:	0.36

Amino Acids

PHE mg:	473
TYR mg:	403
LEU mg:	865
ISO mg:	591
VAL mg:	574
TRY mg:	144
MET mg:	310
CYS mg:	149
ARG mg:	720
HIS mg:	348
THR mg:	471
LYS mg:	909

Minerals

Na mg:	130
Ca mg:	37
Mg mg:	37.39
Zn mg:	0.969
Mn mg:	0.48
K mg:	318
P mg:	120
Fe mg:	1.02
Cu mg:	0.226

Miscellaneous

H2O g:	151.4
CHOL mg:	27
FIBR g:	1.6
GRAMS:	215.8

Whey Cool Vanilla Malted

Serves 1

⅔ cup reduced-fat soy milk (like Westsoy 1% Lite Soy Beverage)
2 tablespoons whey protein powder
1 teaspoon pure vanilla extract
2 tablespoons vanilla Carnation Malt Powder (optional)
4 cubes frozen reduced-fat soy milk

Pour soy milk into an ice cube tray and let it freeze for approximately 6 hours.

In a blender combine the liquid soy milk, whey powder, vanilla extract, and malt powder (if using) and pulse to blend. Add the frozen cubes and process till smooth. Serve immediately.

Nutrition Totals Per Serving

KCal Breakdown: 42.2% Protein; 45.6% Carbohydrate; 12.2% Fat

Calories: 318	Fat: 4 (g)
Protein: 31.0 (g)	Sodium: 367 (mg)
Carbohydrate: 33.5 (g)	Cholesterol: 3 (mg)

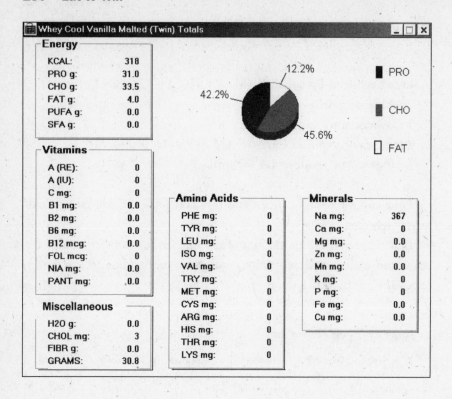

Whey Cool Vanilla Malted (Twin) Totals		

Energy

KCAL:	318
PRO g:	31.0
CHO g:	33.5
FAT g:	4.0
PUFA g:	0.0
SFA g:	0.0

12.2%
42.2%
45.6%

■ PRO
■ CHO
□ FAT

Vitamins

A (RE):	0
A (IU):	0
C mg:	0
B1 mg:	0.0
B2 mg:	0.0
B6 mg:	0.0
B12 mcg:	0.0
FOL mcg:	0
NIA mg:	0.0
PANT mg:	0.0

Amino Acids

PHE mg:	0
TYR mg:	0
LEU mg:	0
ISO mg:	0
VAL mg:	0
TRY mg:	0
MET mg:	0
CYS mg:	0
ARG mg:	0
HIS mg:	0
THR mg:	0
LYS mg:	0

Minerals

Na mg:	367
Ca mg:	0
Mg mg:	0.0
Zn mg:	0.0
Mn mg:	0.0
K mg:	0
P mg:	0
Fe mg:	0.0
Cu mg:	0.0

Miscellaneous

H2O g:	0.0
CHOL mg:	3
FIBR g:	0.0
GRAMS:	30.8

Winner's Circle Salad

Serves 4

1½ cups zucchini in julienne strips (⅓ by 1½ inches)

2 cups carrots in julienne strips (⅓ by 1½ inches)

1 tablespoon frozen orange juice concentrate

1½ teaspoons Dijon mustard

1 teaspoon red wine vinegar

2 tablespoons no-oil Italian dressing

1 teaspoon tamari soy sauce

Pinch of dried thyme

Pinch of pepper

⅓ cup coarsely chopped walnuts

Place zucchini and carrots in a large bowl and mix together. Place remaining ingredients except walnuts into a food processor or blender. Mix until smooth. Add walnuts and pulse until walnuts are coarsely ground. Pour mixture over carrots and zucchini. Toss to coat.

Nutrition Totals Per Serving

KCal Breakdown: 10.5% Protein; 46.5% Carbohydrate; 43.0% Fat

Calories: 90
Protein: 2.6 (g)
Carbohydrate: 11.4 (g)

Fat: 4.7 (g)
Sodium: 180 (mg)
Cholesterol: 0 (mg)

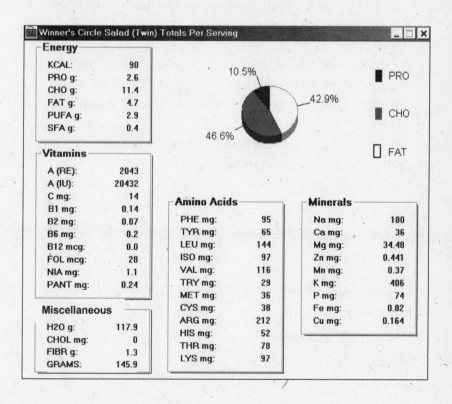

Winner's Circle Salad (Twin) Totals Per Serving		

Energy

KCAL:	90
PRO g:	2.6
CHO g:	11.4
FAT g:	4.7
PUFA g:	2.9
SFA g:	0.4

10.5%
42.9%
46.6%

■ PRO
■ CHO
☐ FAT

Vitamins

A (RE):	2043
A (IU):	20432
C mg:	14
B1 mg:	0.14
B2 mg:	0.07
B6 mg:	0.2
B12 mcg:	0.0
FOL mcg:	28
NIA mg:	1.1
PANT mg:	0.24

Amino Acids

PHE mg:	95
TYR mg:	65
LEU mg:	144
ISO mg:	97
VAL mg:	116
TRY mg:	29
MET mg:	36
CYS mg:	38
ARG mg:	212
HIS mg:	52
THR mg:	78
LYS mg:	97

Minerals

Na mg:	180
Ca mg:	36
Mg mg:	34.48
Zn mg:	0.441
Mn mg:	0.37
K mg:	406
P mg:	74
Fe mg:	0.82
Cu mg:	0.164

Miscellaneous

H2O g:	117.9
CHOL mg:	0
FIBR g:	1.3
GRAMS:	145.9

Ziti Bolognese

Serves 4

1½ cups textured soy protein crumbles (like Yves Veggie Ground
    Round or Boca Burger Recipe Basics) at room temperature
2 cups low-fat spaghetti sauce (tomato and olive oil based)
2 cups (dry) ziti pasta
2 large egg whites
2 tablespoons Parmesan cheese or soy substitute (like Soyco Veggie
    Parmesan)
1 cup fat-free ricotta cheese
1 cup plus 2 tablespoons reduced-fat shredded mozzarella cheese
⅛ teaspoon cracked pepper

Preheat the oven to 350 degrees. In a small bowl combine ½ cup
pasta sauce with the textured crumbles. Set aside. Cook the pasta to the
al dente stage. Drain and rinse with cool water and set it aside.

In a large bowl beat the egg whites with a fork. Add the Parmesan
and pepper. Stir. Add the ricotta and mozzarella and mix well with a
spoon. Add the pasta and stir to combine.

Coat a 2-quart casserole dish with olive oil cooking spray. Fill it in
the following order (making sure to spread out each layer as evenly as
possible):

¼ cup sauce (spread to cover bottom)

half the pasta-and-cheese mixture

½ cup sauce

all of the "meat" mixture

the rest of the pasta-and-cheese mixture

the rest of the sauce (approx. ¾ cup)

2 tablespoons of mozzarella sprinkled over the top

Cover and bake for 25 minutes. Remove lid and bake for 5 more
minutes. Wait 5 to 10 minutes before serving.

Nutrition Totals Per Serving

KCal Breakdown: 42.1% Protein; 42.5% Carbohydrate; 15.4% Fat

Calories: 431
Protein: 43.8 (g)
Carbohydrate: 44.2 (g)

Fat: 7.1 (g)
Sodium: 996 (mg)
Cholesterol: 16 (mg)

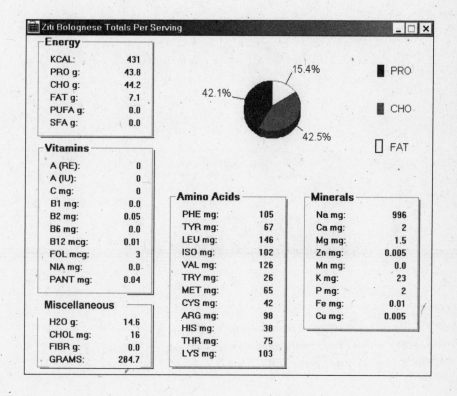

Ziti Bolognese Totals Per Serving

Energy

KCAL:	431
PRO g:	43.8
CHO g:	44.2
FAT g:	7.1
PUFA g:	0.0
SFA g:	0.0

Vitamins

A (RE):	0
A (IU):	0
C mg:	0
B1 mg:	0.0
B2 mg:	0.05
B6 mg:	0.0
B12 mcg:	0.01
FOL mcg:	3
NIA mg:	0.0
PANT mg:	0.04

Miscellaneous

H2O g:	14.6
CHOL mg:	16
FIBR g:	0.0
GRAMS:	284.7

Amino Acids

PHE mg:	105
TYR mg:	67
LEU mg:	146
ISO mg:	102
VAL mg:	126
TRY mg:	26
MET mg:	65
CYS mg:	42
ARG mg:	98
HIS mg:	38
THR mg:	75
LYS mg:	103

Minerals

Na mg:	996
Ca mg:	2
Mg mg:	1.5
Zn mg:	0.005
Mn mg:	0.0
K mg:	23
P mg:	2
Fe mg:	0.01
Cu mg:	0.005

15.4%
42.1%
42.5%

■ PRO
■ CHO
☐ FAT

Section III

GLOSSARY

Adipose tissue: Adipose tissue is connective tissue that functions as the primary storage site for fat in the form of triglycerides. Adipose tissue in people occurs in two different forms: white adipose tissue and brown adipose tissue. Most adult adipose tissue is white.

Aerobic activity: Low-intensity, high-endurance activity that requires oxygen.

Alanine cycle: Some of the pyruvate that is produced is used directly for energy, while the remainder is converted back to alanine, which is eventually converted into glucose and used for energy.

Alpha-linolenic acid: An essential fatty acid found in flaxseed and a number of other plant-seed oils.

Amino acid: A molecule containing ammonia and organic acids that forms the building blocks of all proteins. The human adult requires twenty-two amino acids. Twelve of them can be synthesized by the body (nonessential amino acids), whereas nine must be obtained from foods (essential amino acids).

Ammonia: A toxic metabolic waste product of amino acid metabolism.

Anabolism: The biochemical process in which muscle or other tissue is synthesized; a process of biologic growth.

Anaerobic: Without oxygen.

Anaerobic activity: A high-intensity activity that derives short bursts of energy from lactic acid and ATP.

Angina pectoris: Chest pain or discomfort due to coronary heart disease. Angina occurs when the heart muscle doesn't get as much blood and oxygen as it needs. This usually occurs when one or more of the heart's arteries (coronary arteries) is narrowed or blocked.

Antioxidant: A natural or synthetic chemical or a nutrient that inactivates the damaging portion (active site) of free radicals: Antioxidants also help neutralize chemicals that cause free-radical formation. Phytonutrients such as lycopene, alpha- and beta-carotene, B_1, B_5, B_6, C, E, the minerals selenium, zinc, coenzyme Q_{10}, uric acid, and three enzymes in your body (superoxide dismutase, catalase, and glutathione peroxidase) are all antioxidants. By neutralizing free radicals, antioxidants prevent damage to cell membranes and such genetic material as DNA.

Ascorbic acid: The chemical name for vitamin C.

Atherosclerosis: The process in which deposits of fatty compounds, cholesterol, protein, cellular waste products, calcium, and other substances build up in the inner lining of an artery. This buildup is called plaque.

ATP (adenosine triphosphate): The universal energy molecule. ATP is synthesized in the mitochondria, organelles that metabolize protein, fat, and carbohydrate into energy, stored in the phosophate bonds of ATP. When ATP is split by enzymes, energy is released for various cellular functions, including muscular contraction.

Automatic calorie control: The process of keeping calorie intake at healthy levels by consuming foods high on the satiety index. This is the diet strategy of the Eat to Win Diet to promote excess body fat loss and maintain a healthy body weight.

Beta-carotene (pro-vitamin A): A yellowish pigment found in plants, such as carrots, squash, and pumpkin. An enzyme splits one molecule of beta-carotene in half, forming two molecules of active vitamin A. Beta-carotene is just one of at least ten carotenes found in human blood. Beta-carotene is also a powerful antioxidant that neutralizes a damaging type of activated oxygen called singlet oxygen.

Bile acid: A detergent-like molecule made from cholesterol, which is secreted by the gallbladder into the intestine to assist in the absorption of dietary fats.

Blood lipid: Triglycerides (fat) and cholesterol carried in the blood are usually called blood lipids. Cholesterol is not actually a lipid but a waxy, fatlike compound that has a steroidlike structure with an alcohol chemical group attached.

Blood pressure: The force in the arteries when the heart beats (systolic pressure) and when the heart is at rest (diastolic pressure). Blood pressure is measured in millimeters of mercury (mm Hg).

Blood sugar: Glucose carried in the blood, used for energy by organs and other tissues.

Calorie: A unit of measurement used to express the energy value of food; more correctly called a kilocalorie, since it represents a thousand times the energy of the calorie used to measure chemical reactions in a test tube. One kilocalorie is the amount of heat required to raise one kilogram of water (2.2 pounds) one degree centigrade (almost two degrees Fahrenheit).

Cannibalization: The breakdown of muscle tissue by the body for the purpose of using amino acids for other metabolic purposes.

Catabolism: The biochemical process in which complex molecules are broken down for energy production, recycling of their components, or excretion.

Catecholamines: A group of brain neurotransmitters (chemicals that communicate messages between nerves) including norepinephrine and dopamine. All catecholamines are synthesized from the two amino acids L-phenylalanine and L-tyrosine.

Cell membrane: The outer boundary of a cell. Also called the plasma membrane.

Cholesterol: A sterol manufactured in the liver and other cells found only in animal protein and fats and oils (one exception: spirulina, a blue-green algae, contains cholesterol). The body uses cholesterol to synthesize hormones and cell membranes. High levels of plasma cholesterol (called LDL) are associated with an increased risk of cardiovascular disease. Oxidized cholesterol is suspected as the primary culprit in artery damage.

Chylomicron: A lipoprotein (carrier molecule) in blood plasma that carries fats and cholesterol from the intestines into other body tissues; it is made up of triglycerides surrounded by a protein-fat-phosphorus coating.

Coenzyme Q_{10}: A substance synthesized by the body responsible for the synthesis of adenosine triphosphate (ATP), the universal energy molecule. Research suggests that coenzyme Q_{10} acts as a fat-soluble free-radical neutralizer and helps regulate the electrical conduction system of the heart.

Collagen: A simple protein that is one of the chief components of connective tissue.

Complete protein: An outdated nutritional concept still promoted by the media based on the belief that only animal foods contain all nine essential amino acids in amounts that are sufficient to maintain normal growth rate and body weight.

Complex carbohydrate: A naturally occurring plant, usually a cereal, grain, or fruit, that is high in fiber and starch, and contains small amounts of simple sugars.

Cortisol: A hormone secreted by the adrenal glands that stimulates catabolism.

Creatine: A compound produced in the liver and stored in the muscle fibers, which can combine with phosphorus to form creatine phosphate; this compound is broken down by enzymes to quickly replenish ATP (adenosine triphosphate) during anaerobic exercise.

Creatinine: A metabolic by-product of creatine metabolism.

Cruciferous: A family of vegetables that includes broccoli, Brussels sprouts, cabbage, collard greens, cauliflower, kale, and turnip greens. These vegetables contain substances that may protect against cancer.

Cysteine: A sulfur-containing amino acid with antioxidant properties.

Cytokine: Proteins secreted by cells of the immune system that serve to regulate the immune system.

D-alpha tocopherol: Natural vitamin E. This is the preferred form to use as a dietary supplement because it contains all of the natural isomers, or chemical forms, of vitamin E required by the body to fight diseases such as cancer and atherosclerosis.

Degenerative disease: The gradual deterioration of a biologic system resulting from free-radical damage and other aging biologic processes.

DNA: Deoxyribonucleic acid, the genetic-blueprint double-helix molecular complex in the nucleus of every cell of every living organism.

Docosahexaenoicacid (DHA): An omega-3 fatty acid found primarily in seafood and some plant seeds.

Dopamine: A neurotransmitter that controls fine movement, immune function, insulin regulation, short-term memory, and emotions and drives.

Double-blind: A method of designing a scientific experiment so that neither the experiment's subjects nor the investigator knows what treatment, if any, a subject is getting until after the experiment is over.

Eicosanoid: One of a group of substances containing 20-carbon units used to manufacture prostaglandins and other hormonelike substances. Eicosanoids are manufactured in the body from unsaturated plant oils.

Eicosapentaenoicacid (EPA): An omega-3 fatty acid found in seafood; chemical precursors of EPA are found in seeds.

Electrolyte: Ionized salts in the body fluids. The major electrolytes are made from such common minerals as bicarbonate, calcium, chloride, magnesium, phosphate, potassium, protein, and sodium.

Electron transport system: The metabolic process in which electrons are passed between certain molecules and cofactors releasing energy that is used to regenerate adenosine triphosphate molecules.

Endothelium: The lining the blood vessels, lymphatics, and serous cavities.

Enzymes: Proteins that are capable of inducing chemical changes in other substances without being changed or transformed themselves.

Estrogen: A steroid sex hormone made from cholesterol in the body that promotes secondary female characteristics.

Flavonoids: Compounds present in fruits, vegetables, nuts, and seeds, such as flavonols, flavones, catechins, flavanones, and anthocyanins. The main dietary sources of these compounds in the U.S. diet are tea, onions, fruits, and wine. The main flavonoid in onions is quercetin glucoside, and the main flavonoid in tea is quercetin rutinoside. Flavonoid intake has been inversely linked with coronary heart disease and cancer.

Free radical: A highly chemically reactive atom, molecule, or molecular fragment with a free or unpaired electron.

Free-radical reaction: A cascade of chemical reactions that occurs when a free radical reacts with another molecule in order to gain an electron. The molecule that loses an electron to the free radical then becomes a free radical, repeating the process until the energy of the free radical is spent or the reaction is stopped by an antioxidant.

French paradox: Refers to the lower rates of heart disease among the French even though they consume rich, fatty foods.

Friendly fats: Fats and oils that don't raise blood cholesterol levels or that reduce inflammation in the body. These include fatty acids found in seafood, olives, canola oil, almonds, walnuts, and flaxseed.

Genistein: An isoflavone found in soy foods and beverages that lowers serum cholesterol and inhibits enzymes that promote tumor growth.

Gland: A group of cells that secretes a chemical or hormone.

Gluconeogenesis: The process by which protein is converted to glucose in the body.

Glucose: A simple carbohydrate (monosaccharide) also referred to as dextrose.

Glucose-alanine cycle: Glycogen is broken down to glucose and metabolized to pyruvate, some of which is used directly for energy and the remainder of which is converted to the amino acid alanine. Alanine is returned to the liver and converted to glucose and then stored as glycogen.

Glucose polymer: A processed form of polysaccharides, usually derived from starch, found in many sports drinks.

Glutathione peroxidase: A sulfur-containing enzyme that contains four molecules of selenium; a powerful antioxidant in the body's defense system against free-radical damage.

Glycogen: The storage form of carbohydrate fuel used by animals.

Glycogen-bound water: The water that is stored in the muscles along with glycogen. About 3 grams of water are stored with every gram of glycogen.

Glycogen depletion: The draining of the body's glycogen stores through exercise or underconsumption of carbohydrate or both.

Glycogenolysis: The metabolic process in which glycogen is broken down.

Glycogen replenishment: The replenishing of the body's glycogen stores through carbohydrate and protein consumption.

Glycolysis: The metabolic process in which glucose is converted to lactic acid.

Gout: A painful form of arthritis. Ketogenic diets can lead to an attack of gout in people with the disease.

Gram: A measurement of weight equal to approximately one-twenty-ninth of an ounce.

Halitosis: Bad breath; a side effect of following a ketogenic diet.

High-density lipoproteins (HDLs): Lipoprotein carrier molecules that help prevent cholesterol buildup in the arteries.

High-protein diet: An eating plan that contains 30 percent or more of its total calories as protein.

Homocysteine: A metabolic by-product of protein metabolism that can damage arteries and promote atherosclerosis.

Hormone: One of the numerous substances produced by endocrine glands and other cells that travel to other sites and regulate bodily functions.

Hydrogenation: The chemical process in which unsaturated fatty acids derived from plants are saturated with hydrogen atoms to make them more solid.

Hypertension: High blood pressure.

Hypertriglyceridemia: An elevation of fat carried in the blood.

Hypoglycemia: Blood sugar levels below the normal range, usually below 50mg/dL of blood.

IDL: Intermediate-density lipoproteins; these carrier molecules contain fat and cholesterol and are part of the LDL cholesterol measurement in a blood chemistry profile.

IGF-1 (Insulinlike Growth Factor-1): A family of peptides that play important roles in mammalian growth and development. IGF-1 mediates the anabolic effects of growth hormone. Chronically high levels of IGF-1 have been linked to cancer. High-protein diets elevate blood levels of IGF-1.

Incomplete protein: See complete protein.

Insulin: A hormone secreted by the beta cells of the pancreas that removes glucose from the blood and helps regulate carbohydrate and protein metabolism.

Insulin resistance: A condition in which the body becomes resistant to the effects of the glucose-regulating hormone insulin. Obesity is a leading cause of insulin resistance.

Isoflavone: A phytonutrient found in legumes and vegetables that can prevent sex hormones from stimulating cellular growth that leads to cancer. Soybeans and garbanzo beans are rich sources of isoflavones.

Isoflavones: Compounds found in legumes and grains that inhibit enzymes necessary for the growth of cancer cells. They are often referred to as phytoestrogens or plant estrogens and exhibit powerful anticancer effects in hormone-related cancers such as breast, prostate, endometrial, ovarian, and cervical cancers. Genistein, found in soybeans, has the ability to block the development of cancer at several stages and even return precancerous cells to a normal, healthy state. Isoflavones can also lower blood cholesterol levels.

Ketogenic diet: An eating plan that limits dietary carbohydrates to 40 grams or less each day. This forces the body to convert dietary protein to sugar to compensate for the lack of carbohydrate. This leads to the formation of keto acids (incompletely burned fats) and dehydration.

Ketone: An completely burned fatty acid produced in the liver during starvation (i.e., when carbohydrate intake is low).

Ketosis: The state of dehydration and high blood levels of keto acids found in someone following a very-low-carbohydrate diet.

Kilogram: One one-thousandth of a gram. A postage stamp weighs about a gram. There are approximately 30 grams in 1 ounce.

L-cysteine: An antioxidant sulfur-containing amino acid.

Legume: A member of a plant family that includes beans, peas, and lentils.

Linoleic acid: An essential fatty acid found in vegetable oils and cereals and grains.

Lipid: A fat or oil; a common term for a triglyceride.

Lipolysis: The metabolic process in which triglycerides are broken down into their constituent fatty acids and glycerol. Glycerol can then be used to resynthesize glucose, and fatty acids can be burned in the body for energy.

Lipoprotein: A protein-lipid complex made in the liver that transports fat-soluble compounds (e.g., vitamins, drugs, cholesterol, and fats) in the blood.

L-methionine: A sulfur-containing amino acid with strong antioxidant properties.

LDL cholesterol: Cholesterol carried in the low-density-lipoprotein carrier, which allows the transport of such water-insoluble compounds as cholesterol and fat through the blood, which is a watery fluid.

Low-fat diet: A diet that contains 25 percent or less of its total calories as fat. Healthy low-fat diets do not contain trans (hydrogenated) fats or sugar.

L-phenylalanine: An amino acid used to synthesize the catecholamine neurotransmitters.

L-taurine: A nonessential amino acid that possesses antioxidant properties and helps stabilize the conduction of electrical impulses in the heart, nervous system, and brain.

L-tyrosine: An amino acid that serves as a precursor for the catecholamine neurotransmitters.

Macronutrient: A nutrient, such as carbohydrate, fat, or protein, required by the body in gram quantities.

Maculopathy: An age-related condition in the retina due to atherosclerosis, which causes poor vision and blindness.

Mediterranean diet: The traditional diet of Italy, Spain, Greece, and Crete that emphasizes tomato sauce, olive oil, legumes, garlic, onions, other vegetables, seafood, fruits, whole-grain breads and cereals, and pasta, and limits eggs and meat.

MediterrAsian Diet: The unique dietary style of the Eat to Win Diet that combines the healthiest and most powerful nutritional elements of the Mediterranean and Asian diets.

Metabolic pathway: A sequence of metabolic reactions leading to by-products and final products.

Metabolic rate: The rate at which an individual burns calories; the body's total daily caloric expenditure.

Metabolism: The process of digestion, assimilation, and disposal of fat, protein, carbohydrate, and alcohol.

Methionine: A sulfur-containing amino acid with strong antioxidant properties.

Methylmercury: A dangerous environmental contaminant found in many fish and shellfish. Shark, swordfish, Maine lobster, and sea bass contain high levels of this toxin.

Microtrauma: Small tears in the muscle cells due to exercise stress.

Milligram: A measurement of weight equal to one one-thousandth of a gram.

Mitochondria: The "power plants" inside cells where oxygen and nutrients are metabolized to water, carbon dioxide, and ATP.

Monosaccharide: A simple carbohydrate composed of one sugar molecule, such as glucose.

Monounsaturated fatty acid: A fatty acid that has one double bond commonly found in olives, walnuts, and avocado. Unlike saturated fats, which raise blood cholesterol levels, monounsaturated fatty acids have a neutral effect on blood cholesterol levels.

Muscle mass: Muscle tissue.

Muscle tissue: Tissue that has the ability to move either voluntarily or involuntarily, such as skeletal muscle, cardiac muscle, and smooth muscle.

Narginenin: A phytonutrient found in grapefruit and other fruits and vegetables.

Narginin: A phytonutrient found in grapefruit and other fruits and vegetables.

Net carbs: Carbohydrates that don't raise insulin levels. This term is more a marketing tool than a scientific term.

Neuron: A nerve cell.

Neurotransmitter: A chemical substance that transmits nerve impulses between nerves, muscles, and organs.

Nitrogen: The molecule found in all proteins that must be removed during metabolism in order for protein to be converted to glucose and used for energy.

Nutraceuticals: Commercial products that contain high concentrations of phytonutrients and other compounds thought to prevent or treat diseases; any food that contains nutritional supplements, such as calcium-fortified orange juice.

Omega-3 fatty acid: A family of fats found in seafood and plants that lowers blood triglyceride levels and inflammation.

Omega-6 fatty acid: A family of fats found in vegetable oils that contain essential and other fatty acids.

Omega-9 fatty acid: A family of fats, found in plants, that contribute to good health.

Oxidation: A chemical reaction in which an atom or molecule loses electrons or hydrogen atoms.

Phytic acid (phytates): The storage form of phosphorous in plants that acts as an antioxidant. Phytates bind with metals, such as iron, that can generate toxic free radicals that lead to cancer and cardiovascular disease.

Phytochemical: A number of chemical families with disease-prevention properties found in plants, cereals, and grains.

Phytoestrogen: A compound derived from plants that weakly mimics the effects of the hormone estrogen.

Phytonutrient: Another name for phytochemical.

Phytosterols: Such plant compounds as ergosterol and stigmasterol that help keep cells from growing out of control and protect against colon and skin cancer.

Placebo: An inert compound usually given to a portion of the subjects in a scientific experiment in order to distinguish the psychological effects of the experiment from the physiological effects of the drug being tested.

Potassium: A mineral responsible for transmitting electrical impulses. Potassium is highly active in muscles, brain, and neurons.

Precursor: An intermediate substance in the body's production of another substance.

Prostaglandin: A hormonelike compound derived from linoleic acid, which regulates metabolism, inflammation, and immunity.

Protease inhibitors: Compounds that block the action of proteases—enzymes—that cancer cells use to invade the body and spread to distant sites. Protease inhibitors block the activation of genes that can cause cancer. They also shield DNA from the damaging effects of radiation. Protease inhibitors are effective against a number of health conditions, including cancer, AIDS, cystic fibrosis, acute inflammation, and emphysema.

Pyruvate: A 3-carbon compound that is produced during the oxidation of glucose.

Receptors: Sites on the outside of cells where particular molecules such as hormones can attach. This attachment to the receptor site causes corresponding changes within the cell.

Resveratrol: A compound found in grapes and wine that acts as a weak estrogenlike hormone and is reputed to be responsible for the "French paradox."

Saponins: Compounds, commonly found in grapes and other fruits and vegetables, that possess antioxidant properties and prevent cellular mutations that can lead to cancer, especially in the colon; they also help lower blood cholesterol levels.

Saturated fatty acid: A fatty acid that has no sites of unsaturation or double bonds. Saturated fatty acids tend to be solid at room temperature.

Selenium: An antioxidant trace mineral.

Simple carbohydrate: A simple sugar, such as glucose or fructose.

Sports rehydration drink: A drink designed to replace the water, glucose, and electrolytes lost during vigorous physical activity and sweating.

Synergy: The action of two or more compounds combined such that their effects together are greater than the sum of their individual effects.

Taurine: Taurine is a nonessential amino acid possessing a bipolar chemical structure (+/− charge). Its bipolar nature allows it to function as a charge stabilizer in the conduction of electrical impulses in the nervous system and brain.

Testosterone: A steroid sex hormone made from cholesterol.

Thermogenesis: The state of heightened metabolism or calorie burning. Many foods can increase thermogenesis, including green tea, ginger, and hot spices.

Toxic: Poisonous. Everything, including water and oxygen, is toxic in sufficiently high doses.

Trans fats: The common name for unsaturated fats that have been chemically altered by the addition of hydrogen atoms to create a partially hydrogenated fat that is solid at room temperature. Consumption of trans fats raises blood cholesterol levels and has been linked to increased risk of heart attack and stroke.

Triglycerides: Three fatty acids attached to a 3-carbon backbone. The fats found in foods and stored in adipose tissue.

Type 2 diabetes: A form of diabetes usually caused by obesity and insulin resistence. This form of the disease can be cured with a low-fat, high-complex-carbohydrate diet and exercise.

Unsaturated fats: Fats that contain double bonds between some of their carbon atoms. These double-bond positions are very vulnerable to attack by oxygen and free radicals.

Urea: The final end-product of protein metabolism in humans; a waste product.

Urea cycle: The metabolic process in which two molecules of ammonia are bonded to form the waste product urea.

Uric acid: An antioxidant carried in the blood. High levels of uric acid can cause gouty arthritis.

Vasodilator: A substance that increases blood flow.

Vitamin A: One of the fat-soluble vitamins and an important antioxidant. Also called retinol, it is the form of vitamin A that is found in animals. It is essential to growth, healthy skin and epithelial tissue, and the prevention of night blindness.

Vitamin B$_1$ (thiamin): A member of the B-complex vitamins that is essential for the health of brain and nerve tissue.

Vitamin B$_2$ (riboflavin): A member of the B-complex vitamins that functions as an antioxidant cofactor, taking part in metabolic reactions involving proteins, fats, and carbohydrates.

Vitamin B$_3$ (niacin): A member of the B-complex vitamins that is a particularly important coenzyme in the brain and nerve tissues. It is necessary for the synthesis of DNA, enhances the action of vitamin C and several amino acids, and is required for building the walls of brain cells.

Vitamin B$_5$ (pantothenic acid): A member of the B-complex vitamins that acts as an antioxidant. It is also required for the conversion of choline to the neurotransmitter acetylcholine.

Vitamin B$_6$ (pyridoxine): A member of the B-complex vitamins that acts as an antioxidant. It is necessary for the synthesis of DNA and enhances the action of vitamin C and amino acids in the body and their conversion into neurotransmitters in the brain.

Vitamin B$_{12}$ (cobalamin): A member of the B-complex vitamins that is particularly important in the brain and nerve tissues. It is a powerful water-soluble antioxidant that helps protect against cancer and atherosclerosis.

Vitamin C: One of the most important antioxidant nutrients. Also called ascorbic acid, it is essential in building strong, healthy connective tissue, especially in capillary walls.

Vitamin E: A fat-soluble vitamin chemically known as d-alpha tocopherol. It is a necessary factor in over twenty enzymatic reactions and is essential for the production of the antioxidant enzyme SOD. It also helps prevent the accumulation of lead, which is toxic to the brain.

VLDL: Very-low-density lipoprotein; the carrier for dietary fat in the blood.

Whole grain: A naturally grown carbohydrate food that contains the bran and germ layers of the grain.

Zinc: A mineral that is found in substantial concentrations in the brain. It is a necessary factor in over twenty different enzymatic reactions and is essential for the production of the antioxidant enzyme SOD.

HEALTHY WEIGHTS FOR ADULT MEN AND WOMEN ON THE EAT TO WIN DIET

If you want to know what your healthy weight should be, don't pay attention to current government guidelines because they're based on data from a nation where a majority of people are overweight and obese.

The data in the Eat to Win Healthy Weights for Adult Men and Women tables lists the healthiest and most desirable weights for men and women gathered from research conducted by the Metropolitan Insurance Company in 1959. This was forty-five years prior to the fattening of America—a time when people hadn't yet learned about supersizing meals, and restaurant hamburgers weighed less than a side of beef.

During the 1950s and 1960s, people considered being fat a personal embarrassment and regarded obesity as the inevitable result of gluttony and sloth. Today, many people blame the government or the fast-food chains for their excessive weight and refuse to accept personal responsibility. There is even a national organization exclusively for fat people that promotes the idea that it's healthy and perfectly acceptable to be fat.

Certainly, a lot has changed since 1959, a time when most people took personal pride in their appearance and didn't blame others for their own lack of discipline and restraint. In 1959, even without the advances in diet and nutritional knowledge we now possess in the 21st century, people took personal responsibility for their diets, and it showed.

Your goal is to reach your target weight as depicted in the 1959 Metropolitan Life Insurance Company tables and not the "healthy" weights listed in the U.S. National Center for Health Statistics.

EAT TO WIN HEALTHY WEIGHTS FOR MEN
AGES 25–59, WEIGHT IN POUNDS, WITHOUT SHOES OR CLOTHING

HEIGHT	SMALL FRAME	MEDIUM FRAME	LARGE FRAME
5'1"	106–114	112–123	120–135
5'2"	109–117	115–127	123–138
5'3"	112–120	118–130	126–142
5'4"	115–123	121–133	129–146
5'5"	118–127	124–137	132–150
5'6"	122–131	128–141	136–155
5'7"	126–135	132–146	141–160
5'8"	130–139	136–150	145–164
5'9"	134–144	140–154	149–168
5'10"	138–148	144–159	153–173
5'11"	142–156	148–164	158–178
6'0"	146–156	152–169	162–183
6'1"	150–161	156–174	167–188
6'2"	154–165	161–179	172–193
6'3"	158–169	166–184	176–198

Source: Metropolitan Life Insurance Company

U.S. NATIONAL CENTER FOR HEALTH STATISTICS—MALE
(UNHEALTHY WEIGHTS FOR A FAT NATION)

HEIGHT	18–24 YRS.	25–34 YRS.	35–44 YRS.	45–54 YRS.	55–64 YRS.
5'2"	130	139	146	148	147
5'3"	135	145	149	154	151
5'4"	139	151	155	158	156
5'5"	143	155	159	163	160
5'6"	148	159	164	167	165
5'7"	152	164	169	171	170
5'8"	157	168	174	176	174
5'9"	162	173	178	180	178
5'10"	166	177	183	185	183
5'11"	171	182	188	190	187
6'0"	175	186	192	194	192
6'1"	180	191	197	198	197
6'2"	185	196	202	204	201

EAT TO WIN HEALTHY WEIGHTS FOR WOMEN

AGES 25–59, WEIGHT IN POUNDS, WITHOUT SHOES OR CLOTHING

HEIGHT	SMALL FRAME	MEDIUM FRAME	LARGE FRAME
4'8"	89–95	93–104	101–116
4'9"	91–98	95–107	103–119
4'10"	93–101	98–110	106–122
4'11"	96–104	101–113	109–125
5'0"	99–107	104–116	112–128
5'1"	102–110	107–119	115–131
5'2"	105–113	110–123	118–135
5'3"	108–116	113–127	122–139
5'4"	111–120	117–132	126–143
5'5"	115–124	121–136	130–147
5'6"	119–128	125–140	134–151
5'7"	123–132	129–144	138–155
5'8"	127–136	133–148	142–160
5'9"	131–140	137–152	146–165
5'10"	135–144	141–156	150–170

Source: Metropolitan Life Insurance Company

U.S. NATIONAL CENTER FOR HEALTH STATISTICS—FEMALES
(UNHEALTHY WEIGHTS FOR A FAT NATION)

HEIGHT	18–24 YRS.	25–34 YRS.	35–44 YRS.	45–54 YRS.	55–64 YRS.
4'10"	114	123	133	132	135
4'11"	118	126	136	136	138
5'0"	121	130	139	139	142
5'1"	124	133	141	143	145
5'2"	128	136	144	146	148
5'3"	131	139	146	150	151
5'4"	134	142	149	153	154
5'5"	137	146	151	157	157
5'6"	141	149	154	160	161
5'7"	144	152	156	164	164
5'8"	147	155	159	168	167

BIBLIOGRAPHY

Abbott, W.G., B. Swinburn, G. Ruotolo, et al. Effect of a high-carbohydrate, low-saturated-fat diet on apolipoprotein B, and triglyceride metabolism in Pima Indians. *Journal of Clinical Investigation* 86:642–50, 1990 Aug.

Abernethy, P.J., R. Thayer, A.W. Taylor. Acute and chronic responses of skeletal muscle to endurance and sprint exercise. A review. *Sports Medicine* 10:365–89, 1990 Dec.

Acheson, K.J., J.P. Flatt, E. Jequier. Glycogen synthesis versus lipogenesis after a 500 gram carbohydrate meal in man. *Metabolism* 31:1234–40, 1982 Dec.

Acheson, K.J., Y. Schutz, T. Bessard, K. Anantharaman, J.P. Flatt, E. Jequier. Glycogen storage capacity and de novo lipogenesis during massive carbohydrate overfeeding in man. *American Journal of Clinical Nutrition* 48:240–7, 1988 Aug.

Acheson, K.J., Y. Schutz, T. Bessard, J.P. Flatt, E. Jequier. Carbohydrate metabolism and de novo lipogenesis in human obesity. *American Journal of Clinical Nutrition* 45:78–85, 1987 Jan.

Ackerman, N.R., E.C. Arner, W. Galbraith, R.R. Harris, B.D. Jaffee, W.M. Mackin. Anti-inflammatory consequences of 5-lipoxygenase inhibition. *Advances in Prostaglandin Thromboxane Leukotriene Research* 16:47–62, 1986.

Ackroff, K., A. Sclafani. Effects of the lipase inhibitor orlistat on intake and preference for dietary fat in rats. *American Journal of Physiology* 271:R48–54, 1996 Jul.

Adachi, T., M. Kawamura, K. Hiramori. Relationships between reduction in body weight and reduction in blood pressure and improvement of glucose and lipid metabolism induced by short-term calorie restriction in overweight hypertensive women. *Hypertension Research* 19 (Suppl 1):S57–60, 1996.

Adam, O. Anti-inflammatory diet in rheumatic diseases. *European Journal of Clinical Nutrition* 49:703–17, 1995 Oct.

Adams, S.O., K.E. Grady, C.H. Wolk, C. Mukaida. Weight loss: a comparison of group and individual interventions. *Journal of the American Dietetic Association* 86:485–90, 1986 Apr.

Adams, L.G., et al. Effects of dietary protein and calorie restriction in clinically normal cats and in cats with surgically induced chronic renal failure. *American Journal of Veterinary Research* 54(10) 1653–62, 1993.

Adembri, C., L. Formigli, L. Lobmardo Domenici, S. Brunelleschi, G.P. Novelli. Effect of acetyl-carnitine in a model of muscle ischemia-reperfusion in humans. *Minerva Anestesiology* 57:1018–9, 1991 Oct.

Adibi, S. Metabolism of branch-chain amino acids. *Metabolism* 25(11):1287–1302, 1976.

Adlercreutz, H., H. Markkanen, S. Watanabe. Plasma concentrations of phyto-oestrogens in Japanese men. *Lancet* 342:1209–10, 1993.

Ako, H., D. Okuda, D. Gray. Healthful new oil from macadamia nuts. *Nutrition* 11:286–8, 1995 May–Jun.

Albert, C.M., C.H. Hennekens, CJ OD, et al. Fish consumption and risk of sudden cardiac death [see comments]. *JAMA* 279:23–8, 1998 Jan 7.

Albertazzi, P., F. Pansini, G. Bonaccorsi, L. Zanotti, E. Forini, D. De Aloysio. The effect of dietary soy supplementation on hot flashes. *Obstetrics & Gynecology* 91:6–11, 1998 Jan.

Alford, B.B., A.C. Blankenship, R.D. Hagen. The effects of variations in carbohydrate, protein, and fat content of the diet upon weight loss, blood values, and nutrient intake of adult obese women. *Journal of the American Dietetic Association* 90:534–40, 1990 Apr.

Allison, D.B., R. Zannolli, et al. Weight loss increases and fat loss decreases all-cause mortality rate: results from two independent cohort studies. *International Journal of Obesity and Related Metabolic Disorders* 23(6):603–11, 1999.

American Journal of Clinical Nutrition 79(5):899S–906S, May 2004.

Americans. Washington, DC: US Government Printing Office, 1995. (Homes and Garden Bulletin no. 232.)

Anderson, J.J., P. Rondano, A. Holmes. Roles of diet and physical activity in the prevention of osteoporosis. *Scandinavian Journal of Rheumatology* (Supplement) 103:65–74, 1996.

Anderson, J.W., and others. Health advantages and disadvantages of weight-reducing diets: a computer analysis and critical review. *Journal of the American College of Nutrition* 19:578–90, 2000.2

Andersson, S.O., A. Wolk, R. Bergstríom, E. Giovannucci, C. Lindgren, Baron. Energy, nutrient intake and prostate cancer risk: a population-based case-control study in Sweden. *International Journal of Cancer Research* 68:716–22, 1996.

Ando, K., et al. Impact of aging and life-long calorie restriction on expression of apoptosis-related genes in male F344 rat liver. *Microscopy Research and Technique* 59(4):293–300, 2002.

Angerer, P., C. von Schacky. n-3 polyunsaturated fatty acids and the cardiovascular system. *Current Opinions in Lipidology* 11(1):57–63, 2000.

Anson, R.M., et al. Intermittent fasting dissociates beneficial effects of dietary restriction on glucose metabolism and neuronal resistance to injury from calorie intake. *Proceedings of the National Academy of Sciences USA* 100(10):6216–20, 2003.

Anthony, M.S., T.B. Clarkson, C.L. Hughes, Jr., Morgan, T.M. G.L. Burke. Soybean isoflavones improve cardiovascular risk factors without affecting the reproductive system of peripubertal rhesus monkeys. *Journal of Nutrition* 126:43–50, 1996.

Anton-Kuchly, B., S. Ranganathan, M. Potiron, et al. Effect of a protein-sparing diet on responses to exercise in obese subjects. *Journal of Sports Medicine and Physical Fitness* 33:59–64, 1993 Mar.

Appel, I.J. Nonpharmacologic therapies that reduce blood pressure: a fresh perspective. *Clinical Cardiology* 22(Suppl. III): III–III5, 1999.

Aravanis, C, R.P. Mensink, N. Karalias, B. Christodoulou, A. Kafatos, M.B. Katan. Serum lipids, apoproteins and nutrient intake in rural Cretan boys consuming high-olive-oil diets. *Journal of Clinical Epidemiology* 41:1117–23, 1988.

Archer, J.A., P. Gorden, J. Roth. Defect in insulin binding to receptors in obese man. Amelioration with calorie restriction. *Journal of Clinical Investigation* 55(1):166–74, 1975.

Arenas, J., R. Huertas, Y. Campos, Di AE, J.M. Villalón E. Vilas. Effects of L-carnitine on the pyruvate dehydrogenase complex and carnitine palmitoyl transferase activities in muscle of endurance athletes. FEBS *Letters* 341:91–3, 1994 Mar 14.

Arenas, J., J.R. Ricoy, A.R. Encinas, et al. Carnitine in muscle, serum, and urine of nonprofessional athletes: effects of physical exercise, training, and L-carnitine administration. *Muscle Nerve* 14:598–604, 1991 Jul.

Arnold, L.E., D. Kleykamp, N. Votolato, R.A. Gibson, L. Horrocks. Potential link between dietary intake of fatty acid and behavior: pilot exploration of serum lipids in attention-deficit hyperactivity disorder. *Journal of Child and Adolescent Psychopharmacology* 4(3):171–82, 1994.

Arnon, R., et al. Effects of exogenous apo E-3 and of cholesterol-enriched meals on the cellular metabolism of human chylomicrons and their remnants. *Biochimica et Biophysica Acta* 1085(3):336–42, 1991.

Ashutosh, K., K. Methrotra, J. Fragale-Jackson. Effects of sustained weight loss and exercise on aerobic fitness in obese women. *Journal of Sports Medicine and Physical Fitness* 37:252–7, 1997 Dec.

Assmann, G., G. de Backer, S. Bagnara, et al. International consensus statement on olive oil and the Mediterranean diet: implications for health in Europe. The Olive Oil and the Mediterranean Diet Panel. *European Journal of Cancer Prevention* 6:418–21, 1997 Oct.

Assmann, G., G. de Backer, S. Bagnara, et al. Olive oil and the Mediterranean diet: implications for health in Europe. *British Journal of Nursing* 6:675–7, 1997 Jun 26–Jul 9.

Atkinson, G., T. Reilly. Effects of age and time of day on preferred work rates during prolonged exercise. *Chronobiol International* 12:121–34, 1995 Apr.

Atkinson, R.L., D.L. Kaiser. Effects of calorie restriction and weight loss on glucose and insulin levels in obese humans. *Journal of the American College of Nutrition* 4(4): 411–9, 1985.

Austen, K.F. The role of arachidonic acid metabolites in local and systemic inflammatory processes. *Drugs* 33 Suppl 1:10–7, 1987.

Axel, L., L. Kolman, et al. Origin of a signal intensity loss artifact in fat-saturation MR imaging. *Radiology* 217(3): 911–5, 2000.

Baekey, P.A., J.J. Cerda, C.W. Burgin, E.L. Robbins, R.W. Rice, T.G. Baumgartner. Grapefruit pectin inhibits hypercholesterolemia and atherosclerosis in miniature swine. *Clinical Cardiology* 11:597–600, 1988.

Baggio, G., A. Pagnan, M. Muraca, et al. Olive-oil-enriched diet: effect on serum lipoprotein levels and biliary cholesterol saturation. *American Journal of Clinical Nutrition* 47:960–4, 1988 Jun.

Balage, M., J. Grizard, M. Manin. Effect of calorie restriction on skeletal muscle and liver insulin binding in growing rat. *Hormone and Metabolic Research* 22(4): 207–14, 1990.

Bales, C.W., T.A. Davis, R.E. Beauchene. Long-term protein and calorie restriction: alterations in nucleic acid levels of organs of male rats. *Experimental Gerontology* 23(3):189–96, 1988.

Ball, S.D., et al., Prolongation of satiety after low versus moderately high glycemic index meals in obese adolescents. *Pediatrics* 111(3):488–94 2003.

Ballor, D.L., E.T. Poehlman. Exercise-training enhances fat-free mass preservation during diet-induced weight loss: a meta-analytical finding. *International Journal of Obesity-Related Metabolic Disorders* 18(1):35–40, 1994.

Bangsbo, J., T.E. Graham, B. Kiens, B. Saltin. Elevated muscle glycogen and anaerobic energy production during exhaustive exercise in man. *Journal of Physiology (Lond)* 451:205–27, 1992.

Bangsbo, J., K. Madsen, B. Kiens, E.A. Richter. Muscle glycogen synthesis in recovery from intense exercise in humans. *American Journal of Physiology* 273:E416–24, 1997 Aug.

Barkoukis, H., K.M. Fiedler, E. Lerner. A combined high-fiber, low-glycemic index diet normalizes glucose tolerance and reduces hyperglycemia and hyperinsulinemia in adults with hepatic cirrhosis. *Journal of the American Dietetic Association* 102(10):1503–7; discussion 1507–8 2002.

Barnard, N.D., A. Akhtar, A. Nicholson. Factors that facilitate compliance to lower fat intake. *Archives of Family Medicine* 4:153–8, 1995.

Barnard, N.D., I.W. Scherwitz, D. Ornish. Adherence and acceptability of a low-fat, vegetarian diet among patients with cardiac disease. *Journal of Cardiopulmonary Rehabilitation* 12:423–31, 1992.

Barnard, N.D., A.R. Scialli, P. Bertron, D. Hurlock, K. Edmonds. Acceptability of a therapeutic low-fat, vegan diet in premenopausal women. *Journal of Nutrition Education* 32:314–9, 2002.

Barnes, S., T.G. Peterson, L. Coward. Rationale for the use of genistein-containing soy matrices in chemoprevention trials for breast and prostate cancer. *Journal of Cell Biochemistry* (Supplement) 22:181–7, 1995.

Baron, J.A., A. Schori, et al. A randomized controlled trial of low carbohydrate and low fat/high fiber diets for weight loss. *American Journal of Public Health* 76(11):1293–6, 1986.

Barrett-Connor, E., N.J. Friedlander. Dietary fat, calories, and the risk of breast cancer in postmenopausal women: a prospective population-based study. *Journal of the American College of Nutrition* 12:390–9, 1993.

Barth, C.A., U. Behnke. Nutritional physiology of whey and whey components. *Nahrung* 41:2–12, 1997 Feb.

Baumgaertel, A. Alternative and controversial treatments for attention-deficit/hyperactivity disorder. *Pediatric Clinics of North America* 46(5):977–92, 1999.

Beard, Christopher M., R. James Barnard, David C. Robbins, Jose M. Ordovas, Ernst J. Schaefer. *Arteriosclerosis, Thrombosis, and Vascular Biology* 16:201–207, 1996.

Beck, S.A., K.L. Smith, M.J. Tisdale. Anticachectic and antitumor effect of eicosapentaenoic acid and its effect on protein turnover. *Cancer Research* 51:6089–93, 1991.

Becker, E.F. Inhibition of spontaneous hepatocarcinogenesis in C3H/HeN mice by Edi Pro A, an isolated soy protein. *Carcinogenesis* 2:1213–14, 1981.

Bell, F.P., T.L. Raymond, C.L. Patnode. The influence of diet and carnitine supplementation on plasma carnitine, cholesterol and triglyceride in WHHL (Watanabe-heritable hyperlipidemic), Netherland dwarf and New Zealand rabbits (Oryctolagus cuniculus). *Comparative Biochemistry and Physiology B* 87(3):587–91, 1987.

Bell, J.D., S. Margen, D.H. Calloway. Ketosis, weight loss, uric acid, and nitrogen balance in obese women fed single nutrients at low caloric levels. *Metabolism* 18:193–208, 1969 Mar.

Bellush, L.L., N. Rowland. Preference for high carbohydrate over various high fat diets by diabetic rats. *Physiology and Behavior* 35:319–27, 1985 Sep.

Belluzzi, A., S. Boschi, C. Brignola, A. Munarini, C. Cariani, F. Miglio. Polyunsaturated fatty acids and inflammatory bowel disease. *American Journal of Clinical Nutrition* 71(suppl):339S–42S, 2000.

Bembem, M.G. Age-related alterations in muscular endurance. *Sports Medicine* 25:259–69, 1998 Apr.

Ben, G., L. Gnudi, A. Maran, et al. Effects of chronic alcohol intake on carbohydrate and lipid metabolism in subjects with type II (non-insulin-dependent) diabetes. *American Journal of Medicine* 90:70–6, 1991 Jan.

Berrigan, D., et al. Adult-onset calorie restriction and fasting delay spontaneous tumorigenesis in p53-deficient mice. *Carcinogenesis* 23(5):817–22, 2002.

Berry, E.M., S. Eisenberg, Y. Friedlander, et al. Effects of diets rich in monounsaturated fatty acids on plasma lipoproteins—the Jerusalem Nutrition Study. II. Monounsaturated fatty acids vs carbohydrates. *American Journal of Clinical Nutrition* 56:394–403, 1992 Aug.

Bertelli, A., et al. Protective action of L-carnitine and coenzyme Q10 against hepatic triglyceride infiltration induced by hyperbaric oxygen and ethanol. *Drugs Under Experimental and Clinical Research* 19(2):65–8, 1993.

Bianchi, G.P., et al. Vegetable versus animal protein diet in cirrhotic patients with chronic encephalopathy. A randomized cross-over comparison. *Journal of Internal Medicine* 233(5): 385–92, 1993.

Billeaud, C., D. Bougle, P. Sarda, et al. Effects of preterm infant formula supplementation with alpha-linolenic acid with a linoleate/alpha-linolenate ratio of 6: a multicentric study. *European Journal of Clinical Nutrition* 51:520–27, 1997 Aug.

Binkley, N.C., J.W. Suttie. Vitamin K nutrition and osteoporosis. *Journal of Nutrition* 125:1812–21, 1995 Jul.

Birch, L.L. Children's preferences for high-fat foods. *Nutrition Review* 50:249–55, 1992 Sep.

Birt, D.F. J.C. Pelling, S. Nair, D. Lepley. Diet intervention for modifying cancer risk. *Progressive Clinical Biological Research* 395:223–34, 1996.

Birt, D.F., et al. Influence of diet and calorie restriction on the initiation and promotion of skin carcinogenesis in the SENCAR mouse model. *Cancer Research* 51(7):1851–4, 1991.

Blaak, E.E., J.F. Glatz, et al. Increase in skeletal muscle fatty acid binding protein (FABPC) content is directly related to weight loss and to changes in fat oxidation following a very low calorie diet. *Diabetologia Croatica* 44(11):2013–7, 2001.

Black, A., et al. Calorie restriction and skeletal mass in rhesus monkeys (Macaca mulatta): evidence for an effect mediated through changes in body size. *Journal of Gerontology Series A: Biological Sciences and Medical Sciences* 56(3):B98–107, 2001.

Blomstrand, E. Influence of ingesting a solution of branch-chain amino acids on perceived exertion during exercise. *Acta Physiologica Scandinavia* 159:41–49, 1997.

Boelsma, E., H.F. Hendriks, L. Roza. Nutritional skin care: health effects of micronutrients and fatty acids. *American Journal of Clinical Nutrition* 73(5):853–64, 2001.

Bonjour, J.P., M.A. Schürch, R. Rizzoli. Proteins and bone health. *Pathologie Biologique* (Paris), 45:57–9, 1997 Jan.

Bonjour, J.P., M.A. Schürch, R. Rizzoli. Nutritional aspects of hip fractures. *Journal of Bone and Joint Surgery* 18:139S–144S, 1996 Mar.

Boozer, C.N., A. Brasseur, et al. Dietary fat affects weight loss and adiposity during energy restriction in rats. *American Journal of Clinical Nutrition* 58(6):846–52, 1993.

Bosaeus, I., L. Belfrage, C. Lindgren, H. Andersson. Olive oil instead of butter increases net cholesterol excretion from the small bowel. *European Journal of Clinical Nutrition* 46:111–5, 1992 Feb.

Bosy-Westphal, A., C. Eichhorn, et al. The age-related decline in resting energy expenditure in humans is due to the loss of fat-free mass and to alterations in its metabolically active components. *Journal of Nutrition* 133(7):2356–62, 2003.

Bouche, C., et al. Five-week, low-glycemic index diet decreases total fat mass and improves plasma lipid profile in moderately overweight nondiabetic men. *Diabetes Care* 25(5):822–8, 2002.

Bough, K.J., et al. Seizure resistance is dependent upon age and calorie restriction in rats fed a ketogenic diet. *Epilepsy Research* 35(1):21–8, 1999.

Bough, K.J., P.A. Schwartzkroin, and J.M. Rho. Calorie restriction and ketogenic diet diminish neuronal excitability in rat dentate gyrus in vivo. *Epilepsia* 44(6):752–60, 2003.

Bougnoux, P., S. Koscielny, V. Chajès, P. Descamps, C. Couet, G. Calais. Alpha-linolenic acid content of adipose breast tissue: a host determinant of the risk of early metastasis in breast cancer. *British Journal of Cancer* 70:330–4, 1994.

Boutron, M.C., J. Faivre, P. Marteau, C. Couillault, P. Senesse, V. Quipourt. Calcium, phosphorus, vitamin D, dairy products and colorectal carcinogenesis: a French case-control study. *British Journal of Cancer* 74:145–51, 1996.

Boza, J., J. Jiménez, L. Baró, O. Martínez, Suárez MD, Gil A. Effects of native and hydrolyzed whey protein on intestinal repair of severely starved rats at weaning. *Journal of Pediatric Gastroenterology and Nutrition* 22:186–93, 1996 Feb.

Braet, C., et al., Inpatient treatment of obese children: a multicomponent programme without stringent calorie restriction. *European Journal of Pediatrics* 162(6):391–6, 2003.

Braga, C., C. La Vecchia, S. Franceschi, et al. Olive oil, other seasoning fats, and the risk of colorectal carcinoma. *Cancer* 82:448–53, 1998 Feb 1.

Brand, J.C., et al. Low-glycemic index foods improve long-term glycemic control in NIDDM. *Diabetes Care* 14(2):95–101, 1991.

Brandi, M.L. Natural and synthetic isoflavones in the prevention and treatment of chronic diseases. *Calcified Tissue International* 61 Suppl 1:S5–8, 1997.

Brand-Miller, J., et al. Low-glycemic index diets in the management of diabetes: a meta-analysis of randomized controlled trials. *Diabetes Care* 26(8):226–7, 2003.

Brand-Miller, J.C., P. Petocz, S. Colagiuri. Meta-analysis of low-glycemic index diets in the management of diabetes: response to Franz. *Diabetes Care* 26(12):3363–4; author reply 3364–5, 2003.

Brass, E.P., W.R. Hiatt. Carnitine metabolism during exercise. *Life Sciences* 54:1383–93, 1994.

Brass, E.P., W.R. Hiatt. The role of carnitine and carnitine supplementation during exercise in man and in individuals with special needs [see comments]. *Journal of the American College of Nutrition* 17:207–15, 1998 Jun.

Bravata, D.M., L. Sanders, I. Huang, et al. Efficacy and safety of low-carbohydrate diets: a systematic review. *JAMA* 289:1837–50, 2003.

Bray, G.A., B.M. Popkin. Dietary fat intake does affect obesity! *American Journal of Clinical Nutrition* 68:1157–73, 1998.

Brazelton, T.B. Why children and parents must play while they eat: an interview with T. Berry Brazelton, MD. *Journal of the American Dietetic Association* 93:1385–7, 1993.

Brinker, F. Herb Contraindications and Drug Interactions. 2nd ed. Sandy, Ore: *Eclectic Medical* 71–2, 1998.

Brochu, M., A. Tchernof, et al. Is there a threshold of visceral fat loss that improves the metabolic profile in obese postmenopausal women? *Metabolism* 52(5): 599–604, 2003.

Brockis, J.G., A.J. Levitt, S.M. Cruthers. The effects of vegetable and animal protein diets on calcium, urate and oxalate excretion. *British Journal of Urology* 54(6):590–3, 1982.

Brown, D.J., A.M. Dattner. Phytotherapeutic approaches to common dermatologic conditions. *Archives of Dermatology* 134:1401–4, 1998.

Bruinoff, T.W., C.B. Brouwer, T.M. van Linde-Sibenius, H. Jansen, D.W. Erkelens. Different postprandial metabolism of olive oil and soybean oil: a possible mechanism of the high-density lipoprotein conserving effect of olive oil. *American Journal of Clinical Nutrition* 58:477–83, 1993 Oct.

Bruinsma, K.A., D.L. Taren. Dieting, essential fatty acid intake, and depression. *Nutrition Review* 58(4):98–108, 2000.

Bucholz, A.X., D.A. Scholler. Is a calorie a calorie? *American Journal of Clinical Nutrition* 79:899S–906S, 2004.

Bunker, V.W. The role of nutrition in osteoporosis. *British Journal of Biomedical Science* 51:228–40, 1994 Sep.

Burch, H.B., et al. Hepatic metabolites and cofactors in riboflavin deficiency and calorie restriction. *American Journal of Physiology* 219(2):409–15, 1970.

Burgess, J. I. Stevens, W. Zhang, L. Peck. Long-chain polyunsaturated fatty acids in children with attention-deficit hyperactivity disorder. *American Journal of Clinical Nutrition* 71(suppl):327S–30S, 2000.

Burkinshaw, L., D.B. Morgan. Mass and composition of the fat-free tissues of patients with weight-loss. *Clinical Science* (Lond) 68(4):455–62, 1985.

Burstein, R., A.M., Prentice, G.R. Goldberg, P.R. Murgatroyd, M. Harding, W.A. Coward. Metabolic fuel utilisation in obese women before and after weight loss. *International Journal of Obesity and Related Metabolic Disorders* 20:253–9, 1996 Mar.

Burton, G.W. T.M., R.V. Acuff, et al. Human plasma and tissue alpha-tocopherol concentrations in response to supplementation with deuterated natural and syntheitc vitamin E. *American Journal of Clinical Nutrition* 67:669–84, 1998.

Busetto, L., A. Tregnaghi, et al. Visceral fat loss evaluated by total body magnetic resonance imaging in obese women operated with laparascopic adjustable silicone gastric banding. *International Journal of Obesity and Related Metabolic Disorders* 24(1):60–9, 2000.

Cai, O., H. Wei. Effect of dietary genistein on antioxidant enzyme activities in SENCAR mice. *Nutrition and Cancer* 25:1–7 1996.

Calle-Pascual, A.L., et al. Foods with a low glycemic index do not improve glycemic control of both type 1 and type 2 diabetic patients after one month of therapy. *Diabetes Metabolism Research and Reviews* 14(5):629–33, 1988.

Campaigne, B.N. Body fat distribution in females: metabolic consequences and implications for weight loss. *Medicine and Science in Sports & Exercise* 22(3):291–7, 1990.

Campbell, P.K., K.G. Waymire, et al. Mutation of a novel gene results in abnormal development of spermatid flagella, loss of intermale aggression and reduced body fat in mice. *Genetics* 162(1):307–20, 2002.

Canalis, E. Insulin-like growth factors and osteoporosis [comment]. *Journal of Bone and Joint Surgery* 21:215–6, 1997 Sep.

Capristo, E., et al. Effect of a vegetable-protein-rich polymeric diet treatment on body composition and energy metabolism in inactive Crohn's disease. *European Journal of Gastroenterology and Hepatology* 12(1):5–11, 2000.

Caputo, F.A., R.D. Mattes. Human dietary responses to perceived manipulation of fat content in a midday meal. *International Journal of Obesity and Related Metabolic Disorders* 17:237–40, 1993 Apr.

Carabaza, A., M.D. Ricart, A. Mor, J.J. Guinovart, C.J. Ciudad. Role of AMP on the activation of glycogen synthase and phosphorylase by adenosine, fructose, and glutamine in rat hepatocytes. *Journal of Biological Chemistry* 265:2724–32, 1990 Feb 15.

Carmichael, H.E., B.A. Swinburn, et al. Lower fat intake as a predictor of initial and sustained weight loss in obese subjects consuming an otherwise ad libitum diet. *Journal of the American Dietetic Association* 98(1):35–9, 1998.

Caron, M.F., C.M. White. Evaluation of the antihyperlipidemic properties of dietary supplements. *Pharmacotherapy* 21(4):481–87, 2001.

Carreau, J.P., D. Lapous, J. Raulin. A possible essential metabolite of linoleic acid: lipoic acid, the universal coenzyme of alpha-keto acid oxidation. *Comptes Rendus Academie des Sciences; Hebdomadaires des Seances del'Academie des Sciences D.* 281:941–4, 1975 Sep 29.

Carroll, K.K., E.A. Jacobson, L.A. Eckel, H.L. Newmark. Calcium and carcinogenesis of the mammary gland. *American Journal of Clinical Nutrition* 54:206S–208S, 1991.

Carvalho, M.D., et al. Macrophages take up triacylglycerol-rich emulsions at a faster rate upon co-incubation with native and modified LDL: An investigation on the role of natural chylomicrons in atherosclerosis. *Journal of Cellular Biochemistry* 84(2):309–23, 2002.

Casimirri, F., R. Pasquali, et al. Interrelationships between body weight, body fat distribution and insulin in obese women before and after hypocaloric feeding and weight loss. *Annals of Nutrition and Metabolism* 33(2):79–87, 1989.

Catlett, J.P. Ketotic hypoglycemia. *West Virginia Medical Journal* 79:126–8, 1983 Jun.

Cerrato, P.L. The low-fat approach to weight loss. *Rn* 54(11): 69–71, 1991.

Cerretelli, P., C. Marconi. L-carnitine supplementation in humans. The effects on physical performance. *International Journal of Sports Medicine* 11:1–14, 1990 Feb.

Cha, M.C., J.A. Johnson, et al. High-fat hypocaloric diet modifies carbohydrate utilization of obese rats during weight loss. *American Journal of Physiology, Endocrinology and Metabolism* 280(5):E797–803, 2001.

Chacon, F., et al. Chronobiological features of the immune system. Effect of calorie restriction.m *European Journal of Clinical Nutrition* 56(Suppl 3):S69–72, 2002.

Chajès, V., W. Sattler, A. Stranzl, G.M. Kostner. Influence of n-3 fatty acids on the growth of human breast cancer cells in vitro: relationship to peroxides and vitamin-E. *Breast Cancer Research Treatment* 34:199–212, 1995.

Chan, M.M., M. Nohara, et al. Lecithin decreases human milk fat loss during enteral pumping. *Journal of Pediatric Gastroenterology and Nutrition* 36(5):613–5, 2003.

Chandler, T.J. Physiology of aerobic fitness/endurance. *Instructional Course Lectures* 43:11–5, 1994.

Chandrasekar, B., et al. Calorie restriction attenuates inflammatory responses to myocardial ischemia-reperfusion injury. *American Journal of Physiology Heart and Circulatory Physiology* 280(5):H2094–102, 2001.

Chandrasekar, B., et al. Effects of calorie restriction on transforming growth factor beta 1 and proinflammatory cytokines in murine Sjogren's syndrome. *Clinical Immunology and Immunopathology* 76(3 Pt 1):291–6, 1995.

Chang, S., J. Borensztajn. Uptake of chylomicron remnants and hepatic lipase-treated chylomicrons by a non-transformed murine hepatocyte cell line in culture. *Biochimica et Biophysica Acta* 1256(1)81–7, 1995.

Chang, S., N. Maeda, J. Borensztajn. The role of lipoprotein lipase and apoprotein E in the recognition of chylomicrons and chylomicron remnants by cultured isolated mouse hepatocytes. *Biochemistry Journal* 318(Pt 1):29–34.

Chatterjee, B., et al. Calorie restriction delays age-dependent loss in androgen responsiveness of the rat liver. *FASEB Journal* 3(2):169–73, 1989.

Chaudry, A., S. McClinton, L.E. Moffat, K.W. Wahle. Essential fatty acid distribution in the plasma and tissue phospholipids of patients with benign and malignant prostatic disease. *British Journal of Cancer* 64:1157–60, 1991.

Chaudry, A.A., K.W. Wahle, S. McClinton, L.E. Moffat. Arachidonic acid metabolism in benign and malignant prostatic tissue in vitro: effects of fatty acids and cyclooxygenase inhibitors. *International Journal of Cancer Research* 57:176–80, 1994.

Chen, C., P.F. Williams, G.J. Cooney, J.D. Caterson, J.R. Turtle. The effects of fasting and refeeding on liver glycogen synthase and phosphorylase in obese and lean mice. *Hormone and Metabolic Research* 24:161–6, 1992 Apr.

Chen, Y.Q., B. Liu, D.G. Tang, K.V. Honn. Fatty acid modulation of tumor cell-platelet-vessel wall interaction. *Cancer and Metastasis Reviews* 11(3–4):389–409, 1992 Nov.

Cherry, et al. Calorie restriction delays the crescentic glomerulonephritis of SCG/Kj mice. *Proceedings of the Society for Experimental Biology and Medicine* 218(3):218–22, 1998.

Cho, E., S. Hung, W.C. Willett, et al. Prospective study of dietary fat and the risk of age-related macular degeneration. *American Journal of Clinical Nutrition* 73(2):209–18, 2001.

Cho, C.G., et al. Modulation of glutathione and thioredoxin systems by calorie restriction during the aging process. *Experimental Gerontology* 38(5):539–48, 2003.

Choi, S.Y., et al. Acceleration of uptake of LDL but not chylomicrons or chylomicron remnants by cells that secrete apoE and hepatic lipase. *Journal of Lipid Research* 35(5):848–59, 1994.

Christadoss, P., et al. Suppression of cellular and humoral immunity to T-dependent antigens by calorie restriction. *Cellular Immunology* 88(1):1–8, 1984.

Chung, H.Y., et al. Molecular inflammation hypothesis of aging based on the anti-aging mechanism of calorie restriction. *Microscopy Research and Technique* 59(4):264–72, 2002.

Chung, H.Y., et al. The inflammation hypothesis of aging: molecular modulation by calorie restriction. *Annals of the New York Academy of Sciences* 928:327–35, 2001.

Cicogna, A.C., et al. Effects of protein-calorie restriction on mechanical function of hypertrophied cardiac muscle. *Arquivos Brasileiro de Cardiololgia* 72(4):431–40, 1999.

Clarke, D.H., M.O. Hunt, C.O. Dotson. Muscular strength and endurance as a function of age and activity level. *Research Quarterly for Exercise and Sport* 63:302–10, 1992 Sep.

Clarkson, P.M. Nutritional ergogenic aids: carnitine. *International Journal of Sports Nutrition* 2:185–90, 1992 Jun.

Clifton, P.M., M. Noakes, et al. Very low-fat (12%) and high monounsaturated fat (35%) diets do not differentially affect abdominal fat loss in overweight, nondiabetic women. *Journal of Nutrition* 134(7):1741–5, 2004.

Coderre, L. A.K. Srivastava, J.L. Chiasson. Role of glucocorticoid in the regulation of glycogen metabolism in skeletal muscle. *American Journal of Physiology* 260:E927–32, 1991 Jun.

Coggan, A.R., R.J. Spina, W.M. Kohrt, J.O. Holloszy. Effect of prolonged exercise on muscle citrate concentration before and after endurance training in men. *American Journal of Physiology* 264:E215–20, 1993 Feb.

Cohen, S., et al. Weight gain with risperidone among patients with mental retardation: effect of calorie restriction. *Journal of Clinical Psychiatry* 62(2):114–6, 2001.

Colditz, G.A., W.C. Willett, M.J. Stampfer, et al. Weight as a risk factor for clinical diabetes in women. *American Journal of Epidemiology* 132:501–13, 1990 Sep.

Colman, E., L.I. Katzel, et al. Weight loss reduces abdominal fat and improves insulin action in middle-aged and older men with impaired glucose tolerance. *Metabolism* 44(11):1502–8, 1995.

Conlay, L.A., S.H. Zeisel. Neurotransmitter precursors and brain function. *Neurosurgery* 10:524–9, 1982 Apr.

Conlee, R.K., R.L. Hammer, W.W. Winder, Bracken, M.L., A.G. Nelson, D.W. Barnett. Glycogen repletion and exercise endurance in rats adapted to a high fat diet. *Metabolism* 39:289–94, 1990 Mar.

Conn, H.O. Animal versus vegetable protein diet in hepatic encephalopathy. *Journal of Internal Medicine* 233(5):369–71 1993.

Connolly, J.M., X.H. Liu, D.P. Rose. Dietary linoleic acid-stimulated human breast cancer cell growth and. 1996.

Consolazio, C.F., et al. Metabolic aspects of calorie restriction: nitrogen and mineral balances and vitamin excretion. *American Journal of Clinical Nutrition* 21(8):803–12, 1968.

Consolazio, C.F., et al. Metabolic aspects of calorie restriction: hypohydration effects on body weight and blood parameters. *American Journal of Clinical Nutrition* 21(8):793–802, 1968.

Consolazio, C.F., et al. Thiamin, riboflavin, and pyridoxine excretion during acute starvation and calorie restriction. *American Journal of Clinical Nutrition* 24(9):1060–7, 1971.

Constantin-Teodosiu, D., S. Howell, P.L. Greenhaff. Carnitine metabolism in human muscle fiber types during submaximal dynamic exercise. *Journal of Applied Physiology* 80:1061–4, 1996 Mar.

Cook, C.B., L. Shawar, H. Thompson, C. Prasad. Caloric intake and weight gain of rats depends on endogenous fat preference. *Physiology and Behavior* 61:743–8, 1997 May.

Cooper, C., E.J. Atkinson, D.D. Hensrud, et al. Dietary protein intake and bone mass in women. *Calcified Tissue International* 58:320–5, 1996 May.

Corbett, E.C., Jr. Review: advice on low-fat diets is not better than other weight-reducing diets for sustaining weight loss in obesity. *ACP Journal Club* 137(3):90, 2002.

Corbucci, G.G., G. Montanari, G. Mancinelli, S DI. Metabolic effects induced by

L-carnitine and propionyl-L-carnitine in human hypoxic muscle tissue during exercise. *International Journal of Clinical Pharmacology Research* 10:197–202, 1990.

Cowan, J.C., Vegetable protein nutrition. *Journal of the American Oil Chemists' Society* 56(3):145, 1979.

Cumming, R.G., S.R. Cummings, M.C. Nevitt, et al. Calcium intake and fracture risk: results from the study of osteoporotic fractures. *American Journal of Epidemiology* 145:926–34, 1997 May 15.

Currier, J. Longitudinal studies of the role of NRTIs in fat loss. *AIDS Clinical Care* 14(12):106–7, 2002.

Curtis, C.L., C.E. Hughes, C.R. Flannery, C.B., Little, J.L. Harwood, B. Caterson. N-3 fatty acids specifically modulate catabolic factors involved in articular cartilage degradation. *Journal of Biological Chemistry* 275(2):721–24, 2000.

Danao-Camara, T.C., T.T. Shintani. The dietary treatment of inflammatory arthritis: case reports and review of the literature. *Hawaii Medical Journal* 58(5):126–31, 1999.

Das, U.N. Free radicals: biology and relevance to disease. *Journal of the Association of Physicians of India* 38:495–8, 1990.

Das, U.N. Gamma-linolenic acid, arachidonic acid, and eicosapentaenoic acid as potential anticancer drugs. *Nutrition* 6:429–34, 1990.

Das, U.N. Tumoricidal action of cis-unsaturated fatty acids and their relationship to free radicals and lipid peroxidation. *Cancer Letters* 56:235–43, 1991.

Davie, M., et al. Effect of high and low-carbohydrate diets on nitrogen balance during calorie restriction in obese subjects. *International Journal of Obesity* 6(5):457–62, 1982.

Davies, P., P.J. Bailey, M.M. Goldenberg, A.W. Ford-Hutchinson. The role of arachidonic acid oxygenation products in pain and inflammation. *Annual Review of Immunology* 2:335–57, 1984.

Davies, P., R.J. Bonney, J.L. Humes, E.A. Kuehl, Jr. Synthesis and release of oxygenation products of arachidonic acid by mononuclear phagocytes in response to inflammatory stimuli. *Journal of Inflammation* 2:335–44, 1977 Dec.

Daviglus, M.L., A.R. Dyer, V. Persky, et al. Dietary beta-carotene, vitamin C, and risk of prostate cancer: results from the Western Electric Study. *Epidemiology* 7:472–7, 1996.

de Logeril, M., P. Salen, J.L. Martin, J. Monjaud, J. Delaye, N. Mamelle. Mediterranean diet, traditional risk factors, and the rate of cardiovascular complications after myocardial infarction: final report of the Lyon Diet Heart Study. *Circulation* 99(6):779–85, 1999.

de Lorgeril, M., S. Renaud, N. Mamelle, et al. Mediterranean alpha-linolenic acid-rich diet in secondary prevention of coronary heart disease. *Lancet* 343:1454–9, 1994.

Deal, C.L. Osteoporosis: prevention, diagnosis, and management. *American Journal of Medicine* 102:35S–39S, 1997 Jan 27.

Dean, D.J., G.D. Cartee. Calorie restriction increases insulin-stimulated tyrosine phosphorylation of insulin receptor and insulin receptor substrate-1 in rat skeletal muscle. *Acta Physiologica Scandinavia* 169(2):133–9, 2000.

Dean, D.J., et al. Comparison of the effects of 20 days and 15 months of calorie restriction on male Fischer 344 rats. *Aging (Milano)* 10(4):303–7, 1998.

Decombaz, J., B. Gmuender, G. Sierro, P. Cerretelli. Muscle carnitine after strenuous endurance exercise. *Journal of Applied Physiology* 72:423–7, 1992 Feb.

DeDeckere, E.A., O. Korver, P.M. Verschuren, M.B. Katan. Health aspects of fish and n-3 polyunsaturated fatty acids from plant and marine origin. *European Journal of Clinical Nutrition* 52:749–53, 1998.

Del Boca, J., J.P. Flatt. Fatty acid synthesis from glucose and acetate and the control of lipogenesis in adipose tissue. *European Journal of Biochemistry* 11:127–34, 1969 Nov.

del Mar Grasa, M., C. Cabot, et al. Daily oral oleoyl-estrone gavage induces a dose-dependent loss of fat in Wistar rats. *Obesity Research* 9(3):202–9, 2001.

DeLany, J.P., et al. Long-term calorie restriction reduces energy expenditure in aging monkeys. *Journal of Gerontology Series A: Biological Sciences and Medical Sciences* 54(1):B5–11; discussion B12–3, 1999.

Demling, R.H., L. DeSanti. Effect of a hypocaloric diet, increased protein intake and resistance training on lean mass gains and fat mass loss in overweight police officers. *Annals of Nutrition and Metabolism* 44(1):21–9, 2000.

Dennis, S.C., T.D. Noakes, J.A. Hawley. Nutritional strategies to minimize fatigue during prolonged exercise: fluid, electrolyte and energy replacement. *Journal of Sports Sciences* 15:305–13, 1997 Jun.

Dennis, K.E., A.P. Goldberg. Differential effects of body fatness and body fat distribution on risk factor for cardiovascular disease in women. Impact of weight loss. *Arteriosclerosis, Thrombosis and Vascular Biology* 13(10):1487–94, 1993.

De-Souza, D.A., L.J. Greene. Pharmacological nutrition after burn injury. *Journal of Nutrition* 128:797–803, 1998.

Despres, J.P., M.C. Pouliot, et al. Loss of abdominal fat and metabolic response to exercise training in obese women. *American Journal of Physiology* 261(2 Pt 1):E159–67, 1991.

Dessein, P.H., E.A. Shipton, et al. Beneficial effects of weight loss associated with moderate calorie/carbohydrate restriction, and increased proportional intake of protein and unsaturated fat on serum urate and lipoprotein levels in gout: a pilot study. *Annals of the Rheumatic Diseases* 59(7):539–43, 2000.

Deurenberg, P., J.A. Weststrate, et al. Changes in fat-free mass during weight loss measured by bioelectrical impedance and by densitometry. *American Journal of Clinical Nutrition* 49(1):33–6, 1989.

Deutch, B. Menstrual pain in Danish women correlated with low n-3 polyunsaturated fatty acid intake. *European Journal of Clinical Nutrition* 49(7):508–16, 1995.

Dichi, I., P. Frenhane, J.B. Dichi, et al. Comparison of omega-3 fatty acids and sulfasalazine in ulcerative colitis. *Nutrition* 16:87–90, 2000.

Dietary Protein and Weight Reduction: A Statement for Healthcare Professionals from the Nutrition Committee of the Council on Nutrition, Physical Activity, and Metabolism of the American Heart Association, 104:1869–74, 2001.

Dimitriadis, E., M. Griffin, P. Collins, A. Johnson, D. Owens, G.H. Tomkin. Lipoprotein composition in NIDDM: effects of dietary oleic acid on the composition, oxidisability and function of low and high density lipoproteins. *Diabetologia Croatica* 39(6):667–76, 1996.

Donnelly, J.E., T. Sharp, J. Houmard, et al. Muscle hypertrophy with large-scale weight loss and resistance training. *American Journal of Clinical Nutrition* 58:561–5, 1993 Oct.

Donnelly, J.E., D.J. Jacobsen, et al. Influence of degree of obesity on loss of fat-free mass during very-low-energy diets. *American Journal of Clinical Nutrition* 60(6): 874–8, 1994.

Dornhorst, A., et al. Calorie restriction for treatment of gestational diabetes. *Diabetes* 40 Suppl 2:161–4, 1991.

Doucet, E., P. Imbeault, et al. Physical activity and low-fat diet: is it enough to maintain weight stability in the reduced-obese individual following weight loss by drug therapy and energy restriction? *Obesity Research* 7(4):323–33, 1999.

Doucet, E., P. Imbeault, et al. Appetite after weight loss by energy restriction and a low-fat diet-exercise follow-up. *International Journal of Obesity and Related Metabolic Disorders* 24(7):906–14, 2000.

Douchi, T., S. Kosha, et al. Precedence of bone loss over changes in body composition and body fat distribution within a few years after menopause. *Maturitas* 46(2): 133–8, 2003.

Dreher, M.L., C.V. Maher, P. Kearney. The traditional and emerging role of nuts in healthful diets. *Nutrition Review* 54:241–5, 1996 Aug.

Dreon, D.M., H.A. Fernstrom, P.T. Williams, R.M. Krauss. A very-low-fat diet is not associated with improved lipoprotein profiles in men with a predominance of large, low-density lipoproteins. *American Journal of Clinical Nutrition* 69:411–8, 1999.

Drewnowski, A., M.R. Greenwood. Cream and sugar: human preferences for high-fat foods. *Physiology and Behaviour* 30: 629–33, 1983 Apr.

Drewnowski, A., D.D. Krahn, M.A. Demitrack, K. Nairn, B.A. Gosnell. Taste responses and preferences for sweet high-fat foods: evidence for opioid involvement. *Physiology and Behavior* 51:371–9, 1992 Feb.

Drewnowski, A., C. Kurth, J. Saari, J. Holden-Wiltse. Food preferences in human obesity: carbohydrates versus fats. *Appetite* 18:207–21, 1992 Jun.

Drewnowski, A. Dietary fats: perceptions and preferences. *Journal of the American College of Nutrition* 9:431–5, 1990 Aug.

Drewnowski, A. Sensory preferences for fat and sugar in adolescence and adult life. *Annals of the New York Academy of Sciences* 561:243–50, 1989.

du Toit, P.J., D.J. du Plessis., C.H. van Aswegen. The effect of gamma-linolenic acid and eicosapentaenoic acid on urokinase activity. *Prostaglandins Leukotrienes and Essential Fatty Acids* 51:121–4, 1994.

Dulloo, A.G., C.A. Geissler, T. Horton, A. Collins, D.S. Miller. Normal caffeine consumption: influence on thermogenesis and daily energy expenditure in lean and postobese human volunteers. *American Journal of Clinical Nutrition* 49:44–50, 1989 Jan.

Dulloo, A.G., L. Girardier. Adaptive changes in energy expenditure during refeeding following low-calorie intake: evidence for a specific metabolic component favoring fat storage. *American Journal of Clinical Nutrition* 52:415–20, 1990 Sep.

Dulloo, A.G., J. Jacquet, L. Girardier. Autoregulation of body composition during weight recovery in human: the Minnesota Experiment revisited. *International Journal of Obesity and Related Metabolic Disorders* 20:393–405, 1996 May.

Dulloo, A.G., J. Jacquet, L. Girardier. Poststarvation hyperphagia and body fat overshooting in humans: a role for feedback signals from lean and fat tissues. *American Journal of Clinical Nutrition* 65:717–23, 1997 Mar.

Dulloo, A.G., J. Jacquet. Adaptive reduction in basal metabolic rate in reponse to food deprivation in humans: a role for feedback signals from fat stores. *American Journal of Clinical Nutrition* 68:599–606, 1998 Sep.

Dulloo, A.G., N. Mensi, J. Seydoux, L. Girardier. Differential effects of high-fat diets varying in fatty acid composition on the efficiency of lean and fat tissue deposition during weight recovery after low food intake. *Metabolism* 44:273–9, 1995 Feb.

Dulloo, A.G., D.S. Miller. Obesity: a disorder of the sympathetic nervous system. *World Review of Nutrition and Dietetics* 50:1–56, 1987.

Dulloo, A.G. Human pattern of food intake and fuel-partitioning during weight recovery after starvation: a theory of autoregulation of body composition. *Proceedings of the Nutrition Society* 56:25–40, 1997 Mar.

Durlach, J., et al. Magnesium and ageing. II. Clinical data: aetiological mechanisms and

Dwyer, J.T., B.R. Goldin, N. Saul, L. Gualtieri, S. Barakat, H. Adlercreutz. Tofu and soy drinks contain phytoestrogens. *Journal of the American Dietetic Association* 94:739–43, 1994.

Dyck, D.J., S.J. Peters, P.S. Wendling, A. Chesley, E. Hultman, L.L. Spriet. Regulation of muscle glycogen phosphorylase activity during intense aerobic cycling with elevated FFA. *American Journal of Physiology* 270:E116–25, 1996 Jan.

Dyck, D.J. Dietary fat intake, supplements, and weight loss. *Canadian Journal of Applied Physiology* 25(6):495–523, 2000.

Eaton-Evans, J. Osteoporosis and the role of diet. *British Journal of Biomedical Science* 51:358–70, 1994 Dec.

Ebeling, P., J.A Tuominen, J. Arenas, C. Garcia Benayas, V.A. Koivisto. The association of acetyl-L-carnitine with glucose and lipid metabolism in human muscle in vivo: the effect of hyperinsulinemia. *Metabolism* 46:1454–7, 1997 Dec.

Edwards, R., M. Peet, J. Shay, D. Horrobin. Omega-3 polyunsaturated fatty acid levels in the diet and in red blood cell membranes of depressed patients. *Journal of Affective Disorders* 48:149–155, 1998.

Effect of low-carbohydrate high-protein diets on acid-base balance, stone-forming propensity, and calcium metabolism. *American Journal of Kidney Disease* 2002.

Efficacy and safety of low-carbohydrate diets. *JAMA* 289 (14), 2003.

Elizalde, G., A. Sclafani. Fat appetite in rats: flavor preferences conditioned by nutritive and non-nutritive oil emulsions. *Appetite* 15:189–97, 1990 Dec.

Ells, G.W., K.A. Chisholm, V.A. Simmons, D.F. Horrobin. Vitamin E blocks the cytotoxic effect of gamma-linolenic acid when administered as late as the time of onset of cell death—insight into the mechanism of fatty acid induced cytotoxicity. *Cancer Letters* 98:207–11, 1996.

Engell, D., P. Bordi, M. Borja, C. Lambert, B. Rolls. Effects of information about fat content on food preferences in pre-adolescent children. *Appetite* 30:269–82, 1998 Jun.

Engelman, R.W., N.K. Day, R.A. Good. Calorie intake during mammary development influences cancer risk: lasting inhibition of C3H/HeOu mammary tumorigenesis by peripubertal calorie restriction. *Cancer Research* 54(21):5724–30, 1994.

Epstein, L.H., R.R. Wing, B.C. Penner, M.J. Kress. Effect of diet and controlled exercise on weight loss in obese children. *Journal of Pediatrics* 107:358–61, 1985 Sep.

Erdman, J.W. Control of serum lipids with soy protein. *New England Journal of Medicine* 333:313–4, 1995.

Eriksson, J., T. Valle, et al. Leptin concentrations and their relation to body fat distribution and weight loss—a prospective study in individuals with impaired glucose tolerance. DPS-study group. *Hormone and Metabolic Research* 31(11):616–9, 1999.

Estrada, D.E., H.S. Ewart, T. Tsakiridis, et al. Stimulation of glucose uptake by the natural coenzyme alpha-lipoic acid/thioctic acid: participation of elements of the insulin signaling pathway. *Diabetes* 45:1798–804, 1996 Dec.

Estrada, V., M. Serrano-Rios, et al. Leptin and adipose tissue maldistribution in HIV-infected male patients with predominant fat loss treated with antiretroviral therapy. *Journal of Acquired Immune Deficiency Syndromes* 29(1):32–40, 2002.

Evidence-Based Nutrition Principles and Recommendations for the Treatment and Prevention of Diabetes and Related Complications. *Diabetes Care* 25:148–98, 2002.

Falconer, J.S., J.A. Ross, K.C. Fearon, R.A. Hawkins, O.R. MG, D.C. Carter. Effect of eicosapentaenoic acid and other fatty acids on the growth in vitro of human pancreatic cancer cell lines. *British Journal of Cancer* 69:826–32, 1994.

Felber, J.P., E. Haesler, E Je. Metabolic origin of insulin resistance in obesity with and without type 2 (non-insulin-dependent) diabetes mellitus. *Diabetologia Croatica* 36:1221–9, 1993 Dec.

Fernandes, G., J.T. Venkatraman. Possible mechanisms through which dietary lipids, calorie restriction, and exercise modulate breast cancer. *Advances in Experimental Medicine and Biology* 322:185–201, 1992.

Fernandes, G., E.J. Yunis, R.A. Good. Suppression of adenocarcinoma by the immunological consequences of calorie restriction. *Nature* 263(5577):504–7, 1976.

Fernandes, G. Effects of calorie restriction and omega-3 fatty acids on autoimmunity and aging. *Nutrition Review* 53(4 Pt 2):S72–7; discussion S77–9, 1995.

Fernandes, G., et al. Dietary lipids and calorie restriction affect mammary tumor incidence and gene expression in mouse mammary tumor virus/v-Ha-ras transgenic mice. *Proceedings of the National Academy of Sciences USA* 92(14):6494–8, 1995.

Ferris, S.H., G. Sathananthan, B. Reisberg, S. Gershon. Long-term choline treatment of memory-impaired elderly patients. *Science* 205:1039–40, 1979 Sep 7.

Feskanich, D., W.C. Willett, M.J. Stampfer, G.A Colditz. Milk, dietary calcium, and bone fractures in women: a 12-year prospective study. *American Journal of Public Health* 87:992–7, 1997 Jun.

Feskanich, D., W.C. Willett, M.J. Stampfer, G.A. Colditz. Protein consumption and bone fractures in women. *American Journal of Epidemiology* 143:472–9, 1996 Mar 1.

Feuerstein, G., J.M. Hallenbeck. Leukotrienes in health and disease. *FASEB Journal* 1:186–92, 1987 Sep.

Fiatarone, M.A., O.N. EF, N.D. Ryan, et al. Exercise training and nutritional supplementation for physical frailty in very elderly people [see comments]. *New England Journal of Medicine* 330:1769–75, 1994 Jun 23.

Fielding, R. The role of progressive resistance training and nutrition in the preservation of lean body mass in the elderly. *Journal of the American College of Nutrition* 14(6):587–94, 1995.

Fisher, J.O., L.L. Birch. Fat preferences and fat consumption of 3- to 5-year-old children are related to parental adiposity. *Journal of the American Dietetic Association* 95:759–64, 1995 Jul.

Fisher, W.E., L.G. Boros, W.J. Schirmer. Reversal of enhanced pancreatic cancer growth in diabetes by insulin. *Surgery* 118:453–7, 1995.

Flatt, J.P., E.G. Ball. The role of reduced coenzymes and oxygen in the control of fatty acid synthesis in adipose tissue. *Biochemistry Society Symposium* 24:75–7, 1963.

Flatt, J.P. Body composition, respiratory quotient, and weight maintenance. *American Journal of Clinical Nutrition* 62:1107S–1117S, 1995 Nov.

Flatt, J.P. Carbohydrate balance and body-weight regulation. *Proceedings of the Nutrition Society* 55:449–65, 1996 Mar.

Flatt, J.P. Carbohydrate balance and food intake regulation [letter; comment]. *American Journal of Clinical Nutrition* 62:155–7, 1995 Jul.

Flatt, J.P. Conversion of carbohydrate to fat in adipose tissue: an energy-yielding and, therefore, self-limiting process. *Journal of Lipid Research* 11:131–43, 1970 Mar.

Flatt, J.P. Dietary fat, carbohydrate balance, and weight maintenance: effects of exercise. *American Journal of Clinical Nutrition* 45:296–306, 1987 Jan.

Flatt, J.P. Energy metabolism and the control of lipogenesis in adipose tissue. *Hormone and Metabolic Research* 2 Suppl 2:93–101, 1970.

Flatt, J.P. Glycogen levels and obesity. *International Journal of Obesity and Related Metabolic Disorders* 20 Suppl 2:S1–11, 1996 Mar.

Flatt, J.P. How NOT to approach the obesity problem. *Obesity Research* 5:632–3, 1997 Nov.

Flatt, J.P. Importance of nutrient balance in body weight regulation. *Diabetes Metabolism Research and Reviews* 4:571–81, 1988 Sep.

Flatt, J.P. Integration of the overall response to exercise. *International Journal of Obesity and Related Metabolic Disorders* 19 Suppl 4:S31–40, 1995 Oct.

Flatt, J.P. McCollum Award Lecture: diet, lifestyle, and weight maintenance. *American Journal of Clinical Nutrition* 62:820–36, 1995 Oct.

Flatt, J.P. On the maximal possible rate of ketogenesis. *Diabetes* 21:50–3, 1972 Jan.

Flatt, J.P. Role of the increased adipose tissue mass in the apparent insulin insensitivity of obesity. *American Journal of Clinical Nutrition* 25:1189–92, 1972 Nov.

Flatt, J.P. The difference in the storage capacities for carbohydrate and for fat, and its implications in the regulation of body weight. *Annals of the New York Academy of Sciences* 499:104–23, 1987.

Flatt, J.P. Use and storage of carbohydrate and fat. *American Journal of Clinical Nutrition* 61:952S–959S, 1995 Apr.

Flegal, K.M., M.D. Carroll, R.J. Kuczmarski, C.L. Johnson. Overweight and obesity in the United States: prevalence and trends, 1960–1994. *International Journal of Obesity* 22:39–47, 1998.

Fleming, R.M. The effect of high-, moderate-, and low-fat diets on weight loss and cardiovascular disease risk factors. *Preventative Cardiology* 5(3):110–8, 2002.

Fleming, R.M. Caloric intake, not carbohydrate or fat consumption, determines weight loss. *American Journal of Medicine* 114(1):78, 2003.

Fogelholm, G.M., R. Koskinen, J. Laakso, T. Rankinen, I. Ruokonen. Gradual and rapid weight loss: effects on nutrition and performance in male athletes. *Medicine & Science in Sports & Exercise* 25:371–7, 1993 Mar.

Fogelholm, G.M., H.T. Sievanen, et al. Assessment of fat-mass loss during weight reduction in obese women. *Metabolism* 46(8):968–75, 1997.

Fogteloo, J., et al. The decline in plasma leptin in response to calorie restriction predicts the effects of adjunctive leptin treatment on body weight in humans. *European Journal of Internal Medicine* 14(7): 415–8, 2003.

Foreyt, J.P., R.S. Reeves, L.S. Darnell, J.C. Wohlleb, A.M. Gotto. Soup consumption as a behavioral weight loss strategy. *Journal of the American Dietetic Association* 86:524–6, 1986 Apr.

Foster, G.D., T.A. Wadden, Z.V. Kendrick, K.A. Letizia, D.P. Lander, A.M. Conill. The energy cost of walking before and after significant weight loss. *Medicine & Science in Sports & Exercise* 27:888–94, 1995 Jun.

Franco-Maside, A., L. Caamaño, M.J. Go, R. Cacabelos. Brain mapping activity and mental performance after chronic treatment with CDP-choline in Alzheimer's disease. Methods Find *Experimental Clinical Pharmacology* 16:597–607, 1994 Oct.

Franke, A.A., L.J. Custer. Daidzein and genistein concentrations in human milk after soy consumption. *Clinical Chemistry* 42:955–64, 1996.

Franson, R.C., J.S. Saal, J.A. Saal. Human disc phospholipase A2 is inflammatory. *Spine Journal* 17:S129–32, 1992 Jun.

Fraser, R., A.G. Bosanquet, W.A. Day. Filtration of chylomicrons by the liver may influence cholesterol metabolism and atherosclerosis. *Atherosclerosis Journal* 29(2): 113–23, 1978.

Freyssenet, D., P. Berthon, C. Denis, J.C. Barthelemy, C.Y. Guezennec, J.C. Chatard. Effect of a 6-week endurance training programme and branched-chain amino acid supplementation on histomorphometric characteristics of aged human muscle. *Archives of Physiology and Biochemistry* 104:157–62, 1996.

Fried, P.I., P.A. McClean, E.A. Phillipson, N. Zamel, F.T. Murray, E.B. Marliss. Effect of ketosis on respiratory sensitivity to carbon dioxide in obesity. *New England Journal of Medicine* 294:1081–6, 1976 May 13.

Friedberg, C.E., M.J.E.M. Janssen, R.J. Heine, D.E. Grobbee. Fish oil and glycemic control in diabetes: a meta-analysis. *Diabetes Care* 21:494–500, 1998.

Friedewald, W.T., T.J. Thom. Decline of coronary heart disease mortality in the United States. *Israel Journal of Medical Sciences* 22:307–12, 1986.

Friedman, J.E., J.E. Caro, W.J. Pories, J.L. Azevedo, Jr., G.L. Dohm. Glucose metabolism in incubated human muscle: effect of obesity and non-insulin-dependent diabetes mellitus. *Metabolism* 43:1047–54, 1994 Aug.

Friedmann, B., W. Kindermann. Energy metabolism and regulatory hormones in women and men during endurance exercise. *European Journal of Applied Physiology* 59:1–9, 1989.

Frieri, G., M.T. Pimpo, A. Palombieri, et al. Polyunsaturated fatty acid dietary supplementation: an adjuvant approach to treatment of Helicobacter pylori infection. *Nutrition Research* 20(7):907–16, 2000.

Friolet, R., H. Hoppeler, S. Krähenbühl. Relationship between the coenzyme A and the carnitine pools in human skeletal muscle at rest and after exhaustive exercise under normoxic and acutely hypoxic conditions. *Journal of Clinical Investigation* 94:1490–5, 1994 Oct.

Fritsché, R., J.J. Pahud, S. Pecquet, A. Pfeifer. Induction of systemic immunologic tolerance to beta-lactoglobulin by oral administration of a whey protein hydrolysate. *Journal of Allergy and Clinical Immunology* 100:266–73, 1997 Aug.

Fukagawa, N.K., J.W. Anderson, G. Hageman, V.R. Young, K.L. Minaker. High-carbohydrate, high-fiber diets increase peripheral insulin sensitivity in healthy young and old adults. *American Journal of Clinical Nutrition* 52:524–8, 1990 Sep.

Fukutake, M., M. Takahashi, K. Ishida, H. Kawamura, T. Sugimura. Quantification of genistein and genistin in soybeans and soybean products. 1996.

Funkhouser, A.B., B. Laferrere, et al. Measurement of percent body fat during weight loss in obese women. Comparison of four methods. *Annals of the New York Academy of Sciences* 904: 539–41, 2000.

Gallina, D.L., et al. Dissociated response of plasma albumin and transferrin to protein-calorie restriction in squirrel monkeys (Saimiri sciureus). *American Journal of Clinical Nutrition* 46(6):941–8, 1987.

Garg, A., S.M. Grundy. High-carbohydrate, low-fat diet? Negative [comment]. *Hospital Practice* (Office Edition), 27 Suppl 1:11–4; discussion 14–6, 1992 Feb.

Garland, C., R.B. Shekelle, E. Barrett-Connor, M.H. Criqui, A.H. Rossof, O. Paul. Dietary vitamin D and calcium and risk of colorectal cancer: a 19-year prospective study in men. *Lancet* 1:307–9, 1985.

Garland, L.G., S.T. Hodgson. Inhibition of leukotriene production by inhibitors of lipoxygenation. *Advanced Prostaglandin Thromboxane Leukotriene Research* 22:33–48, 1994.

Garriga, J., R. Cussó. Effect of starvation on glycogen and glucose metabolism in different areas of the rat brain. *Brain Research* 591:277–82, 1992 Sep 25.

Garrow, J.S. Is body fat distribution changed by dieting? *Acta Medica Scandinavia Supplement* 723:199–203, 1988.

Garrow, J. Flushing away the fat. Weight loss during trials of orlistat was significant, but over half was due to diet. *British Medical Journal* 317(7162):830–1, 1998.

Gausseres, N., et al. Whole-body protein turnover in humans fed a soy protein-rich vegetable *European Journal of Clinical Nutrition* 51(5):308–11, 1997.

Gausseres, N., et al. Calorie restriction increases insulin-stimulated glucose transport in skeletal muscle from IRS-1 knockout mice. *Diabetes* 48(10):1930–6, 1999.

Geerling, B.J., A. Badart-Smook, C. van Deursen, et al. Nutritional supplementation with N-3 fatty acids and antioxidants in patients with Crohn's disease in remission: effects on antioxidant status and fatty acid profile. *Inflammatory Bowel Disease* 6(2):77–84, 2000.

Geerling, B.J., A.C. Houwelingen, A. Badart-Smook, R.W. Stockbrügger, R.J.M. Brummer. Fat intake and fatty acid profile in plasma phospholipids and adipose tissue in patients with Crohn's disease, compared with controls. *American Journal of Gastroenterology* 94(2):410–7, 1999.

Giacco, R., et al. Long-term dietary treatment with increased amounts of fiber-rich low-glycemic index natural foods improves blood glucose control and reduces the number of hypoglycemic events in type 1 diabetic patients. *Diabetes Care* 23(10):1461–6, 2000.

Giamberardino, M.A., I. Dragani, R. Valente, Lisa F. Di, R. Saggini, L. Vecchiet. Effects of prolonged L-carnitine administration on delayed muscle pain and CK release after eccentric effort. *International Journal of Sports Medicine* 17:320–4, 1996 Jul.

Gilbertson, H.R., et al. Effect of low-glycemic-index dietary advice on dietary quality and food choice in children with type 1 diabetes. *American Journal of Clinical Nutrition* 77(1):83–90, 2003.

Gilbertson, H.R., et al. The effect of flexible low glycemic index dietary advice versus measured carbohydrate exchange diets on glycemic control in children with type 1 diabetes. *Diabetes Care* 24(7):1137–43, 2001.

Gillette, C.A., et al. Energy availability and mammary carcinogenesis: effects of calorie restriction and exercise. *Carcinogenesis* 18(6):1183–8, 1997.

Giovanella, B.C., et al. Calorie restriction: effect on growth of human tumors heterotransplanted in nude mice. *Journal of the National Cancer Institute* 68(2):249–57, 1982.

Giovannucci, E., E.B. Rimm, A. Ascherio, M.J. Stampfer, G.A. Colditz, W.C. Willett. Alcohol, low-methionine—low-folate diets, and risk of colon cancer in men. *Journal of the National Cancer Institute* 87:265–73, 1995.

Giovannucci, E., E.B. Rimm, Y. Liu, M.J. Stampfer, W.C. Willett. A prospective study of tomato products, lycopene, and prostate cancer risk. *Journal of the National Cancer Institute* 94:391–8, 2002.

Giovannucci, E., M.J. Stampfer, G.A. Colditz, E.B. Rimm, D. Trichopoulos, B.A.

Rosner. Folate, methionine, and alcohol intake and risk of colorectal adenoma. *Journal of the National Cancer Institute* 85:875–84, 1993.

Giovannucci, E. How is individual risk for prostate cancer assessed? *Hematology Oncology Clinics of North America* 10:537–48, 1996.

Giovenali, P., D. Fenocchio, G. Montanari, et al. Selective trophic effect of L-carnitine in type I and IIa skeletal muscle fibers. *Kidney International* 46:1616–9, 1994 Dec.

Girard, N., et al. Long-term calorie restriction protects rat pituitary growth hormone-releasing hormone binding sites from age-related alterations. *Neuroendocrinology* 68(1):21–9, 1998.

GISSI-Prevenzione Investigators. Dietary supplementation with n-3 polyunsaturated fatty acids and vitamin E after myocardial infarction: results of the GISSI-Prevenzione trial. *Lancet* 354:447–455, 1999.

Glauber, H., P. Wallace, K. Griver, G. Brechtel. Adverse metabolic effect of omega-3 fatty acids in non-insulin-dependent diabetes mellitus. *Annals of Internal Medicine* 108:663–8, 1988.

Gmoshinskiï, I.V., V.K. Mazo, S.N. Zorin. The effect of a protein concentrate from milk whey and its fractions on the macromolecular permeability of the intestinal barrier in rats with experimental food anaphylaxis. *Vopr Pitan*:3–6, 1996.

Goetzl, E.J. Oxygenation products of arachidonic acid as mediators of hypersensitivity and inflammation. *Medical Clinics of North America* 65:809–28, 1981 Jul.

Goforth, H.W., Jr., D.A. Arnall, B.L. Bennett, P.G. Law. Persistence of supercompensated muscle glycogen in trained subjects after carbohydrate loading. *Journal of Applied Physiology* 82:342–7, 1997 Jan.

Golay, A., J.P. Felber. Evolution from obesity to diabetes. *Diabetes Metabolism* 20:3–14, 1994 Jan–Feb.

Goldstein, M.R. Nuts, nuts good for your heart . . . ? [letter; comment]. *Archives of Internal Medicine* 152:2507–2511, 1992 Dec.

González, E.R. Studies show the obese may prefer fats to sweets [news]. JAMA, 250:579, 583, 1983 Aug 5.

Gooderham, M.H., H. Adlercreutz, S.T. Ojala, K. Wï, B.J. Holub. A soy protein isolate rich in genistein and daidzein and its effects on plasma isoflavone concentrations, platelet aggregation, blood lipids and *Journal of Nutrition* 126:2000–6, 1996.

Goodpaster, B.H., D.E. Kelley, et al. Effects of weight loss on regional fat distribution and insulin sensitivity in obesity. *Diabetes* 48(4):839–47, 1999.

Gorin, A.A., Phelan, S., Wing, R.R., Hill, J.O. Promoting long-term weight control: does dieting consistency matter? International *Journal of Obesity and Related Metabolic Disorders*. 2004 Feb; 28(2): 278–81

Gosker, H.R., M.P. Engelen, et al. Muscle fiber type IIX atrophy is involved in the loss of fat-free mass in chronic obstructive pulmonary disease. *American Journal of Clinical Nutrition* 76(1):113–9, 2002.

Graham, G.G., W.C. Maclean, Jr. Role of vegetable protein in human nutrition. *Journal of Pediatrics* 98(4):666, 1981.

Grammatikos, S.I., P.V. Subbaiah, T.A. Victor, W.M. Miller. n-3 and n-6 fatty acid processing and growth effects in neoplastic and non-cancerous human mammary epithelial cell lines. *British Journal of Cancer* 70:219–27, 1994.

Granström E. The arachidonic acid cascade. The prostaglandins, thromboxanes and leukotrienes. *Journal of Inflammation* 8 Suppl:S15–25, 1984 Jun.

Greenhaff, P. Renal dysfunction accompanying oral creatine supplements. *Lancet* 352:233–34, 1998.

Grey, N.J., I. Karl, D.M. Kipnis. Physiologic mechanisms in the development of starvation ketosis in man. *Diabetes* 24:10–6, 1975 Jan.

Grieve, D.J., et al. Comparison of effects of chylomicrons and chylomicron remnants on agonist-induced endothelium-dependent relaxation in rat aorta. *Biochemical Society Transactions* 25(3):399S, 1997.

Grieve, D.J., et al. Effects of chylomicrons and chylomicron remnants on endothelium-dependent relaxation of rat aorta. *European Journal of Pharmacology* 348(2–3):181–90, 1998.

Griffiths, A.J., S.M. Humphreys, M.L. Clark, B.A. Fielding, K.N. Frayn. Immediate metabolic availability of dietary fat in combination with carbohydrate. *American Journal of Clinical Nutrition* 59:53–9, 1994.

Griffiths, D.E., K. Cain, R.L. Hyams. Oxidative phosphorylation: a new biological function for lipoic acid. *Biochemical Society Transactions* 5:205–7, 1977.

Grimaldi, A., C. Sachon, F. Bosquet, R. Doumith. Intolerance to carbohydrates: the seven questions. *Revue de Medecine Interne* 11:297–307, 1990 Jul–Aug.

Gulliford, M.C., E.J. Bicknell, J.H. Scarpello. Differential effect of protein and fat ingestion on blood glucose responses to high- and low-glycemic-index carbohydrates in noninsulin-dependent diabetic subjects. *American Journal of Clinical Nutrition* 50(4):773–7, 1989.

Gumaste, V.V. Vegetable protein diet and hepatic encephalopathy. *Gastroenterology* 105(5):1578–9, 1993.

Gurr, M.I., R.T. Jung, et al. Adipose tissue cellularity in man: the relationship between fat cell size and number, the mass and distribution of body fat and the history of weight gain and loss. *International Journal of Obesity* 6(5):419–36, 1982.

Gwinup, G. Weight loss without dietary restriction: efficacy of different forms of aerobic exercise. *American Journal of Sports Medicine* 15:275–9, 1987 May–Jun.

Hackney, A.C. Endurance training and testosterone levels. *Sports Medieine* 8:117–27, 1989 Aug.

Haenszel, W., M. Kurihara. Studies of Japanese migrants. I. Mortality from cancer and other diseases among Japanese in the United States. *Journal of the National Cancer Institute* 40:43–68, 1968 Jan.

Hale, P.J., B.M. Singh, et al. Following weight loss in massively obese patients correction of the insulin resistance of fat metabolism is delayed relative to the improvement in carbohydrate metabolism. *Metabolism* 37(5):411–7, 1988.

Hamilton-Fairley, D., et al. Response of sex hormone binding globulin and insulin-like growth factor binding protein-1 to an oral glucose tolerance test in obese women with polycystic ovary syndrome before and after calorie restriction. *Clinical Endocrinology* (Oxf) 39(3):363–7, 1993.

Hanai T., T. Hashimoto, K. Nishiwaki, et al. Comparison of prostanoids and their precursor fatty acids in human hepatocellular carcinoma and noncancerous reference tissues. *Journal of Surgical Research* 54:57–60, 1993.

Hansen, B.C. Introduction. Symposium: Calorie restriction: effects on body composition, insulin signaling and aging. *Journal of Nutrition* 131(3):900S–2S, 2001.

Hansen, B.C., N.L. Bodkin, H.K. Ortmeyer. Calorie restriction in nonhuman primates: mechanisms of reduced morbidity and mortality. *Journal of Toxicology Science* 52(2 Suppl):56–60, 1999.

Hardin, C.D., T.M. Roberts. Differential regulation of glucose and glycogen metabolism in vascular smooth muscle by exogenous substrates. *Journal of Molecular and Cellular Cardiology* 29:1207–16, 1997 Apr.

Hardman, A.E., C. Williams, S.A. Wootton. The influence of short-term endurance training on maximum oxygen uptake, submaximum endurance and the ability to perform brief, maximal exercise. *Journal of Sports Sciences* 4:109–16, 1986 Autumn.

Hardman, A.E., C. Williams. Increased dietary carbohydrate and endurance during single-leg cycling using a limb with normal muscle glycogen concentration. *Journal of Sports Sciences* 7:127–38, 1989 Summer.

Hargreaves, M. Carbohydrate and lipid requirements of soccer. *Journal of Sports Sciences* 12 Spec No:S13–6, 1994 Summer.

Harney, J.P., J. Madara, H. I'Anson. Effects of acute inhibition of fatty acid oxidation on latency to seizure and concentrations of beta hydroxybutyrate in plasma of rats maintained on calorie restriction and/or the ketogenic diet. *Epilepsy Research* 49(3):239–46, 2002.

Harper, C.R., T.A. Jacobson. The fats of life: the role of omega-3 fatty acids in the prevention of coronary heart disease. *Archives of Internal Medicine* 161(18):2185–2192, 2001.

Harris, W.S. N-3 fatty acids and serum lipoproteins: human studies. *American Journal of Clinical Nutrition* 65:1645S–1654S, 1997.

Harvey-Berino, J. The efficacy of dietary fat vs. total energy restriction for weight loss. *Obesity Research* 6(3):202–7, 1998.

Haskin, C.L., S.B. Milam, I.L. Cameron. Pathogenesis of degenerative joint disease in the human temporomandibular joint. *Critical Reviews in Oral Biology & Medicine* 6:248–77, 1995.

Havel, P.J., S. Kasim-Karakas, et al. Relationship of plasma leptin to plasma insulin and adiposity in normal weight and overweight women: effects of dietary fat content and sustained weight loss. *Journal of Clinical Endocrinology & Metabolism* 81(12):4406–13, 1996.

Hawrylewicz, E.J., J.J. Zapata, W.H. Blair. Soy and experimental cancer: animal studies. *Journal of Nutrition* 125:698S–708S, 1995.

Hayashi, N., T. Tsuguhiko, H. Yamamori, et al. Effect of intravenous omega-6 and omega-3 fat emulsions on nitrogen retention and protein kinetics in burned rats. *Nutrition* 15(2):135–139, 1999.

Hayashi, Y., S. Fukushima, S. Kishimoto, et al. Anticancer effects of free polyunsaturated fatty acids in an oily lymphographic agent following intrahepatic arterial administration to a rabbit bearing VX-2 tumor. *Cancer Research* 52:400–5, 1992.

Haymond, M.W., C. Howard, E. Ben-Galim, D.C. DeVivo. Effects of ketosis on glucose flux in children and adults. *American Journal of Physiology* 245:E373–8, 1983 Oct.

He, Q., E.S. Engelson, et al. Preferential loss of omental-mesenteric fat during growth hormone therapy of HIV-associated lipodystrophy. *Journal of Applied Physiology* 94(5):2051–7, 2003.

Heaney, R.P. Pathophysiology of osteoporosis. *American Journal of Medical Sciences* 312:251–6, 1996 Dec.

Heatherton, T.F., J. Polivy, C.P. Herman. Restraint, weight loss, and variability of body weight. *Journal of Abnormal Psychology* 100:78–83, 1991 Feb.

Heber, D., J.M. Ashley, D.A. Leaf, R.J. Barnard. Reduction of serum estradiol in postmenopausal women given free access to low-fat high-carbohydrate diet. *Nutrition* 7:137–9; discussion 139–40, 1991 Mar–Apr.

Heffernan, M.A., A.W. Thorburn, et al. Increase of fat oxidation and weight loss in obese mice caused by chronic treatment with human growth hormone or a modified C-terminal fragment. *International Journal of Obesity and Related Metabolic Disorders* 25(10):1442–9, 2001.

Heilbronn, L.K., M. Noakes, et al. Energy restriction and weight loss on very-low-fat diets reduce C-reactive protein concentrations in obese, healthy women. *Arteriosclerosis, Thrombosis and Vascular Biology* 21(6):968–70, 2001.

Heilbronn, L.K., E. Ravussin. Calorie restriction and aging: review of the literature and implications for studies in humans. *American Journal of Clinical Nutrition* 78(3):361–9, 2003.

Heilbronn, L.K., M. Noakes, P.M. Clifton. The effect of high- and low-glycemic index energy restricted diets on plasma lipid and glucose profiles in type 2 diabetic subjects with varying glycemic control. *Journal of the American College of Nutrition* 21(2):120–7, 2002.

Heinonen, O.J. Carnitine and physical exercise. *Sports Medicine* 22:109–32, 1996 Aug.

Heleniak, E.P., B. Aston Prostaglandins, brown fat and weight loss. *Medical Hypotheses* 28(1):13–33, 1989.

Heller, A., T. Koch, J. Schmeck, K. van Ackern. Lipid mediators in inflammatory disorders. *Drugs* 55:487–96, 1998 Apr.

Hendel, H.W., A. Gotfredsen, et al. Change in fat-free mass assessed by bioelectrical impedance, total body potassium and dual energy X-ray absorptiometry during prolonged weight loss. *Scandinavian Journal of Clinical Lab Investigation* 56(8): 671–9, 1996.

Hendrich, S., K.W. Lee, X. Xu, H.J. Wang, P.A. Murphy. Defining food components as new nutrients. *Journal of Nutrition* 124:1789S–1792S, 1994.

Hernandez, M., et al. The protein efficiency ratios of 30:70 mixtures of animal: vegetable protein are similar or higher than those of the animal foods alone *Journal of Nutrition* 126(2):574–81, 1996.

Hersey W.C.R., J.E. Graves, M.I. Pollock, et al. Endurance exercise training improves body composition and plasma insulin responses in 70- to 79-year-old men and women. *Metabolism* 43:847–54, 1994 Jul.

Hibbeln, J.R., N. Salem, Jr. Dietary polyunsaturated fatty acids and depression: when cholesterol does not satisfy. *American Journal of Clinical, Nutrition* 62(1):1–9, 1995.

Hickner, R.C., J.S. Fisher, P.A. Hansen, et al. Muscle glycogen accumulation after endurance exercise in trained and untrained individuals. *Journal of Applied Physiology* 83:897–903, 1997 Sep.

Hietanen, E., H. Bartsch, J.C. Bé, A.M. Camus, S. McClinton. Diet and oxidative stress in breast, colon and prostate cancer patients: a case-control study. *European Journal of Clinical Nutrition* 48:575–86, 1994.

Higashi, K., T. Ishikawa, H. Shige, et al. Olive oil increases the magnitude of postprandial chylomicron remnants compared to milk fat and safflower oil. *Journal of the American College of Nutrition* 16:429–34, 1997 Oct.

Higgs, G.A, K.E. Eakins, S. Moncada, J.R. Vane. Arachidonic acid metabolism in inflammation and the mode of action of anti-inflammatory drugs. *Agents Actions* (Suppl):167–75, 1979.

Higgs, G.A. The role of eicosandoids in inflammation. *Progress in Lipid Research* 25:555–61, 1986.

Hill, D.E., et al. The influence of protein-calorie versus calorie restriction on the body composition and cellular growth of muscle and liver in weanling rats. *Johns Hopkins Med Journals* 127(3):146–63, 1970.

Hill, J.O., M. DiGirolamo. Preferential loss of body fat during starvation in dietary obese rats. *Life Sciences* 49(25):1907–14, 1991.

Himeno, Y., R.W. Engelman, and R.A. Good. Influence of calorie restriction on oncogene expression and DNA synthesis during liver regeneration. *Proceedings of the National Academy of Sciences USA* 89(12):5497–501, 1992.

Honn, K.V., K.K. Nelson, C. Renaud, R. Bazaz, C.A. Diglio, J. Timar. Fatty acid modulation of tumor cell adhesion to microvessel endothelium and experimental metastasis. *Prostaglandins* 44(5):413–29, 1992.

Honorie, E.K., J.K. Williams, M.S. Anthony, T.B. Clarkson. Soy isoflavones enhance coronary vascular reactivity in atherosclerotic female macaques. *Fertility and Sterility* 67:148–54, 1997.

Hood, DaT, R. Amino acid metabolism during exercise and following endurance training. *Sports Medicine* 9(1):23–25, 1990.

Hopewell, J.W, M.E. Robbins, G.J. van den Aardweg, G.M. Morris, G.A. Ross, Whitehouse. The modulation of radiation-induced damage to pig skin by essential fatty acids. *British Journal of Cancer* 68:1–7, 1993.

Hopewell, J.W., G.J. van den Aardweg, G.M. Morris, M. Rezvani, M.E. Robbins, G.A. Ross, Amelioration of both early and late radiation-induced damage to pig skin by essential fatty *International Journal of Radiation Oncology, Biology, Physics* 30:1119–25, 1994.

Hoppel, C.L, S.M. Genuth. Urinary excretion of acetylcarnitine during human diabetic and fasting ketosis. *American Journal of Physiology* 243:E168–72, 1982 Aug.

Hori, N., et al. Long-term potentiation is lost in aged rats but preserved by calorie restriction. *Neuroreport* 3(12):1085–8, 1992.

Horrobin, D.F, C.N. Bennett. Depression and bipolar disorder: relationships to impaired fatty acid and phospholipid metabolism and to diabetes, cardiovascular disease, immunological abnormalities, cancer, ageing and osteoporosis. *Prostaglandins, Leukotrienes and Essential Fatty Acids* 60(4):217–34, 1999.

Horrobin, D.F. The membrane phospholipid hypothesis as a biochemical basis for the neurodevelopmental concept of schizophrenia. *Schizophrenia Research* 30(3): 193–208, 1998.

Houmard, J.A., W.S. Wheeler, M.R. McCammon, et al. An evaluation of waist to hip ratio measurement methods in relation to lipid and carbohydrate metabolism in men. *International Journal of Obesity* 15:181–8, 1991 Mar.

Houtkooper, L. Food selection for endurance sports. *Medicine & Science in Sports & Exercise* 24:S349–59, 1992 Sep.

Howard, A.N. The historical development, efficacy and safety of very-low-calorie diets. *International Journal of Obesity* 5:195–208, 1981.

Howell, T.J., D.E. MacDougall, P.J. Jones. Phytosterols partially explain differences in cholesterol metabolism caused by corn or olive oil feeding. *Journal of Lipid Research* 39:892–900, 1998 Apr.

Hrboticky, N., B. Zimmer, P.C. Weber. Alpha-Linolenic acid reduces the lovastatin-induced rise in arachidonic acid and elevates cellular and lipoprotein eicosapentaenoic and docosahexaenoic acid levels in Hep G2 cells. *Journal of Nutritional Biochemistry* 7:465–471, 1996.

Hrelia, S., A. Bordoni, P. Biagi, C.A. Rossi, L. Bernardi, D.F. Horrobin. Gamma-Linolenic acid supplementation can affect cancer cell proliferation via modification of fatty acid composition. *Biochemical Biophysical Research Communications* 225:441–7, 1996.

Hu, F.B., M.I. Stampfer, J.E. Manson, et al. Dietary intake of alpha-linolenic acid and risk of fatal ischemic heart disease among women. *American Journal of Clinical Nutrition* 69:890–897, 1999.

Hu, F.B., M.J. Stampfer, E.B. Rjimm, J.E. Manson, A. Ascherio, G.A. Colditz, B.A. Rosner, D. Spiegelman, E.E. Speizer, E.M. Sacks, C.H. Hennekens, W.C. Willett. A prospective study of egg consumption and risk of cardiovascular disease in men and women. JAMA 281:1387–1394, 1999.

Huang, Z, S.E. Hankinson, G.A. Colditz, et al. Dual effects of weight and weight gain on breast cancer risk [see comments]. *JAMA* 278:1407–11, 1997 Nov 5.

Hubbard, N.E., K.L. Erickson. Role of dietary oleic acid in linoleic acid-enhanced metastasis of a mouse mammary tumor. *Cancer Letters* 56(2):165–71, 1991.

Huertas, R., Y. Campos, E. Di, et al. Respiratory chain enzymes in muscle of endurance athletes: effect of L-carnitine. *Biochemical and Biophysical Research Communications* 188:102–7, 1992 Oct 15.

Hultin, M.,T. Olivecrona. Conversion of chylomicrons into remnants. *Atherosclerosis* 141 Suppl 1:S25–9, 1998.

Hursting, S.D., et al. Calorie restriction induces a p53-independent delay of spontaneous carcinogenesis in p53-deficient and wild-type mice. *Cancer Research* 57(14):2843–6, 1997.

Hursting, S.D., et al. Calorie restriction, aging, and cancer prevention: mechanisms of action and applicability to humans. *Annual Review of Medicine* 54:131–52, 2003.

Hursting, S.D., S.N. Perkins, J.M. Phang, Calorie restriction delays spontaneous tumorigenesis in p53-knockout transgenic mice. *Proceedings of the National Academy of Sciences USA* 91(15):7036–40, 1994.

Hutchins, A.M., J.L. Slavin, J.W. Lampe. Urinary isoflavonoid phytoestrogen and lignan excretion after consumption of fermented and unfermented soy products. *Journal of the American Dietetic Association* 95:545–51, 1995.

Hyun, Y., O. Ishiko, et al. Probucol decreases total body fat loss in VX2-carcinoma-induced cachectic rabbits. *Oncology Reports* 8(6):1309–11, 2001.

Ibayashi, H., et al. Systemic triglyceride storage disease with normal carnitine: a putative defect in long-chain fatty acid metabolism. *Journal of Neurological Sciences* 85(2):149–59, 1988.

Itatsu, S., Y. Kudo, T. Iguchi, Y. Takeda. [Studies on the bone metabolisms in either after natural menopause or surgical menopause: implications of IGF-IGFBP system for postmenopausal osteoporosis]. *Nippon Sanka Fujinka Gakkai Zasshi* 47:1329–36, 1995 Dec.

Ito, H., et al. Effects of increased physical activity and mild calorie restriction on heart rate variability in obese women. *Japanese Heart Journal* 42(4):459–69, 2001.

Ivy, J.L., M.C. Lee, J.T. Brozinick, Jr., M.J. Reed. Muscle glycogen storage after different amounts of carbohydrate ingestion. *Journal of Applied Physiology* 65:2018–23, 1988 Nov.

Jarvi, A.E., et al. Improved glycemic control and lipid profile and normalized fibrinolytic activity on a low-glycemic index diet in type 2 diabetic patients. *Diabetes Care* 22(1):10–8, 1999.

Jayanthi, S., G. Jayanthi, P. Varalakshmi. Effect of DL alpha-lipoic acid on some carbohydrate metabolising enzymes in stone forming rats. *Biochemistry International* 25:123–36, 1991 Sep.

Jeejeebhoy, K.N., Vegetable proteins: are they nutritionally equivalent to animal protein. *European Journal of Gastroenterology and Hepatology* 12(1):1–2, 2000.

Jeffery, R.W., et al. A randomized trial of counseling for fat restriction versus calorie restriction in the treatment of obesity. *International Journal of Obesity and Related Metabolic Disorders* 19(2):132–7, 1995.

Jeffery, R.W., P.D. Thompson, R.R. Wing. Effects on weight reduction of strong monetary contracts for calorie restriction or weight loss. *Behavior Research and Therapy* 16(5):363–9, 1978.

Jenkins, D.J., D.G. Popovich, C.W. Kendall, et al. Effect of a diet high in vegetables, fruit, and nuts on serum lipids. *Metabolism* 46:530–7, 1997 May.

Jenkins, D.J.A., T.M.S. Wolever, A.V. Roa, et al. Effect on blood lipids of very high intakes of fiber in diets in saturated fat and cholesterol. *New England Journal of Medicine* 329:21–7, 1993.

Jenkins, D.J., et al. Effect of high vegetable protein diets on urinary calcium loss in middle-aged men and women. *European Journal of Clinical Nutrition* 57(2):376–82, 2003.

Jenkins, D.J., et al. Hypocholesterolemic effect of vegetable protein in a hypocaloric diet. *Atherosclerosis* 78(2–3):99–107, 1989.

Jenkins, D.J., et al. Low glycemic index carbohydrate foods in the management of hyperlipidemia. *American Journal of Clinical Nutrition* 42(4):604–17, 1985.

Jenkins, D.J., et al. Low glycemic index foods and reduced glucose, amino acid, and endocrine responses in cirrhosis. *American Journal of Gastroenterology* 84(7):732–9, 1989.

Jenkins, D.J., et al. Low glycemic index: lente carbohydrates and physiological effects of altered food frequency. *American Journal of Clinical Nutrition* 59(3 Suppl):706S–9S, 1994.

Jenkins, D.J., et al. Low-glycemic index diet in hyperlipidemia: use of traditional starchy foods. *American Journal of Clinical Nutrition* 46(1):66–71, 1987.

Jenkins, D.J., et al. Low-glycemic-index starchy foods in the diabetic diet. *American Journal of Clinical Nutrition* 48(2):248–54, 1988.

Jenkins, D.J., et al. Metabolic effects of a low-glycemic-index diet. *American Journal of Clinical Nutrition* 46(6):968–75, 1987.

Jenkins, D.J., et al. The effect on serum lipids and oxidized low-density lipoprotein of supplementing self-selected low-fat diets with soluble-fiber, soy, and vegetable protein foods. *Metabolism* 49(1): 67–72, 2000.

Jensen, J., R. Aslesen, J.L. Ivy, O. Brørs. Role of glycogen concentration and epinephrine on glucose uptake in rat epitrochlearis muscle. *American Journal of Physiology* 272:E649–55, 1997 Apr.

Jensen, J., H. Oftebro, B. Breigan, et al. Comparison of changes in testosterone concentrations after strength and endurance exercise in well trained men. *European Journal of Applied Physiology* 63:467–71, 1991.

Jenski, I.J., M. Zerouga, W. Stillwell. Omega-3 fatty acid-containing liposomes in cancer therapy. *Proceedings of the Society for Experimental Biology and Medicine* 210:227–33, 1995.

Jeppesen, J., P. Schaaf, C. Jones, M.Y. Zhou, Y.D. Chen, G.M. Reaven. Effects of low-fat, high-carbohydrate diets on risk factors for ischemic heart disease in post-menopausal women. *American Journal of Clinical Nutrition* 65(4):1027–33, 1997 Apr.

Jerusalinsky, D., E. Kornisiuk, I. Izquierdo. Cholinergic neurotransmission and synaptic plasticity concerning memory processing. *Neurochemical Research* 22:507–15, 1997 Apr.

Jeschke, M.G., D.N. Herndon, C. Ebener, R.E. Barrow, K.W. Jauch. Nutritional intervention high in vitamins, protein, amino acids, and omega-3 fatty acids improves protein metabolism during the hypermetabolic state after thermal injury. *Archives of Surgery* 136:1301–6, 2001.

Jeukendrup, A.E., W.H. Saris, A.J. Wagenmakers. Fat metabolism during exercise: a review. Part I: fatty acid mobilization and muscle metabolism. *International Journal of Sports Medicine* 19:231–44, 1998 May.

Jiang, W.G., S. Hiscox, M.B. Hallett, D.F. Horrobin, R.E. Mansel, M.C. Puntis. Regulation of the expression of E-cadherin on human cancer cells by gamma-linolenic acid (GLA). *Cancer Research* 55:5043–8, 1995.

Jimenez-Cruz, A., et al. A flexible, low-glycemic index Mexican-style diet in overweight and obese subjects with type 2 diabetes improves metabolic parameters during a 6-week treatment period. *Diabetes Care* 26(7):1967–70, 2003.

Jimenez-Cruz, A., H. Seimandi-Mora, M. Bacardi-Gascon. Effect of low glycemic index diets in hyperlipidemia. *Nutrition Hospital* 18(6):331–5, 2003.

Johnson, R.H., J.L. Walton. Fitness, fatness, and post-exercise ketosis. *Lancet* 1:566–8, 1971 Mar 20.

Johnson S.L., L. McPhee, I.L. Birch. Conditioned preferences: young children prefer flavors associated with high dietary fat. *Physiology and Behavior* 50:1245–51, 1991 Dec.

Johnston, C.S., S.L. Tjonn, et al. High-protein, low-fat diets are effective for weight loss and favorably alter biomarkers in healthy adults. *Journal of Nutrition* 134(3): 586–91, 2004.

Jolly, C.A., et al. Calorie restriction modulates Th-1 and Th-2 cytokine-induced immunoglobulin secretion in young and old C57BL/6 cultured submandibular glands. *Aging (Milano)* 11(6):383–9, 1999.

Jones, A.L., et al. Uptake and processing of remnants of chylomicrons and very low density lipoproteins by rat liver. *Journal of Lipid Research* 25(11):1151–8, 1984.

Jones, L.M., A. Goulding, et al. DEXA: a practical and accurate tool to demonstrate total and regional bone loss, lean tissue loss and fat mass gain in paraplegia. *Spinal Cord* 36(9):637–40, 1998.

Jones, P.R., D.A. Edwards. Areas of fat loss in overweight young females following an 8-week period of energy intake reduction. *Annals of Human Biology* 26(2): 151–62, 1999.

Joossens, J.V., J. Geboers. Nutrition and cancer. *Biomedical Pharmacotherapy* 40:127–38, 1986.

Juhaeri, J. Stevens, et al. Associations of weight loss and changes in fat distribution with the remission of hypertension in a bi-ethnic cohort: the Atherosclerosis Risk in Communities Study. *Preventive Medicine* 36(3):330–9, 2003.

Juhl, A., J. Marniemi, R. Huupponen, A. Virtanen, M. Rastas, T. Ronnemaa. Effects of diet and simvastatin on serum lipids, insulin, and antioxidants in hypercholesterolemic men; a randomized controlled trial. *JAMA* 2887(5):598–605, 2002.

Kabir, M., et al. Four-week low-glycemic index breakfast with a modest amount of soluble fibers in type 2 diabetic men. *Metabolism* 51(7):819–26, 2002.

Kagan, A., G.G. Rhoads, P.D. Zeegen, M.Z. Nichaman. Coronary heart disease among men of Japanese ancestry in Hawaii. The Honolulu Heart study. *Israel Journal of Medical Sciences* 7:1573–7, 1971 Dec.

Kanders, B.S., P.T. Lavin, M.B. Kowalchuk, I. Greenberg, G.L. Blackburn. An evaluation of the effect of aspartame on weight loss. *Appetite* 11 (Suppl 1):73–84, 1988.

Kanter, M.M., M.H. Williams. Antioxidants, carnitine, and choline as putative ergogenic aids. *International Journal of Sports Nutrition* 5 (Suppl):S120–31, 1995 Jun.

Kapadia, C.R., M.F. Colpoys, Z.M. Jlang, D.W. Wilmore. Maintainence of skeletal muscle intracellular glutamine during standard surgical trauma. *JPEN Journal of Paranteral and Enteral Nutrition* 9:583–9, 1985.

Karch, P.B., J.R. Beaton. Diet and body weight loss in the rat during calorie restriction. *Canadian Journal of Physiology and Pharmacology* 46(1):101–7, 1968.

Karhunen, L.J., R.I. Lappalainen, S.M. Haffner, et al. Serum leptin, food intake and preferences for sugar and fat in obese women. *International Journal of Obesity and Related Metabolic Disorders* 22:819–21, 1998 Aug.

Karmali, R.A., L. Adams, J.R. Trout. Plant and marine n-3 fatty acids inhibit experimental metastasis of rat mammary adenocarcinoma cells. *Prostaglandins, Leukotrienes and Essential Fatty Acids* 48:309–14, 1993.

Karmann, H., N. Mrosovsky, A. Heitz, Y. Le Maho. Protein sparing on very low calorie diets: ground squirrels succeed where obese people fail. *International Journal of Obesity and Related Metabolic Disorders* 18:351–3, 1994 May.

Karpe, F., et al. Chylomicron/chylomicron remnant turnover, in humans: evidence for margination of chylomicrons and poor conversion of larger to smaller chylomicron remnants. *Journal of Lipid Research* 38(5):949–61, 1997.

Karvonen, H.M., et al. Effect of alpha-linolenic acid-rich Camelina sativa oil on serum fatty acid composition and serum lipids in hypercholesterolemic subjects. *Metabolism* 51(10):1253–60, 2002.

Katan, M.B., S.M. Grundy, W.C. Willett. Should a low-fat, high-carbohydrate diet be recommended for everyone? Beyond low-fat diets. *New England Journal of Medicine* 337:563–6, 1997.

Katdare, M., H. Singhal, H. Newmark, M.P. Osborne, N.T. Telang. Prevention of mammary preneoplastic transformation by naturally-occurring tumor inhibitors. *Cancer Letters* 111:141–7, 1997.

Kawamura, M., et al. Blood pressure is reduced by short-time calorie restriction in overweight hypertensive women with a constant intake of sodium and potassium. *Journal of Hypertension Supplement* 11 (Suppl 5):S320–1, 1993.

Kawamura, M., et al. Factors that affect calorie-sensitive and calorie-insensitive reduction in blood pressure during short-term calorie restriction in overweight hypertensive women. *Hypertension* 27(3 Pt 1):408–13, 1996.

Keim, N.L., M.D. Van Loan, et al. Weight loss is greater with consumption of large morning meals and fat-free mass is preserved with large evening meals in women on a controlled weight reduction regimen. *Journal of Nutrition* 127(1):75–82, 1997.

Keim, N.L., T.F. Barbieri, et al. Physiological and biochemical variables associated with body fat loss in overweight women. *International Journal of Obesity* 15(4):283–93, 1991.

Keler, T. C.S. Barker, S. Sorof. Specific growth stimulation by linoleic acid in hepatoma cell lines transfected with the target protein of a liver carcinogen. *Proceedings of the National Academy of Sciences USA* 89:4830–4, 1992.

Kelley, D.E., et al. Relative effects of calorie restriction and weight loss in noninsulin-dependent diabetes mellitus. *Journal of Clinical Endocnology and Metabolism* 77(5):1287–93, 1993.

Kendall, A., D.A. Levitsky, et al. Weight loss on a low-fat diet: consequence of the imprecision of the control of food intake in humans. *American Journal of Clinical Nutrition* 53(5):1124–9, 1991.

Kennedy, A.R. The evidence for soybean products as cancer preventive agents. *Journal of Nutrition* 125:733S–743S, 1995.

Kern, D.L., L. McPhee, I. Fisher, S. Johnson, L.L. Birch. The postingestive consequences of fat condition preferences for flavors associated with high dietary fat. *Physiology and Behavior* 54:71–6, 1993 Jul.

Keshavarzian, A., et al. Dietary protein supplementation from vegetable sources in the management of chronic portal systemic encephalopathy. *American Journal of Gastroenterology* 79(12):945–9, 1984.

Kida, Y., A. Esposito-Del Puente, C. Bogardus, D.M. Mott. Insulin resistance is associated with reduced fasting and insulin-stimulated glycogen synthase phosphatase activity in human skeletal muscle. *Journal of Clinical Investigation* 85:476–81, 1990 Feb.

Kim, J.G., I.Y. Lee. Serum insulin-like growth factor binding protein profiles in postmenopausal women: their correlation with bone mineral density. *American Journal of Obstetrics and Gynecology* 174:1511–7, 1996 May.

Kim, Y.L., J.B. Mason. Nutrition chemoprevention of gastrointestinal cancers: a critical review. *Nutrition Review* 54:259–79, 1996.

Kim, H.J., et al. Modulation of redox-sensitive transcription factors by calorie restriction during aging. *Mechanics of Ageing Development* 123(12):1589–95, 2002.

Kim, K.R., S.Y. Nam, et al. Low-dose growth hormone treatment with diet restriction accelerates body fat loss, exerts anabolic effect and improves growth hormone secretory dysfunction in obese adults. *Hormone Research* 51(2):78–84, 1999.

King, R.A., J.L. Broadbent, R.J. Head. Absorption and excretion of the soy isoflavone genistein in fats. *Journal of Nutrition* 126:176–82, 1996.

Kinscherf, R. V. Hack, T. Fischbach, et al. Low plasma glutamine in combination with high glutamate levels indicate risk for loss of body cell mass in healthy individuals: the effect of N-acetyl-cysteine. *Journal of Molecular Medicine* 74:393–400, 1996 Jul.

Kiritsakis, A., P. Markakis. Olive oil: a review. *Advances in Food and Nutrition Research* 31:453–82, 1987.

Kitazato, H., et al. Effects of chronic intake of vegetable protein added to animal or fish protein on renal hemodynamics. *Nephron* 90(1):31–6, 2002.

Klein, R.F. Alcohol-induced bone disease: impact of ethanol on osteoblast proliferation. *Alcoholism: Clinical and Experimental Research* 21:392–9, 1997 May.

Klein, S., R.R. Wolfe. Carbohydrate restriction regulates the adaptive response to fasting. *American Journal of Physiology* 262:E631–6, 1992 May.

Klem, M.L., Wing, R.R., McGuire, M.T., Seagle, H.M., Hill, J.O. A descriptive study of individuals successful at long-term maintenance of substantial weight loss. *American Journal of Clinical Nutrition*, 1997, 66, 239–246.

Knopp, R.H., C.E. Walden, B.M. Retzlaff, et al. Long-term cholesterol lowering effects of 4 fat-restricted diets in hypercholesterolemic and combined hyperlipidemic men: The Dietary Alternatives Study. *JAMA* 278:1509–15, 1997.

Kobayashi, S., M.A. Venkatachalam. Differential effects of calorie restriction on glomeruli and tubules of the remnant kidney. *Kidney International* 42(3):710–7, 1992.

Kockx, M., R. Leenen, et al. Relationship between visceral fat and PAI-1 in overweight men and women before and after weight loss. *Journal of Thrombosis and Haemostasis* 82(5):1490–6, 1999.

Kohrt, W.M., M. Landt, S.J. Birge Jr. Serum leptin levels are reduced in response to exercise training, but not hormone replacement therapy, in older women. *Journal of Clinical Endocrinology & Metabolism* 81:3980–5, 1996 Nov.

Kolonel, L.N., J.H. Hankin, A.M. Nomura. Multiethnic studies of diet, nutrition, and cancer in Hawaii. *Princess Takamatsu Symposium* 16:29–40, 1985.

Kolonel, L.N., J.H. Hankin, C.N. Yoshizawa. Vitamin A and prostate cancer in elderly men: enhancement of risk. *Cancer Research* 47:2982–5, 1987.

Kolonel, L.N. Nutrition and prostate cancer. *Cancer Causes and Control* 7:83–44, 1996.

Komandi, K., E. Dworschak. Measurement of some antinutritive factors in meat products containing texturated vegetable protein (TVP). *Nahrung* 32(7):643–8, 1988.

Konig, W., K.D. Bremm, H.J. Brom, et al. The role of leukotriene-inducing and -metabolizing enzymes in inflammation. *International Archives of Allergy and Applied Immunology* 82:526–31, 1987.

Korcok, M. Hunger strikers may have died of fat, not protein, loss. JAMA 246(17):1878–9, 1981.

Koubova, J., L. Guarente. How does calorie restriction work? *Genes Development* 17(3):313–21, 2003.

Krahn, D.D., B.A. Gosnell. Fat-preferring rats consume more alcohol than carbohydrate-preferring rats. *Alcohol* 8:313–6, 1991 Jul–Aug.

Kral, T.V.E., L.S. Roe, B.J. Rolls. Combined effects of energy density and portion size on energy intake in women. *American Journal of Clinical Nutrition* 79:962–8, 2004.

Kral, T.V., B.J. Rolls. Energy density and portion size: their independent and combined effects on energy intake. *Physiology and Behavior* 82(1):131–8, 2004.

Kral, T.V., L.S. Roe, et al. Does nutrition information about the energy density of meals affect food intake in normal-weight women? *Appetite* 39(2):137–45, 2002.

Krauss, R.M., R.H. Eckel, B. Howard, L.J. Appel, S.R. Daniels, R.J. Deckelbaum, et al. AHA Scientific Statement: AHA dietary guidelines revision 2000: A statement for healthcare professionals from the nutrition committee of the American Heart Association. *Circulation* 102(18):2284–2299, 2000.

Krebs, J.D., S. Evans, et al. Changes in risk factors for cardiovascular disease with body fat loss in obese women. *Diabetes, Obesity and Metabolism* 4(6):379–87, 2002.

Kreitzman, S.N., A.Y. Coxon, K.F. Szaz. Glycogen storage: illusions of easy weight loss, excessive weight regain, and distortions in estimates of body composition. *American Journal of Clinical Nutrition* 56:292S–293S, 1992 Jul.

Kreitzman, S.N., A.Y. Coxon, et al. Dependence of weight loss during very-low-calorie diets on total energy expenditure rather than on resting metabolic rate, which is associated with fat-free mass. *American Journal of Clinical Nutrition* 56(1 Suppl):258S–261S, 1992.

Kremer, J.M. N-3 fatty acid supplements in rheumatoid arthritis. *American Journal of Clinical Nutrition* (Suppl 1):349S–351S, 2000.

Kris-Etherton, P., R.H. Eckel, B.V. Howard, S. St. Jeor, T.L. Bazzare. AHA science advisory: Lyon diet heart study. Benefits of a Mediterranean-style, National Cholesterol Education Program/American Heart Association Step I dietary pattern on cardiovascular disease. *Circulation* 103:1823–1825, 2001.

Kris-Etherton, P.M., J.A. Derr, V.A. Mustad, F.H. Seligson, T.A. Pearson. Effects of a milk chocolate bar per day substituted for a high-carbohydrate snack in young men on an NCEP/AHA Step 1 Diet. *American Journal of Clinical Nutrition* 60:1037S–1042S, 1994 Dec.

Kris-Etherton, P.M., D.S. Taylor, S. Yu-Poth, et al. Polyunsaturated fatty acids in the food chain in the United States. *American Journal of Clinical Nutrition* 71(1 Suppl):179S–188S, 2000.

Kritchevsky, D. and D.M. Klurfeld. Gallstone formation in hamsters: effect of varying animal and vegetable protein levels. *American Journal of Clinical Nutrition* 37(5):802–4, 1983.

Kritchevsky, D., D.M. Klurfeld. Influence of vegetable protein on gallstone formation in hamsters. *American Journal of Clinical Nutrition* 32(11):2174–6, 1979.

Kritchevsky, D., et al. Atherogenicity of animal and vegetable protein. Influence of the lysine to arginine ratio. *Atherosclerosis* 41(2–3): 429–31, 1982.

Kritchevsky, D. Vegetable protein and atherosclerosis. *Journal of the American Oil Chemists' Society* 56(3):135–40, 1979.

Kubo, C., et al. Effects of calorie restriction on immunologic functions and development of autoimmune disease in NZB mice. *Proceedings of the Society for Experimental Biology and Medicine* 201(2):192–9, 1992.

Kuroki, E., M. Iida, T. Matsumoto, K. Aoyagi, K. Kanamoto, M. Fujishima. Serum n3 polyunsaturated fatty acids are depleted in Crohn's disease. *Digestive Diseases and Sciences* 42(6):1137–1141, 1997.

la Vecchia, C., E. Negri, S. Franceschi, A. Decarli, A. Giacosa, L. Lipworth. Olive oil, other dietary fats, and the risk of breast cancer (Italy). *Cancer Causes and Control* 6:545–50, 1995 Nov.

Laaksonen, D.E., J. Nuutinen, et al. Changes in abdominal subcutaneous fat water content with rapid weight loss and long-term weight maintenance in abdominally obese men and women. *International Journal of Obesity and Related Metabolic Disorders* 27(6):677–83, 2003.

Lakin, J.A., S.N. Steen, R.A. Oppliger. Eating behaviors, weight loss methods, and nutrition practices among high school wrestlers. *Journal of Community Health Nursing* 7:223–34, 1990.

Lamarche, B., J.P. Despres, et al. Is body fat loss a determinant factor in the improvement of carbohydrate and lipid metabolism following aerobic exercise training in obese women? *Metabolism* 41(11):1249–56, 1992.

Lamartiniere, C.A., J.B. Moore, N.M. Brown, R. Thompson, M.J. Hardin, S. Barnes. Genistein suppresses mammary cancer in rats. *Carcinogenesis* 16:2833–40, 1995.

Lambert, M.S., K.M. Botham, P.A. Mayes. Modification of the fatty acid composition of dietary oils and fats on incorporation into chylomicrons and chylomicron remnants. *British Journal of Nutrition* 76(3):435–45, 1996.

Lands, W.E. Control of prostaglandin biosynthesis. *Progress in Lipid Research* 20:875–83, 1981.

Lane, M.A., D.K. Ingram, G.S. Roth. Calorie restriction in nonhuman primates: effects on diabetes and cardiovascular disease risk. *Toxicological Sciences* 52(2 Suppl):41–8, 1999.

Lane, M.A., D.K. Ingram, and G.S. Roth. Effects of aging and long-term calorie restriction on DHEA and DHEA sulfate in rhesus monkeys. *Annals of the New York Academy of Sciences* 774:319–22, 1995.

Lane, M.A., et al. Calorie restriction lowers body temperature in rhesus monkeys, consistent with a postulated anti-aging mechanism in rodents. *Proceedings of the National Academy of Sciences USA* 93(9):4159–64, 1996.

Lane, M.A., et al. Dehydroepiandrosterone sulfate: a biomarker of primate aging slowed by calorie restriction. *Journal of Clinical Endocrinology and Metabolism* 82(7):2093–6, 1997.

Lane, M.A., et al. Short-term calorie restriction improves disease-related markers in older male rhesus monkeys (Macaca mulatta). *Mechanics of Ageing Development* 112(3):185–96, 2000.

Langendonk, J.G., H. Pijl, et al. Circadian rhythm of plasma leptin levels in upper and lower body obese women: influence of body fat distribution and weight loss. *Journal of Clinical and Endocrinology and Metabolism* 83(5):1706–12, 1998.

Langfort, J., W. Pilis, R. Zarzeczny, K. Nazar, U.S.H. Kaciuba. Effect of low-carbohydrate-ketogenic diet on metabolic and hormonal responses to graded exercise in men. *Journal of Physiology and Pharmacology* 47:361–71, 1996 Jun.

Lanska, D.J., M.J. Lanska, et al. A prospective study of body fat distribution and weight loss. *International Journal of Obesity* 9(4):241–6, 1985.

Lauritsen, K., L.S. Laursen, K. Bukhave, J. Rask-Madsen. Does vitamin E supplementation modulate in vivo arachidonate metabolism in human inflammation? *Annual Review of Pharmacology and Toxicology* 61:246–9, 1987 Oct.

Lavoie, C., F. Pe, J.L. Chiasson. Role of the sympathoadrenal system in the regulation of glycogen metabolism in resting and exercising skeletal muscles. *Hormone and Metabolic Research* 24:266–71, 1992 Jun.

Lawrence, J.C. Jr., P.J. Roach. New insights into the role and mechanism of glycogen synthase activation by insulin. *Diabetes* 46:541–7, 1997 Apr.

Leaf, A., K.B. Frisa. Eating for health or for athletic performance? *American Journal of Clinical Nutrition* 49:1066–1069, 1989.

Lean, M.E., T.S. Han, T. Prvan, P.R. Richmond, A. Avenell. Weight loss with high and low carbohydrate 1200 kcal diets in free living women. *European Journal of Clinical Nutrition* 51:243–8, 1997 Apr.

Lee, I.M., J.E. Manson, C.H. Hennekens, R.S. Paffenbarger, Jr. Body weight and mortality. A 27-year follow-up of middle-aged men [see comments]. *JAMA* 270:2823–8, 1993 Dec 15.

Leenen, R., K. van der Kooy, J.C. Seidell, P. Deurenberg, H.P. Koppeschaar. Visceral fat accumulation in relation to sex hormones in obese men and women undergoing weight loss therapy. *Journal of Endocrinology and Metabolism* 78:1515–20, 1994 Jun.

Leenen, R., K. van der Kooy, et al. Visceral fat accumulation in obese subjects: relation to energy expenditure and response to weight loss. *American Journal of Physiology* 263(5 pt 1):E913–9, 1992.

Leenen, R., K. van der Kooy, et al. Relative effects of weight loss and dietary fat modification on serum lipid levels in the dietary treatment of obesity. *Journal of Lipid Research* 34(12):2183–91, 1993.

Leenen, R., K. van der Kooy, et al. Visceral fat loss measured by magnetic resonance imaging in relation to changes in serum lipid levels of obese men and women. *Arteriosclerosis Thrombosis and Vascular Biology* 13(4):487–94, 1993.

Leenen, R., K. van der Kooy, et al. Visceral fat accumulation in relation to sex hormones in obese men and women undergoing weight loss therapy. *Journal of Clinical Endocrinology and Metabolism* 78(6):1515–20, 1994.

Lefkowith, J.B., S. Klahr. Polyunsaturated fatty acids and renal disease. *Proceedings of the Society for Experimental Biology and Medicine* 213:13–23, 1996 Oct.

Lehmann, R., A. Vokac, et al. Loss of abdominal fat and improvement of the cardiovascular risk profile by regular moderate exercise training in patients with NIDDM. *Diabetologia Croatica* 38(11):1313–9, 1995.

Leitzmann, M.F., Meir J. Stampfer, et al. Dietary intake of n-3 and n-6 fatty acids and the risk of prostate cancer. *American Journal of Clinical Nutrition* 80(1):204–16, 2004 Jul.

Leung, L.H. Pantothenic acid as a weight-reducing agent: fasting without hunger, weakness and ketosis. *Medical Hypotheses* 44:403–5, 1995 May.

Lewis, G.P. Biochemistry, pathophysiology and pharmacology of slow-reacting substances/leukotrienes. *Agents Actions* 11:569–71, 1981 Dec.

Lewis, R.A., K.F. Austen, R.J. Soberman. Leukotrienes and other products of the 5-lipoxygenase pathway. Biochemistry and relation to pathobiology in human diseases. *New England Journal of Medicine* 323:645–55, 1990 Sep 6.

Lewis, R.A., K.F. Austen. The biologically active leukotrienes. Biosynthesis, metabolism, receptors, functions, and pharmacology. *Journal of Clinical Investigation* 73:889–97, 1984 Apr.

Li, Y., et al. Visceral fat: higher responsiveness of fat mass and gene expression to calorie restriction than subcutaneous fat. *Experimental Biology and Medicine (Maywood)* 228(10):1118–23, 2003.

Liao, S. Androgen action: molecular mechanism and medical application. *Journal of the Formosan Medical Association* 93:741–51, 1994.

Lichtenstein, A.H., L.M. Ausman, et al. Short-term consumption of a low-fat diet beneficially affects plasma lipid concentrations only when accompanied by weight loss. Hypercholesterolemia, low-fat diet, and plasma lipids. *Arteriosclerosis Thrombosis and Vascular Biology* 14(11):1751–60, 1994.

Lichtenstein, K.A., K.M. Delaney, et al. Incidence of and risk factors for lipoatrophy (abnormal fat loss) in ambulatory HIV-1-infected patients. *Journal of Acquired Immune Deficiency Syndromes* 32(1):48–56, 2003.

Lim, C.F., et al. Transport of thyroxine into cultured hepatocytes: effects of mild non-thyroidal illness and calorie restriction in obese subjects. *Clinical Endocrinology (Oxf)* 40(1):79–85, 1994.

Lin, S.J., P.A. Defossez, and L. Guarente. Requirement of NAD and SIR2 for lifespan extension by calorie restriction in Saccharomyces cerevisiae. *Science* 289(5487):2126–8, 2000.

Lipkin M., H. Newmark. Calcium and the prevention of colon cancer. *Journal of Cellular Biochemistry* (Supplement) 22:65–73, 1995.

Lipworth, L., M.E. Martínez, J. Angell, C.C. Hsieh, D. Trichopoulos. Olive oil and human cancer: an assessment of the evidence. *American Journal of Preventive Medicine* 26:181–90, 1997 Mar–Apr.

Lissner L., D.A. Levitsky, B.J. Strupp, H.J. Kalkwarf, D.A. Roe. Dietary fat and the regulation of energy intake in human subjects. *American Journal of Clinical Nutrition* 46:886–892, 1987.

Liu, X.H., J.M. Connolly, D.P. Rose. Eicosanoids as mediators of linoleic acid-stimulated invasion and type IV. 1996.

Lockwood, K., S. Moesgaard, K. Folkers. Partial and complete regression of breast cancer in patients in relation to dosage of coenzyme Q10. *Biochemical and Biophysical Research Communications* 199:1504–8, 1994.

Lockwood, K., S. Moesgaard, T. Hanioka, K. Folkers. Apparent partial remission of breast cancer in "high risk" patients supplemented with nutritional antioxidants, essential fatty acids and. *Molecular Aspects of Medicine* 15:s231–40, 1994.

Lok, E., et al. Calorie restriction and cellular proliferation in various tissues of the female Swiss Webster mouse. *Cancer Letters* 51(1):67–73, 1990.

Lorenz-Meyer, H., P. Bauer, C. Nicolay, B. Schulz, J. Purrmann, W.E. Fleig, et al. Omega-3 fatty acids and low carbohydrate diet for maintenance of remission in Crohn's disease. A randomized controlled multicenter trial. Study Group Members (German Crohn's disease Study Group). *Scandinavian Journal of Gastroenterology* 31(8):778–785, 1996.

Lovejoy, J.C., G.A. Bray, et al. Consumption of a controlled low-fat diet containing olestra for 9 months improves health risk factors in conjunction with weight loss in obese men: the Ole' Study. *International Journal of Obesity and Related Metabolic Disorders* 27(10):1242–9, 2003.

Luscombe, N.D., M. Noakes, and P.M. Clifton. Diets high and low in glycemic index versus high monounsaturated fat diets: effects on glucose and lipid metabolism in NIDDM. *European Journal of Clinical Nutrition* 53(6):473–8, 1999.

Lynch, N.A., B.J. Nicklas, et al. Reductions in visceral fat during weight loss and walking are associated with improvements in VO(2 max). *Journal of Applied Physiology* 90(1):99–104, 2001.

Macconi, D., et al. Selective dietary restriction of protein and calorie intakes prevents spontaneous proteinuria in male MWF rats. *Experimental Nephrology* 5(5): 404–13, 1997.

Madhavi, N., U.N. Das. Effect of n-6 and n-3 fatty acids on the survival of vincristine sensitive and resistant human cervical carcinoma cells in vitro. *Cancer Letters* 84:31–41, 1994.

Mahfouz-Cercone, S., J.E. Johnson, and G.U. Liepa. Effect of dietary animal and vegetable protein on gallstone formation and biliary constituents in the hamster. *Lipids* 19(1): 5–10, 1984.

Mai, V., et al. Calorie restriction and diet composition modulate spontaneous intestinal tumorigenesis in Apc(Min) mice through different mechanisms. *Cancer Research* 63(8): 1752–5, 2003.

Maki, K.C., M.H. Davidson, et al. Consumption of diacylglycerol oil as part of a reduced-energy diet enhances loss of body weight and fat in comparison with consumption of a triacylglycerol control oil. *American Journal of Clinical Nutrition* 76(6):1230–6, 2002.

Malmsten, C. Arachidonic acid metabolism and inflammation. A brief introduction. *Scandinavian Journal of Rheumatology* (Suppl) 53:31–45, 1984.

Malmsten, C.L. Arachidonic acid metabolism in inflammation and hypersensitivity reactions: a brief introduction. *Cephalalgia* 6 Suppl 4:13–6, 1986.

Malmsten, C.L. Leukotrienes: mediators of inflammation and immediate hypersensitivity reactions. *Critical Reviews in Immunology* 4:307–34, 1984.

Malmsten, C.L. Prostaglandins, thromboxanes, and leukotrienes in inflammation. *American Journal of Medicine* 80:11–7, 1986 Apr 28.

Mamo, J.C. and J.R. Wheeler, Chylomicrons or their remnants penetrate rabbit thoracic aorta as efficiently as do smaller macromolecules, including low-density lipoprotein, high-density lipoprotein, and albumin. *Coronary Artery Disease* 5(8):695–705, 1994.

Mani, U.V., S. Bhatt, N.C. Mehta, S.N. Pradhan, V. Shah, I. Mani. Glycemic index of traditional Indian carbohydrate foods. *Journal of the American College of Nutrition* 9:573–7, 1990 Dec.

Mann, J. Meta-analysis of low-glycemic index diets in the management of diabetes: response to Franz. *Diabetes Care* 26(12):3364; author reply 3364–5, 2003.

Manson, J.E., G.A. Colditz, M.J. Stampfer, et al. A prospective study of obesity and risk of coronary heart disease in women [see comments]. *New England Journal of Medicine* 322:882–9, 1990 Mar 29.

Manson. J.E., M.J. Stampfer, C.H. Hennekens, W.C. Willett. Body weight and longevity. A reassessment. JAMA 257:353–8, 1987 Jan 16.

Manson, J.E., W.C. Willett, M.J. Stampfer, et al. Body weight and mortality among women [see comments]. *New England Journal of Medicine* 333:677–85, 1995 Sep 14.

Marangella, M., et al. Effect of animal and vegetable protein intake on oxalate excretion in idiopathic calcium stone disease. *British Journal of Urology* 63(4):348–51, 1989.

Margaritis, J., F. Tessier, E. Prou, P. Marconnet, J.F. Marini. Effects of endurance training on skeletal muscle oxidative capacities with and without selenium supplementation. *Journal of Trace Elements in Medicine and Biology* 11:37–43, 1997 Apr.

Marin, P., I. Ho-K, S. Jansson, M. Krotkiewski, G. Holm, P. Björntorp. Uptake of glucose carbon in muscle glycogen and adipose tissue triglycerides in vivo in humans. *American Journal of Physiology* 263:E473–80, 1992 Sep.

Markovic, T.P., L.V. Campbell, et al. Beneficial effect on average lipid levels from energy restriction and fat loss in obese individuals with or without type 2 diabetes. *Diabetes Care* 21(5): 695–700, 1998.

Marks, B.L., J.M. Rippe. The importance of fat free mass maintenance in weight loss programmes. *Sports Medicine* 22(5): 273–81, 1996.

Marnett, L.J., C.L. Wilcox. Stimulation of prostaglandin biosynthesis by lipoic acid. *Biochimica et Biophysica Acta* 487:222–30, 1977 Apr 26.

Marquart, L.F. J. Sobal. Weight loss beliefs, practices and support systems for high school wrestlers *Journal of Adolescent Health* 15:410–5, 1994 Jul.

Martin, M.A., et al. Protein calorie restriction has opposite effects on glucose metabolism and insulin gene expression in the fetal and adult rat endocrine pancreas. *American Journal of Physiology Endocrinology and Metabolism* 2003.

Martin-Du Pan, R.C., R.J. Wurtman. [The role of nutrition in the synthesis of neurotransmitters and in cerebral functions: clinical implications]. *Schweizerische Medizinische Wochenschrift* 111:1422–34, 1981 Sep 26.

Martin-Moreno, J.M., W.C. Willett, L. Gorgojo, et al. Dietary fat, olive oil intake and breast cancer risk. *International Journal of Cancer Research* 58:774–80, 1994 Sep 15.

Martins, I.J., et al. Effects of particle size and number on the plasma clearance of chylomicrons and remnants. *Journal of Lipid Research* 37(12):2696–705, 1996.

Martinuzzi, A., L. Vergani, M. Rosa, C. Angelini. L-carnitine uptake in differentiating human cultured muscle. *Biochimica et Biophysica Acta* 1095:217–22, 1991 Nov 12.

Mataix, J. Recent findings in olive oil research. *European Journal of Clinical Nutrition* 47 Suppl 1:S82–4, 1993 Sep.

Mathieson, P.W. and D.K. Peters. Fat cell loss and mesangiocapillary glomerulonephritis: chicken, egg or both? *Nephron Clinical Practice* 96(2): c33–4, 2004.

Matkovic, V., J.Z. Ilich, M. Skugor, et al. Leptin is inversely related to age at menarche in human females. *Journal of Clinical Endocrinology and Metabolism* 82:3239–45, 1997 Oct.

Mattes, R.D. Fat preference and adherence to a reduced-fat diet. *American Journal of Clinical Nutrition* 57:373–81, 1993 Mar.

Mattison, J.A., et al. Calorie restriction in rhesus monkeys. *Experimental Gerontology* 38(1–2):35–46, 2003.

Mavri, A., M.C. Alessi, et al. Subcutaneous abdominal, but not femoral fat expression of plasminogen activator inhibitor-1 (PAI-1) is related to plasma PAI-1 levels and insulin resistance and decreases after weight loss. *Diabetologia Croatica* 44(11): 2025–31, 2001.

Mayo, M.J., J.R. Grantham, et al. Exercise-induced weight loss preferentially reduces abdominal fat. *Medicine & Science in Sports & Exercise* 35(2):207–13, 2003.

Mayser, P., U. Mrowietz, P. Arenberger, P. Bartak, J. Buchvald, E. Christophers, et al. Omega-3 fatty acid-based lipid infusion in patients with chronic plaque psoriasis: results of a double-blind, randomized, placebo controlled, multicenter trial. *Journal of the American Academy of Dermatology* 38(4):539–547, 1998.

McCarty, M.F. Anabolic effects of insulin on bone suggest a role for chromium picolinate in preservation of bone density. *Medical Hypotheses* 45:241–6, 1995 Sep.

McCarty, M.F. Optimizing exercise for fat loss. *Medical Hypotheses* 44(5):325–30, 1995.

McCarty, M.F. Pre-exercise administration of yohimbine may enhance the efficacy of exercise training as a fat loss strategy by boosting lipolysis. *Medical Hypotheses* 58(6): 491–5, 2002.

McCrory, M.A., P.J. Fuss, E. Saltzman, S.B. Roberts. Dietary determinants of energy intake and weight regulation in healthy adults. *Journal of Nutrition* 130(2S Suppl):276S–279S, 2000 Feb.

McGuffin M, Hobbs C, Upton R, et al. eds. *Botanical Safety Handbook*, Boca Raton, FL: CRC Press; 1997.

McGuire, M.T., Wing, R.R., Klem, M.L., Seagle, H.M., Hill, J.O. Long-term maintenance of weight loss: Do people who lose weight through various weight loss methods use different behaviors to maintain their weight? *International Journal of Obesity*, 1998, *22*, 572–577.

McGuire, M.T., Wing, R.R., Klem, M.L., Lang, W., Hill, J.O. What predicts weight regain among a group of successful weight losers? (1999). *Journal of Consulting and Clinical Psychology*, *67*, 177–185.

McLellan, T.M., I. Jacobs. Muscle glycogen utilization and the expression of relative exercise intensity. *International Journal of Sports Medicine* 12:21–6, 1991 Feb.

McManus, K., L. Antinoro, et al. A randomized controlled trial of a moderate-fat, low-energy diet compared with a low fat, low-energy diet for weight loss in overweight adults. *International Journal of Obesity and Related Metabolic Disorders* 25(10):1503–11, 2001.

Meckling, K.A., C. O'Sullivan, et al. Comparison of a low-fat diet to a low-carbohydrate diet on weight loss, body composition, and risk factors for diabetes and cardiovascular disease in free-living, overweight men and women. *Journal of Clinical Endocrinology and Metabolism* 89(6):2717–23, 2004.

Mee, J.F., O.F. KJ P. Reitsma, R. Mehra. Effect of a whey protein concentrate used as a colostrum substitute or supplement on calf immunity, weight gain, and health. *Journal of Dairy Science* 79:886–94, 1996 May.

Meezan, E., E. Meezan, J. Meezan, S. Manzella, L. Rodn. Alkylglycosides as artificial primers for glycogen biosynthesis. *Cell and Molecular Biology* (Noisy-le-grand), 43:369–81, 1997 May.

Mela, D.J., D.A. Sacchetti, Sensory preferences for fats: relationships with diet and body composition. *American Journal of Clinical Nutrition* 53:908–15, 1991 Apr.

Mela, D.J. Understanding fat preference and consumption: applications of behavioural sciences to a nutritional problem. *Proceedings of the Nutrition Society* 54:453–64, 1995 Jul.

Mengeaud, V., J.L. Nano, S. Fournel, P. Rampal. Effects of eicosapentaenoic acid, gamma-linolenic acid and prostaglandin El on three human colon carcinoma cell lines. Prostaglandins *Leukotrienes and Essential Fatty Acids* 47:313–9, 1992.

Menozzi, R., M. Bondi, et al. Resting metabolic rate, fat-free mass and catecholamine excretion during weight loss in female obese patients. *British Journal of Nutrition* 84(4): 515–20, 2000.

Mensink, R.P., M.J. de Groot, L.T. van den Broeke, A.P. Severijnen-Nobels, P.N. Demacker, M.B. Katan. Effects of monounsaturated fatty acids v complex carbohydrates on serum lipoproteins and apoproteins in healthy men and women. *Metabolism* 38: 172–8, 1989 Feb.

Mensink, R.P., M.B. Katan. An epidemiological and an experimental study on the effect of olive oil on total serum and HDL cholesterol in healthy volunteers. *European Journal of Clinical Nutrition* 43 Suppl 2:43–8, 1989.

Merry, B.J. Calorie restriction and age-related oxidative stress. *Annals of the New York Academy of Sciences* 908:180–98, 2000.

Merry, B.J. Molecular mechanisms linking calorie restriction and longevity. *International Journal of Biochemistry and Cell Biology* 34(11):1340–54, 2002.

Mertens, D.J., T. Kavanagh, et al. Exercise without dietary restriction as a means to long-term fat loss in the obese cardiac patient. *Journal of Sports Medicine and Physical Fitness* 38(4): 310–6, 1998.

Messina, M.J., V. Persky, K.D. Setchell, S. Barnes. Soy intake and cancer risk: a review of the in vitro and in vivo data. *Nutrition and Cancer* 21:113–31, 1994.

Metz, J.A. J.J. Anderson, P.N. Gallagher, Jr. Intakes of calcium, phosphorus, and protein, and physical-activity level are related to radial bone mass in young adult women [see comments]. *American Journal of Clinical Nutrition* 58:537–42, 1993 Oct.

Mikkelsen, P.B., S. Toubro, and A. Astrup. Effect of fat-reduced diets on 24-h energy expenditure: comparisons between animal protein, vegetable protein, and carbohydrate. *American Journal of Clinical Nutrition* 72(5):1135–41, 2000.

Milan, G., M. Granzotto, et al. Resistin and adiponectin expression in visceral fat of obese rats: effect of weight loss. *Obesity Research* 10(11): 1095–103.

Miller, C.C., C.A. McCreedy, A.D. Jones, V.A. Ziboh. Oxidative metabolism of dihomogammalinolenic acid by guinea pig epidermis: evidence of generation of anti-inflammatory products. *Prostaglandins* 35: 917–38, 1988 Jun.

Miller, J.B., E. Pang, and L. Bramall. Rice: a high or low glycemic index food? *American Journal of Clinical Nutrition* 56(6):1034–6, 1992.

Miraglia del, G.E., N. Santoro, et al. Inadequate leptin level negatively affects body fat loss during a weight reduction programme for childhood obesity. *Acta Paediatrica* 91(2):132–5, 2002.

Mirkin, G. Nuts do not prevent heart attacks [letter; comment]. *Archives of Internal Medicine* 153: 125, 1993 Jan 11.

Mitchell, E.A., M.G. Aman, S.H. Turbott, M. Manku. Clinical characteristics and serum essential fatty acid levels in hyperactive children. *Clinical Pediatrics (Phila)* 26:406–411, 1987.

Mitchell, S.L., L.H. Epstein. Changes in taste and satiety in dietary-restrained women following stress. *Physiology and Behavior* 60: 495–9, 1996 Aug.

Miyata, T., R. Kawai, S. Taketomi, S.M. Sprague. Possible involvement of advanced glycation end-products in bone resorption. *Nephrology Dialysis Transplantation* 11 (Suppl 5) 54–7, 1996.

Mizushima, S., E.H. Moriguchi, P. Ishikawa, et al. Fish intake and cardiovascular risk among middle-aged Japanese in Japan and Brazil. *Journal of Cardiovascular Risk* 4: 191–9, 1997 Jun.

Mizutani, H., et al. Calorie restriction prevents the occlusive coronary vascular disease of autoimmune (NNZW × BXSB) F1 mice. *Proceedings of the National Academy of Sciences USA* 91(10):4402–6, 1994.

Moeller, L.E., C.T. Peterson, et al. Isoflavone-rich soy protein prevents loss of hip lean mass but does not prevent the shift in regional fat distribution in perimenopausal women. *Menopause* 10(4):322–31, 2003.

Mohs, R.C., K.L. Davis, J.R. Tinklenberg, L.E. Hollister, J.A. Yesavage, B.S. Kopell. Choline chloride treatment of memory deficits in the elderly. *American Journal of Psychiatry* 136: 1275–7, 1979 Oct.

Mokdad, et al. The continuing epidemic of obesity in the United States. *JAMA* 284: 1650–51, 2000.

Montori, V.M., A. Farmer, P.C. Wollan, S.F. Dinneen. Fish oil supplementation in type 2 diabetes: a quantitative systematic review. *Diabetes Care* 23: 1407–15, 2000.

Moore, T.L., T.D. Weiss. Mediators of inflammation. *Seminars in Arthritis and Rheumatism* 14: 247–62, 1985 May.

Moriguti, J.C., E. Ferriolli, and J.S. Marchini. Urinary calcium loss in elderly men on a vegetable: animal (1:1) high-protein diet. *Gerontology* 45(5):274–8, 1999.

Morrison, L. Diet and coronary atherosclerosis. *JAMA* 173:884–8, 1960.

Moustafa, A.e.-H., I.H. Borai, and S. Shoukry. Effect of calorie restriction and protein deficiency on protein metabolism in rats. *Zeitschrift fur Ernahrungswissenschaft* 19(3):166–72, 1980.

Mueller-Cunningham, W.M., R. Quintana, et al. An ad libitum, very low-fat diet results in weight loss and changes in nutrient intakes in postmenopausal women. *Journal of the American Dietetic Association* 103(12):1600–6, 2003.

Mullan, I.M., E.E. Holton, Z.M. Vickers. Preference for and consumption of fat-free and full-fat cheese by children. *Journal of the American Dietetic Association* 96: 603–4, 1996 Jun.

Muller, C., E. Assimacopoulos-Jeannet, F. Mosimann, et al. Endogenous glucose production, gluconeogenesis and liver glycogen concentration in obese non-diabetic patients. *Diabetologia Croatica* 40: 463–8, 1997 Apr.

Mundy, G.R. Cytokines and growth factors in the regulation of bone remodeling. *Journal of Bone and Mineral Research* 8 (Suppl 2):S505–10, 1993 Dec.

Mura, C.V., et al. Effects of calorie restriction and aging on the expression of antioxidant enzymes and ubiquitin in the liver of Emory mice. *Mechanics of Ageing Development* 91(2):115–29, 1996.

Murdoch, S.J., S.E. Kahn, et al. PLTP activity decreases with weight loss: changes in PLTP are associated with changes in subcutaneous fat and FFA but not IAF or insulin sensitivity. *Journal of Lipid Research* 44(9):1705–12, 2003.

Muthukumar, A.R., et al. Calorie restriction decreases proinflammatory cytokines and polymeric Ig receptor expression in the submandibular glands of autoimmune prone (NZB × NZW)F1 mice. *Journal of Clinical Immunology* 20(5):354–61, 2000.

Mynarcik, D.C., M.A. McNurlan, et al. Association of severe insulin resistance with both loss of limb fat and elevated serum tumor necrosis factor receptor levels in HIV lipodystrophy. *Journal of Acquired Immune Deficiency Syndromes* 25(4):312–21, 2000.

Nagamatsu, M., K.K. Nickander, J.D. Schmelzer, et al. Lipoic acid improves nerve blood flow, reduces oxidative stress, and improves distal nerve conduction in experimental diabetic neuropathy. *Diabetes Care* 18: 1160–7, 1995 Aug.

Nakamura, E., et al. A strategy for identifying biomarkers of aging: further evaluation of hematology and blood chemistry data from a calorie restriction study in rhesus monkeys. *Experimental Gerontology* 33(5):421–43, 1998.

Nakamura, M., M. Tanaka, et al. Association between basal serum and leptin levels and changes in abdominal fat distribution during weight loss. *Journal of Atherosclerosis and Thrombosis* 6(1):28–32, 2000.

Nakamura, Y., et al., Egg consumption, serum cholesterol, and cause-specific and all-cause mortality: the National Integrated Project for Prospective Observation of Non-communicable Disease and Its Trends in the Aged, 1980 (NIPPON DATA80). *American Journal of Clinical Nutrition* 80(1):58–63, 2004.

Nakano, Y., et al. Calorie restriction reduced blood pressure in obesity hypertensives by improvement of autonomic nerve activity and insulin sensitivity. *Journal of Cardiovascular Pharmacology* 38 Suppl 1:S69–74, 2001.

Nakatani, A., D.H. Han, P.A. Hansen, et al. Effect of endurance exercise training on muscle glycogen supercompensation in rats. *Journal of Applied Physiology* 82:711–5, 1997 Feb.

Nakielny, S., D.G. Campbell, P. Cohen. The molecular mechanism by which adrenalin inhibits glycogen synthesis. *European Journal of Biochemistry* 199:713–22, 1991 Aug 1.

Nal, ecz K.A., ecz M.J. Nal. Carnitine—a known compound, a novel function in neural cells. *Acta Neurobiologice Experimentalis* (Warszawa) (Warsz), 56:597–609, 1996.

Nara, M., T. Kanda, et al. Reduction of leptin precedes fat loss from running exercise in insulin-resistant rats. *Experimental and Clinical Endocrinology and Diabetes* 107(7): 431–4, 1999.

Naranjo, W.M., et al. Protein calorie restriction affects nonhepatic IGF-I production and the lymphoid system: studies using the liver-specific IGF-I gene-deleted mouse model. *Endocrinology* 143(6):2233–41, 2002.

Narayanan, I., B. Singh, et al. Fat loss during feeding of human milk. *Archives of Disease in Childhood* 59(5):475–7, 1984.

Narisawa, T., Y. Fukaura, K. Yazawa, C. Ishikawa, Y. Isoda, Y. Nishizawa. Colon cancer prevention with a small amount of dietary perilla oil high in alpha-linolenic acid in an animal model. *Cancer* 73:2069–75, 1994.

Narisawa, T., M. Takahashi, H. Kotanagi, H. Kusaka, Y. Yamazaki, H. Koyama. Inhibitory effect of dietary perilla oil rich in the n-3 polyunsaturated fatty acid alpha-linolenic acid on colon carcinogenesis in rats. *Japanese Journal of Cancer Research* 82:1089–96, 1991.

Naughton, D.P., A.E. Fisher. Life extension properties of superoxide dismutase mimics arise from "Calorie Restriction". *Chemico-Biological Interactions* 10(3):197–8, 2003.

Neïchev, K., E. Slavcheva, L. Abrashev, P. Todorova, I. Mitov, D. Veselinova. [The immunomodulating properties of a glucomacropeptide from whey. I. The stimulation of resistance in mice]. *Acta Microbiologica Bulgarica* 25:54–61, 1990.

Nelson, R.G., M.L. Sievers, W.C. Knowler, et al. Low incidence of fatal coronary heart disease in Pima Indians despite high prevalence of non-insulin-dependent diabetes. *Circulation* 81:987–995, 1990.

Neoptolemos, J.P., D. Husband, C. Imray, S. Rowley, N. Lawson. Arachidonic acid and docosahexaenoic acid are increased in human colorectal cancer. *Gut* 32:278–81, 1991.

Nestel, P.J., S.E. Pomeroy, T. Sasahara, et al. Arterial compliance in obese subjects is improved with dietary plant n-3 fatty acid from flaxseed oil despite increased LDL oxidizability. *Arteriosclerosis Thrombosis and Vascular Biology* 17(6)1163–1170, 1997 Jul.

Nettleton, J.A. Are n-3 fatty acids essential nutrients for fetal and infant development? *Journal of the American Dietetic Association* 93:58–64, 1993 Jan.

Nettleton, J.A. Omega-3 fatty acids: comparison of plant and seafood sources in human nutrition. *Journal of the American Dietetic Association* 91:331–7, 1991 Mar.

Nettleton, J.A., D.M. Hegsted. The effects of protein and calorie restriction on tissue nitrogen content and protein catabolism. *Nutrition and Metabolism* 17(3):166–80, 1974.

Newberne, P.M., A.E. Rogers. The role of nutrients in cancer causation. *Princess Takamatsu Symposium* 16:205–22, 1985.

Newcomer, L.M., I.B. King, K.G. Wicklund, J.L. Stanford. The association of fatty acids with prostate cancer risk. *Prostate Journal* 47(4):262–268, 2001.

Newmark, H.L., M. Lipkin. Calcium, vitamin D, and colon cancer. *Cancer Research* 52:2067s–2070s, 1992.

Nicklas, B.J., E.M. Rogus, A.P. Goldberg. Exercise blunts declines in lipolysis and fat oxidation after dietary-induced weight loss in obese older women. *American Journal of Physiology* 273:E149–55, 1997 Jul.

Nicklas, B.J., E.M. Rogus, et al. Exercise blunts declines in lipolysis and fat oxidation after dietary-induced weight loss in obese older women. *American Journal of Physiology* 273(1 Pt 1):E149–55, 1997.

Nindl, B.C., K.E. Friedl, et al. Regional fat placement in physically fit males and changes with weight loss. *Medicine & Science in Sports & Exercise* 28(7): 786–93, 1996.

Niskanen, L.K., S. Haffner, et al. Serum leptin in obesity is related to gender and body fat topography but does not predict successful weight loss. *European Journal of Endocrinology* 137(1):61–7, 1997.

Nissen, S., J.C. Fuller, Jr., J. Sell, P.R. Ferket, D.V. Rives. The effect of beta-hydroxy-beta-methylbutyrate on growth, mortality, and carcass qualities of broiler chickens. *Poultry Science Journal* 73:137–55, 1994 Jan.

Nissen, S., R. Sharp, M. Ray, et al. Effect of leucine metabolite beta-hydroxy-beta-methylbutyrate on muscle metabolism during resistance-exercise training. *Journal of Applied Physiology* 81:2095–104, 1996 Nov.

Nordestgaard, B.G., A. Tybjaerg-Hansen. IDL, VLDL, chylomicrons and atherosclerosis. *European Journal of Epidemiology* 8 Suppl 1:92–8, 1992.

Nordheim, K., V.I. NK. Glycogen and lactate metabolism during low-intensity exercise in man. *Acta Physiologica Scandinavia* 139:475–84, 1990 Jul.

Obin, M., et al. Calorie restriction increases light-dependent photoreceptor cell loss in the neural retina of fischer 344 rats. *Neurobiology of Aging* 21(5):639–45, 2000.

Obin, M., et al. Calorie restriction modulates age-dependent changes in the retinas of Brown Norway rats. *Mechanics of Ageing Development* 114(2):133–47, 2000.

O'Brien, T., T.T. Nguyen, J. Buithieu, B.A. Kottke. Lipoprotein compositional changes in the fasting and postprandial state on a high-carbohydrate low-fat and a high-fat diet in subjects with noninsulin-dependent diabetes mellitus. *Journal of Clinical Endocrinology & Metabolism* 77:1345–51, 1993 Nov.

Obstetrics & Gynecology 94:395–398, 1999; and, *American Journal of Public Health* 86:195–199, 1999.

O'Dea, K., A.J. Sinclair. Increased proportion of arachidonic acid in plasma lipids after 2 weeks on a diet of tropical seafood. *American Journal of Clinical Nutrition* 36:868–72, 1982 Nov.

O'Dea, K., A.J. Sinclair. The effects of low-fat diets rich in arachidonic acid on the composition of plasma fatty acids and bleeding time in Australian aborigines. *Journal of Nutritional Science and Vitaminology* (Tokyo) 31:441–53, 1985 Aug.

O'Dea, K., R.M. Spargo, Metabolic adaptation to a low carbohydrate-high protein ('traditional') diet in Australian Aborigines. *Diabetologia Croatica* 23:494–8, 1982 Dec.

Odent, M. Land food . . . sea food . . . brain food. *Midwifery Today Childbirth Education* 18–20, 1996 Winter.

Odland, L.M., G.I. Heigenhauser, D. Wong, M.G. Hollidge-Horvat, L.L. Spriet. Effects of increased fat availability on fat-carbohydrate interaction during prolonged exercise in men. *American Journal of Physiology* 274:R894–902, 1998 Apr.

O'Hara, W., C. Allen, R.J. Shephard. Loss of body fat during an arctic winter expedition. *Canadian Journal of Physiology and Pharmacology* 55:1235–41, 1977 Dec.

O'Hara, W., C. Allen, R.J. Shephard. Treatment of obesity by exercise in the cold. *Canadian Medical Association Journal* 117:773–8, 786, 1977 Oct 8.

Ohisalo, J.J., J.M. Kaartinen, et al. Weight loss normalizes the inhibitory effect of N6-(phenylisopropyl) adenosine on lipolysis in fat cells of massively obese human subjects. *Clinical Science (Lond)* 83(5):589–92, 1992.

Okamoto, M., F. Misunobu, K. Ashida, T. Mifune, Y. Hosaki, H. Tsugeno, et al. Effects of perilla seed oil supplementation on leukotriene generation by leucocytes in patients with asthma associated with lipometabolism. *International Archives of Allergy and Immunology* 122(2):137–142, 2000.

Okamoto, M. F. Misunobu, K. Ashida, T. Mifune, Y. Hosaki, H. Tsugeno, et al. Effects of dietary supplementation with n-3 fatty acids compared with n-6 fatty acids on bronchial asthma. *Internal Medicine* 39(2): 107–111, 2000.

Okita, M., A. Watanabe, and H. Nagashima. A vegetable protein-rich diet for the treatment of liver cirrhosis. *Acta Medicinae Okayama* 39(1):59–65, 1985.

Ornish, D., L.W. Scherwitz, J.H. Billings, et al. Intensive lifestyle changes for reversal of coronary heart disease. *JAMA* 280:2001–7, 1998.

Ornish, D.M., K.L. Lee, W.R. Fair, E.B. Pettengill, P.R. Carroll. Dietary trial in prostate cancer: early experience and implications for clinical trial design. *Urology* 57(4 Suppl 1):200–1 2001.

Orth, M., C. Luley, H. Wieland. Effects of VLDL, chylomicrons, and chylomicron remnants on platelet aggregability. *Thrombosis Research* 79(3):297–305, 1995.

Packard, P.T., R.R. Recker. Caffeine does not affect the rate of gain in spine bone in young women. *Osteoporosis International* 6:149–52, 1996.

Pagliacci, M.C., M. Smacchia, G. Migliorati, F. Grignani, C. Riccardi, Nicoletti. Growth-inhibitory effects of the natural phyto-oestrogen genistein in MCF-7 human breast cancer cells. *European Journal of Cancer* 30A 11:1675–82, 1994.

Pagnan, A., R. Corrocher, G.B. Ambrosio, et al. Effects of an olive-oil-rich diet on erythrocyte membrane lipid composition and cation transport systems. *Clinical Science* 76:87–93, 1989 Jan.

Pahlavani, M.A., et al. Melatonin fails to modulate immune parameters influenced by calorie restriction in aging Fischer 344 rats. *Experimental Biology and Medicine (Maywood)* 227(3):201–7, 2002.

Palli, D., A. Decarli, F. Cipriani, D. Forman, D. Amadori. Plasma pepsinogens, nutrients, and diet in areas of Italy at varying gastric cancer risk. *Cancer Epidemiology Biomarkers and Prevention* 1:45–50, 1991.

Pan, X.M., et al. Exposure to cigarette smoke delays the plasma clearance of chylomicrons and chylomicron remnants in rats. *American Journal of Physiology* 273(1 Pt 1):G158–63, 1997.

Pandalai, P.K., M.J. Pilat, K. Yamazaki, H. Naik, K.J. Pienta. The effects of omega-3 and omega-6 fatty acids on in vitro prostate cancer growth. *Anticancer Research* 16:815–20, 1996.

Papet, I., P. Ostaszewski, F. Glomot, et al. The effect of a high dose of 3-hydroxy-3-methylbutyrate on protein metabolism in growing lambs. *British Journal of Nutrition* 77:885–96, 1997 Jun.

Pariza, M.W. Calorie restriction, ad libitum feeding, and cancer. *Proceedings of the Society for Experimental Biology and Medicine* 183(3):293–8, 1986.

Pariza, M.W. Dietary fat, calorie restriction, ad libitum feeding, and cancer risk. *Nutrition Review* 45(1):1–7, 1987.

Parker, B., M. Noakes, et al. Effect of a high-protein, high-monounsaturated fat weight loss diet on glycemic control and lipid levels in type 2 diabetes. *Diabetes Care* 25(3):425–30, 2002.

Parks, E.J., J.B. German, P.A. Davis, et al. Reduced oxidative susceptibility of LDL from patients participating in an intensive atherosclerosis treatment program. *American Journal of Clinical Nutrition* 69:778–85, 1998.

Pascale, R.W., R.R. Wing, et al. Effects of a behavioral weight loss program stressing calorie restriction versus calorie plus fat restriction in obese individuals with NIDDM or a family history of diabetes. *Diabetes Care* 18(9):1241–8, 1995.

Pasman, W.J., M.A. van Baak, A.E. Jeukendrup, A. de Haan. The effect of different dosages of caffeine on endurance performance time. *International Journal of Sports Medicine* 16:225–30, 1995 May.

Pasquali, R., F. Casimirri, et al. Body fat distribution and weight loss in obese women. *American Journal of Clinical Nutrition* 49(1):185–7, 1989.

Pathophysiological consequences of magnesium deficit in the elderly. *Magnesium Research* 6(4):379–94, 1993.

Payne, A.M., S.L. Dodd, C. Leeuwenburgh. Life-long calorie restriction in Fischer 344 rats attenuates age-related loss in skeletal muscle-specific force and reduces extracellular space. *Journal of Applied Physiology* 95(6):2554–62, 2003.

Peak, M., M. al-Habori, L. Agius. Regulation of glycogen synthesis and glycolysis by insulin, pH and cell volume. Interactions between swelling and alkalinization in mediating the effects of insulin. *Biochemistry Journal* 282 (Pt 3):797–805, 1992 Mar 15.

Peebles, E.D., T. Pansky, et al. Effects of dietary fat and eggshell cuticle removal on egg water loss and embryo growth in broiler hatching eggs. *Poultry Science Journal* 77(10):1522–30, 1998.

Pelkman, C.L., V.K. Fishell, et al. Effects of moderate-fat (from monounsaturated fat) and low-fat weight-loss diets on the serum lipid profile in overweight and obese men and women. *American Journal of Clinical Nutrition* 79(2):204–12, 2004.

Perez, C., F. Lucas, A. Sclafani. Carbohydrate, fat, and protein condition similar flavor preferences in rats using an oral-delay procedure. *Physiology and Behavior* 57:549–54, 1995 Mar.

Perez-Jimenez, F., A. Espino, F. Lopez-Segura, et al. Lipoprotein concentrations in normolipidemic males consuming oleic acid-rich diets from two different sources: olive oil and oleic acid-rich sunflower oil. *American Journal of Clinical Nutrition* 62:769–75, 1995 Oct.

Perkins, S.N., et al. Calorie restriction reduces ulcerative dermatitis and infection-related mortality in p53-deficient and wild-type mice. *Journal of Investigative Dermatology* 111(2):292–6, 1998.

Peters Futre, E.M., T.D. Noakes, R.I. Raine, S.E. Terblanche. Muscle glycogen repletion during active postexercise recovery. *American Journal of Physiology* 253:E305–11, 1987 Sep.

Peterson, G., S. Barnes. Genistein inhibits both estrogen and growth factor-stimulated proliferation of human breast cancer cells. *Cell Growth and Differentiation* 7:1345–51, 1996.

Petrakis, N.L., S. Barnes, E.B. King, et al. Stimulatory influence of soy protein isolate on breast secretion in pre- and postmenopausal women. *Cancer Epidemiology Biomarkers and Prevention* 5:785–94, 1996.

Petroni, A., M. Blasevich, M. Salami, N. Papini, G.E. Montedoro, C. Galli. Inhibition of platelet aggregation and eicosanoid production by phenolic components of olive oil. *Thrombosis Research* 78:151–60, 1995 Apr 15.

Petroni, A., M. Blasevich, M. Salami, M. Servili, G.E. Montedoro, C. Galli. A phenolic antioxidant extracted from olive oil inhibits platelet aggregation and arachidonic acid metabolism in vitro. *World Review of Nutrition and Dietetics* 75:169–72, 1994.

Phinney, S.D., B.R. Bistrian, R.R. Wolfe, G.L. Blackburn. The human metabolic response to chronic ketosis without caloric restriction: physical and biochemical adaptation. *Metabolism* 32:757–68, 1983 Aug.

Piatti, P.M., F. Monti, I. Fermo, et al. Hypocaloric high-protein diet improves glucose oxidation and spares lean body mass: comparison to hypocaloric high-carbohydrate diet. *Metabolism* 43:1481–7, 1994 Dec.

Pinckard, R.N. The "new" chemical mediators of inflammation. *Monographs in Pathology* 38–53, 1982.

Pirozzo, S. and P. Glasziou. Weight loss. The role of low fat diets. *Australian Family Physician* 29(6):566–9, 2000.

Pitsikas, N. and S. Algeri. Deterioration of spatial and nonspatial reference and working memory in aged rats: protective effect of life-long calorie restriction. *Neurobiology of Aging* 13(3):369–73, 1992.

Pocino, M., L. Baute, and I. Malave. Calorie restriction modifies the delayed-type hypersensitivity response to the hapten trinitrobenzenesulfonic acid and to hapten-modified syngeneic spleen cells. *Cellular Immunology* 109(2):261–71, 1987.

Poetschke, H.L., et al. Effects of calorie restriction on thymocyte growth, death and maturation. *Carcinogenesis* 21(11):1959–64, 2000.

Poirier, P., C. Catellier, et al. Role of body fat loss in the exercise-induced improvement of the plasma lipid profile in non-insulin-dependent diabetes mellitus. *Metabolism* 45(11): 1383–7, 1996.

Popkess-Vawter, S. and J. Turner. Beyond calories and fat grams: am I deserving of successful weight loss? *Nutrition* 17(4):362–3, 2001.

Potter, S.M. Soy protein and serum lipids. *Current Opinions in Lipidology* 7:260–4, 1996.

Powell, D.M., et al. Effect of short-term feed restriction and calorie source on hormonal and metabolic responses in geldings receiving a small meal. *Journal of Animal Science* 78(12): 3107–13, 2000.

Powell, J.J., et al. The effects of different percentages of dietary fat intake, exercise, and calorie restriction on body composition and body weight in obese females. *American Journal of Health Promotion* 8(6):442–8, 1994.

Powers, S.K., D. Criswell. Adaptive strategies of respiratory muscles in response to endurance exercise. *Medicine & Science in Sports & Exercise* 28:1115–22, 1996 Sep.

Poynten, A.M., T.P. Markovic, et al. Fat oxidation, body composition and insulin sensitivity in diabetic and normoglycaemic obese adults 5 years after weight loss. *International Journal of Obesity and Related Metabolic Disorders* 27(10):1212–8, 2003.

Prasad, C., A.J. delaHoussaye, A. Prasad, H. Mizuma. Augmentation of dietary fat preference by chronic, but not acute, hypercorticosteronemia. *Life Sciences* 56:1361–71, 1995 Mar 10.

Prasad, K. Dietary flaxseed in prevention of hypercholesterolemic atherosclerosis. *Atherosclerosis* 132(1):69–76, 1997.

Preisinger, E., G. Leitner, E. Uher, et al. [Nutrition and osteoporosis: a nutritional analysis of women in postmenopause]. *Wien Klinische Wochenschrift* 107:418–22, 1995.

Prestamo, G., et al. Soybean vegetable protein (Tofu) preserved with high pressure *Journal of Agricultural and Food Chemistry* 48(7):2943–7, 2000.

Prior, J.C., S.I. Barr, R. Chow, R.A. Faulkner. Prevention and management of osteoporosis: consensus statements from the Scientific Advisory Board of the Osteoporosis Society of Canada. 5. Physical activity as therapy for osteoporosis. *Canadian Medical Association Journal* 155:940–4, 1996 Oct 1.

Prisco, D, R. Paniccia, B. Bandinelli, et al. Effect of medium term supplementation with a moderate dose of n–3 polyunsaturated fatty acid on blood pressure in mild hypertensive patients. *Thrombosis Research* 91:105–112, 1998.

Pritchard, R.S., J.A. Baron, M. Gerhardsson de Verdier. Dietary calcium, vitamin D, and the rissk of colorectal cancer in Stockholm, Sweden. *Cancer Epidemiology, Biomarkers & Prevention* 5:897–900, 1996.

Purasiri, P., A. Murray, S. Richardson, S.D. Heys, D. Horrobin, O. Eremin. Modulation of cytokine production in vivo by dietary essential fatty acids in patients with colorectal cancer. *Clinical Science* 87:711–7, 1994.

Purnell, J.Q., S.E. Kahn, et al. Effect of weight loss with reduction of intra-abdominal fat on lipid metabolism in older men. *Journal of Clinical Endocrinology and Metabolism* 85(3): 977–82, 2000.

Quinn, M., et al. Nitrogen, water and electrolyte metabolism on protein and protein-free low-calorie diets in man. I. Water restriction. *Metabolism* 3(1):49–67, 1954.

Raben, A., B. Kiens, E.A. Richter, et al. Serum sex hormones and endurance performance after a lacto-ovo vegetarian and a mixed diet. *Medicine & Science in Sports & Exercise* 24:1290–7, 1992 Nov.

Raben, A., N.D. Jensen, et al. Spontaneous weight loss during 11 weeks' ad libitum intake of a low fat/high fiber diet in young, normal weight subjects. *International Journal of Obesity and Related Metabolic Disorders* 19(12):916–23. 1995.

Raines, E.W., R. Ross. Biology of atherosclerotic plaque formation: possible role of growth factors in lesion development and the potential impact of soy. *Journal of Nutrition* 125:624S–630S, 1995.

Rains, T.M., N.F. Shay. Zinc status specifically changes preferences for carbohydrate and protein in rats selecting from separate carbohydrate-, protein-, and fat-containing diets. *Journal of Nutrition* 125:2874–9, 1995 Nov.

Rainwater, D.L., B.D. Mitchell, A.G. Comuzzie, S.M. Haffner. Relationship of low-density lipoprotein particle size and measures of adiposity. *International Journal of Obesity and Related Metabolic Disorders* 23:180–9, 1999.

Rao, G.N. Influence of diet on tumors of hormonal tissues. *Progress in Clinical and Biological Research* 394:41–56, 1996.

Rao, K.S., Dietary calorie restriction, DNA-repair and brain aging. *Molecular and Cellular Biochemistry* 253(1–2):313–8, 2003.

Rao, M.N., A.B. Morrison, Evaluation of protein in foods. XII. Effects of calorie restriction. *Canadian Journal of Biochemistry* 44(10):1365–75, 1966.

Rasmussen, O., F.F. Lauszus, C. Christiansen, C. Thomsen, K. Hermansen. Differential effects of saturated and monounsaturated fat on blood glucose and insulin responses in subjects with non-insulin-dependent diabetes mellitus. *American Journal of Clinical Nutrition* 63:249–53, 1996 Feb.

Rasmussen, O.W., C. Thomsen, K.W. Hansen, M. Vesterlund, E. Winther, K. Hermansen. Effects on blood pressure, glucose, and lipid levels of a high-monounsaturated fat diet compared with a high-carbohydrate diet in NIDDM subjects. *Diabetes Care* 16:1565–71, 1993 Dec.

Rattan, S.I., et al. Dietary calorie restriction does not affect the levels of protein elongation factors in rat livers during ageing. *Mechanics of Ageing Development* 58(1):85–91, 1991.

Ready, A.E. B. Naimark, J. Ducas, et al. Influence of walking volume on health benefits in women post-menopause. *Medicine & Science in Sports & Exercise* 28:1097–105, 1996 Sep.

Reddy, S.T., C.Y. Wang, K. Sakhaee, I. Brinkley, C.Y. Pak. Effect of low-carbohydrate high-protein diets on acid-base balance, stone-forming propensity, and calcium metabolism. *American Journal of Kidney Disease* 40: 265–74, 2002.

Reddy, B.S., J.R. Pleasants, B.S. Wostmann. Effect of protein-calorie restriction on brain amino acid pool in neonatal rats. *Proceedings of the Society for Experimental Biology and Medicine* 136(3): 949–53, 1971.

Reichmann, H., N. van Lindeneiner. Carnitine analysis in normal human red blood cells, plasma, and muscle tissue. *European Neurology* 34:40–3, 1994.

Reinli, K., G. Block. Phytoestrogen content of foods—a compendium of literature values. *Nutrition and Cancer* 26:123–48, 1996.

Remesar, X., P. Guijarro, et al. Oral oleoyl-estrone induces the rapid loss of body fat in Zucker lean rats fed a hyperlipidic diet. *International Journal of Obesity and Related Metabolic Disorders* 24(11): 1405–12, 2000.

Ren, J.M. S. Broberg, K. Sahlin, E. Hultman. Influence of reduced glycogen level on glycogenolysis during short-term stimulation in man. *Acta Physiological Scandinavia* 139:467–74, 1990 Jul.

Richardson, A.J., B.K. Puri. The potential role of fatty acids in attention-deficit/hyperactivity disorder. *Prostaglandins Leukotrienes and Essential Fatty Acids* 63(½):79–87, 2000.

Richter, F., H.L. Newmark, A. Richter, D. Leung, M. Lipkin. Inhibition of Western-diet induced hyperproliferation and hyperplasia in mouse colon by two sources of calcium. *Carcinogenesis* 16:2685–9, 1995.

Ricketts, C.D. Fat preferences, dietary fat intake and body composition in children. *European Journal of Clinical Nutrition* 51:778–81, 1997 Nov.

Rico, H., P. Relea, R. Crespo, et al. Biochemical markers of nutrition in type-I and type-II osteoporosis. *Journal of Bone and Joint Surgery* (British Volume) 77:148–51, 1995 Jan.

Rissanen, P., S. Makimattila, et al. Effect of weight loss and regional fat distribution on plasma leptin concentration in obese women. *International Journal of Obesity and Related Metabolic Disorders* 23(6):645–9, 1999.

Robertson, T.L., H. Kato, G.G. Rhoads, et al. Epidemiologic studies of coronary heart disease and stroke in Japanese men living in Japan, Hawaii and California. Incidence of myocardial infarction and death from coronary heart disease. *American Journal of Cardiology* 39:239–43, 1977 Feb.

Robinson, D.R. Prostaglandins and the mechanism of action of anti-inflammatory drugs. *American Journal of Medicine* 75:26–31, 1983 Oct 31.

Roche, H.M., A. Zampelas, J.M. Knapper, et al. Effect of long-term olive oil dietary intervention on postprandial triacylglycerol and factor VII metabolism. *American Journal of Clinical Nutrition* 68:552–60, 1998 Sep.

Rock, C.L., C. Thomson, et al. Reduction in fat intake is not associated with weight loss in most women after breast cancer diagnosis: evidence from a randomized controlled trial. *Cancer* 91(1):25–34, 2001.

Rockwood, G.A., S.J. Bhathena. High-fat diet preference in developing and adult rats. *Physiology and Behavior* 48:79–82, 1990 Jul.

Rohan, T.E., G.R. Howe, J.D. Burch, M. Jain. Dietary factors and risk of prostate cancer: a case-control study in Ontario, Canada. *Cancer Causes and Control* 6:145–54, 1995.

Rolls, B.J., D.L. Miller. Is the low-fat message giving people a license to eat more? *Journal of the American College of Nutrition* 16:535–43, 1997 Dec.

Rolls, B.J. and E.A. Bell. Intake of fat and carbohydrate: role of energy density. *European Journal of Clinical Nutrition* 53(Suppl 1):S166–73, 1999.

Rose, D.P., L.A. Cohen. Effects of dietary menhaden oil and retinyl acetate on the growth of DU 145 human prostatic adenocarcinoma cells transplanted into athymic nude mice. *Carcinogenesis* 9:603–5, 1988.

Rose, D.P., J.M. Connolly, X.H. Liu. Effects of linoleic acid and gamma-linolenic acid on the growth and. 1995.

Rose, D.P., J.M. Connolly, J. Rayburn, M. Coleman. Influence of diets containing eicosapentaenoic or docosahexaenoic acid on. 1995.

Rose, D.P., M.A. Hatala. Dietary fatty acids and breast cancer invasion and metastasis. 1994.

Rosen, C.J., L.R. Donahue, S.J. Hunter. Insulin-like growth factors and bone: the osteoporosis connection. *Proceedings of the Society for Experimental Biology and Medicine* 206:83–102, 1994 Jun.

Rosen, J.C., J. Gross, D. Loew, E.A. Sims. Mood and appetite during minimal-carbohydrate and carbohydrate-supplemented hypocaloric diets. *American Journal of Clinical Nutrition* 42:371–9, 1985 Sep.

Ross, R., L Le, E.B. Marliss, D.V. Morris, R. Gougeon. Adipose tissue distribution changes during rapid weight loss in obese adults. *International Journal of Obesity* 15:733–9, 1991 Nov.

Ross, R.K., H. Shimizu, A. Paganini-Hill, G. Honda, B.E. Henderson. Case-control studies of prostate cancer in blacks and whites in southern California. *Journal of the National Cancer Institute* 78:869–74, 1974.

Ross, R., I. Janssen. Is abdominal fat preferentially reduced in response to exercise-induced weight loss? *Medicine and Science in Sports and Exercise* 31(11 Suppl):S568–72, 1999.

Roth, E. Oxygen free radicals and their clinical implications. *Acta Chirurgica Hungarica* 36:302–5, 1997.

Roth, G.S., D.K. Ingram, M.A. Lane. Calorie restriction in primates: will it work and how will we know? *Journal of the American Geriatrics Society* 47(7):896–903, 1999.

Roubenoff, R. Sarcopenic obesity: does muscle loss cause fat gain? Lessons from rheumatoid arthritis and osteoarthritis. *Annals of the New York Academy of Sciences* 904:553–7, 2000.

Roust, L.R., B.A. Kottke, M.D. Jensen. Serum lipid responses to a eucaloric high-complex carbohydrate diet in different obesity phenotypes. *Mayo Clinic Proceedings* 69:930–6, 1994 Oct.

Rudolf, M.C, R.S. Sherwin. Maternal ketosis and its effects on the fetus. *Clinical Endocrinology & Metabolism* 12:413–28, 1983 Jul.

Ruiz-Gutierrez, V., N. Morgado, J.L. Prada, F Pe-Je, F.J. Muriana. Composition of human VLDL triacylglycerols after ingestion of olive oil and high oleic sunflower oil. *Journal of Nutrition* 128:570–6, 1998 Mar.

Russell, S.T., T.P. Zimmerman, et al. "Induction of lipolysis in vitro and loss of body fat in vivo by zinc-alpha2-glycoprotein." *Biochimica et Biophysica Acta* 1636(1):59–68, 2004.

Ryan, A.S., R.E. Pratley, D. Elahi, A.P. Goldberg. Resistive training increases fat-free mass and maintains RMR despite weight loss in postmenopausal women. *Journal of Applied Physiology* 79:818–23, 1995 Sep.

Ryan, A.S., R.E. Pratley, A.P. Goldberg, D. Elahi. Resistive training increases insulin action in postmenopausal women. *Journals of Gerontology Series A: Biological Sciences and Medical Sciences* 51:M199–205, 1996 Sep.

Ryan, A.S., R.E. Pratley, et al. Resistive training increases fat-free mass and maintains RMR despite weight loss in postmenopausal women. *Journal of Applied Physiology* 79(3):818–23, 1995.

Saad, M.E., S. Lillioja, B.L. Nyomba, C. Castillo, R. Ferraro, M. De Gregorio. Racial differences in the relation between blood pressure and insulin resistance. *New England Journal of Medicine* 324:733–9, 1991.

Safer, D.J. Diet, behavior modification, and exercise: a review of obesity treatments from a long-term perspective. *Southern Medical Journal* 84:1470–4, 1991 Dec.

Sahlin, K. Muscle carnitine metabolism during incremental dynamic exercise in humans. *Acta Physiological Scandinavia* 138:259–62, 1990 Mar.

Saitoh, S., T. Matsuo, K. Tagami, H. Chang, K. Tokuyama, M. Suzuki. Effects of short-term dietary change from high fat to high carbohydrate diets on the storage and utilization of glycogen and triacylglycerol in untrained rats. *European Journal of Applied Physiology* 74:13–22, 1996.

Saldanha Aoki, M., A.L. Rodriguez Amaral Almeida, et al. Carnitine supplementation fails to maximize fat mass loss induced by endurance training in rats. *Annals of Nutrition and Metabolism* 48(2):90–4, 2004.

Saltzman, E., The low glycemic index diet: not yet ready for prime time. *Nutrition Review* 57(9 Pt 1):297, 1999.

Salyers, A.A., J.F. Sperry, T.D. Wilkins, A.R. Walker, N.J. Richardson. Neutral steroid concentrations in the faeces of North American White and South African Black populations at different risks for cancer of the colon. SBM. *South African Medical Journal* 51:823–7, 1977.

Samuelsson, B. An elucidation of the arachidonic acid cascade. Discovery of prostaglandins, thromboxane and leukotrienes. *Drugs* 33 Suppl 1:2–9, 1987.

Samuelsson, B. Arachidonic acid metabolism: role in inflammation. *Zeitschrift fur Rheumatologic* 50 Suppl 1:3–6, 1991.

Samuelsson, B. Leukotrienes: a new class of mediators of immediate hypersensitivity reactions and inflammation. *Advanced Prostaglandin Thromboxane Leukotiene Research* 11:1–13, 1983.

Sanchez, C.J., E. Hooper, P.J. Garry, J.M. Goodwin, J.S. Goodwin. The relationship between dietary intake of choline, choline serum levels, and cognitive function in healthy elderly persons. *Journal of the American Geriatrics Society* 32:208–12, 1984 Mar.

Santos, M.S., A.H. Lichtenstein, et al. Immunological effects of low-fat diets with and without weight loss. *Journal of the American College of Nutrition* 22(2):174–82, 2003.

Sarwar, G., The protein efficiency ratios of animal: vegetable protein mixtures. *Journal of Nutrition* 126(9):2278–9, 1996.

346 Bibliography

Satabin, P., B. Bois-Joyeux, M. Chanez, C.Y. Guezennec, J. Peret. Post-exercise glycogen resynthesis in trained high-protein or high-fat-fed rats after glucose feeding. *European Journal of Applied Physiology* 58:591–5, 1989.
Sauer, L.A., R.T. Dauchy. The effect of omega-6 and omega-3 fatty acids on 3H-thymidine incorporation in hepatoma 7288CTC perfused in situ. *British Journal of Cancer* 66:297–303, 1992.
Scally, M.C., A. Hodge. A report of hypothyroidism induced by an over-the-counter fat loss supplement (Tiratricol). *International Journal of Sport Nutrition and Exercise Metabolism* 13(1):112–6, 2003.
Schürch, M.A., R. Rizzoli, D. Slosman, L. Vadas, P. Vergnaud, J.P. Bonjour. Protein supplements increase serum insulin-like growth factor-I levels and attenuate proximal femur bone loss in patients with recent hip fracture. A randomized, double-blind, placebo-controlled trial. *Annals of Internal Medicine* 128:801–9, 1998 May 15.
Schaefer, E.J., A.H. Lichtenstein, S., Lamon-Fava, et al. Body weight and low-density lipoprotein cholesterol changes after consumption of a low-fat ad libitum diet [see comments]. *JAMA* 274:1450–5, 1995 Nov 8.
Schaefer, E.J., A.H. Lichtenstein, S. Lamon-Fava, et al. Body weight and low-density lipoprotein cholesterol changes after consumption of a low-fat ad libitum diet. *JAMA* 274:1450–5, 1995.
Schmolke, G. [Leukotrienes]. *Medizinische Monatsschrift für Pharmazeuten* 14:226–8, 1991 Aug.
Schooff, M. Are low-fat diets better than other weight-reducing diets in achieving long-term weight loss? *American Family Physician* 67(3):507–8, 2003.
Schröder, J.M. Inflammatory mediators and chemoattractants. *Clinical Dermatology* 13:137–50, 1995 Mar–Apr.
Schutz, Y., J.P. Flatt, E. Je. Failure of dietary fat intake to promote fat oxidation: a factor favoring the development of obesity [see comments]. *American Journal of Clinical Nutrition* 50:307–14, 1989 Aug.
Schwartz, M.W., J.D. Brunzell. Regulation of body adiposity and the problem of obesity. *Arteriosclerosis Thrombosis and Vascular Biology* 17:233–8, 1997.
Sclafani, A., K. Ackroff. Deprivation alters rats' flavor preferences for carbohydrates and fats. *Physiology and Behavior* 53:1091–9, 1993 Jun.
Scrofano, M.M., et al. Aging, calorie restriction and ubiquitin-dependent proteolysis in the livers of Emory mice. *Mechanisms of Ageing and Development* 101(3):277–96, 1998.
Scrofano, M.M., et al. The effects of aging and calorie restriction on plasma nutrient levels in male and female Emory mice. *Mechanisms of Ageing and Development* 105(1–2):31–44, 1998.
Sebastian, A., et al. Dietary ratio of animal to vegetable protein and rate of bone loss and risk of fracture in postmenopausal women. *American Journal of Clinical Nutrition* 74(3):411–2, 2001.
Sellmeyer, D.E., et al. A high ratio of dietary animal to vegetable protein increases the rate of bone loss and the risk of fracture in postmenopausal women. Study of Osteoporotic Fractures Research Group. *American Journal of Clinical Nutrition* 73(1):118–22, 2001.
Serra, F, G.P. Diaspri, A. Gasbarrini, et al. [Effect of CDP-choline on senile mental deterioration. Multicenter experience on 237 cases]. *Minerva Medica* 81:465–70, 1990 Jun.
Shapses, S.A., S. Heshka, et al. Effect of calcium supplementation on weight and fat loss in women. *Journal of Clinical Endocrinology and Metabolism* 89(2):632–7, 2004.
Sharman, M.J., J.S. Volek. Weight loss leads to reductions in inflammatory biomarkers after a very low-carbohydrate and low-fat diet in overweight men. *Clinical Science* (Lond), 2004.
Shephard, R.J. Physical activity and reduction of health risks: how far are the benefits independent of fat loss? *Journal of Sports Medicine and Physical Fitness* 34(1):91–8, 1994.

Sheppard, L., A.R. Kristal, et al. Weight loss in women participating in a randomized trial of low-fat diets. *American Journal of Clinical Nutrition* 54(5):821–8, 1991.

Shi, X., C.V. Gisolfi. Fluid and carbohydrate replacement during intermittent exercise. *Sports Medicine* 25:157–172, 1998.

Shick, S.M., R.R. Wing, et al. Persons successful at long-term weight loss and maintenance continue to consume a low-energy, low-fat diet. *Journal of the American Dietetic Association* 98(4):408–13, 1998.

Shils, M.E., J.A. Olson, M. Shike, A.C. Ross. *Modern Nutrition in Health and Disease*, 9th ed. Baltimore, MD: Williams & Wilkins; 90–92, 1377–8, 1999.

Shoda, R., K. Matsueda, S. Yamato, N. Umeda. Therapeutic efficacy of N-3 polyunsaturated fatty acid in experimental Crohn's disease. *Journal of Gastroenterology* 30(Suppl 8):98–101, 1995.

Siddique, H., A.A. El-Zarok, Effect of olive oil and sunflower oil on serum lipids and myocardial triglycerides in rats. *Planta Medica* 10:46–49, 1980.

Signoret, J.L., A. Whiteley, F. Lhermitte. Influence of choline on amnesia in early Alzheimer's disease [letter]. *Lancet* 2:837, 1978 Oct 14.

Simons, L.A., et al. Chylomicrons and chylomicron remnants in coronary artery disease: a case-control study. *Atherosclerosis* 65(1–2):181–9, 1987.

Simopoulos, A.P. Essential fatty acids in health and chronic disease. *American Journal of Clinical Nutrition* 70(30 Suppl):560S–569S, 1999.

Simopoulos, A.P. Human requirement for N-3 polyunsaturated fatty acids. *Poult Science* 79(7):961–970, 2000.

Simpson, R.J., A. Hammacher, D.K. Smith, J.M. Matthews, L.D. Ward. Interleukin-6: structure-function relationships. *Protein Science* 6:929–55, 1997 May.

Simpson, D.S., A case study of the introduction of vegetable protein into school meals. *Journal of the American Oil Chemists' Society* 56(3):192–4, 1979.

Simpson, D.S. A case study of the introduction of vegetable protein into school meals. *Journal of the American Oil Chemists' Society* 56(3):192–4, 1979.

Sinclair, A.J., L. Johnson, K OD, R.T. Holman. Diets rich in lean beef increase arachidonic acid and long-chain omega 3 polyunsaturated fatty acid levels in plasma phospholipids. *Lipids* 29:337–43, 1994 May.

Siow, B.L. Cerebral ageing, neurotransmitters and therapeutic implications. *Singapore Medical Journal* 26:151–3, 1985 Apr.

Sirtori, C.R., E. Gatti, E. Tremoli, et al. Olive oil, corn oil, and n-3 fatty acids differently affect lipids, lipoproteins, platelets, and superoxide formation in type II hypercholesterolemia. *American Journal of Clinical Nutrition* 56:113–22, 1992 Jul.

Sirtori, C.R., E. Tremoli, E. Gatti, et al. Controlled evaluation of fat intake in the Mediterranean diet: comparative activities of olive oil and corn oil on plasma lipids and platelets in high-risk patients. *American Journal of Clinical Nutrition* 44:635–42, 1986 Nov.

Sitaram, N., H. Weingartner, E.D. Caine, J.C. Grillin Choline: Selective enhancement of serial learning and encoding of low imagery words in man. *Life Sciences* 22:1555–60, 1978 May 1.

Sitton, S.C. Role of craving for carbohydrates upon completion of a protein-sparing fast. *Psychological Reports* 69:683–6, 1991 Oct.

Skottova, N., et al. Lipoprotein lipase enhances removal of chylomicrons and chylomicron remnants by the perfused rat liver. *Journal of Lipid Research* 36(6):1334–44, 1995.

Skov, A.R., S. Toubro, et al. Changes in renal function during weight loss induced by high vs low-protein low-fat diets in overweight subjects. *International Journal of Obesity and Related Metabolic Disorders* 23(11):1170–7, 1999.

Skutches, C.L., O.E. Owen G.A. Reichard, Jr. Acetone and acetol inhibition of insulin-stimulated glucose oxidation in adipose tissue and isolated adipocytes. *Diabetes* 39:450–5, 1990 Apr.

Smith, U. Carbohydrates, fat, and insulin action. *American Journal of Clinical Nutrition* 59:686S–689S, 1994 Mar.

So F.V., N. Guthrie, A.E. Chambers, M. Moussa, K.K. Carroll, Inhibition of human breast cancer cell proliferation and delay of mammary tumorigenesis by flavonoids and citrus juices. *Nutrition and Cancer* 26:167–81, 1996.

Solomon, C.G., J.E. Manson, Obesity and mortality: a review of the epidemiologic data. *American Journal of Clinical Nutrition* 66:1044S–1050S, 1997 Oct.

Sonnichsen, A.C., W.O. Richter, et al. Benefit from hypocaloric diet in obese men depends on the extent of weight-loss regarding cholesterol, and on a simultaneous change in body fat distribution regarding insulin sensitivity and glucose tolerance. *Metabolism* 41(9):1035–9, 1992.

Soroka, N., et al. Comparison of a vegetable-based (soya) and an animal-based low-protein diet in predialysis chronic renal failure patients. *Nephron* 79(2):173–80, 1998.

Sossin, K., F. Gizis, L.F. Marquart, Sobal, J. Nutrition beliefs, attitudes, and resource use of high school wrestling coaches. *International Journal Sports Nutrition* 7:219–28, 1997 Sep.

Souba, W.W.R.J.S., D.W. Wilmore. Glutamine metabolism by the intestinal tract. *JPEN Journal of Parenteral and Enteral Nutrition* 9:608–17, 1985.

Southgate, J., E. Pitt, Trejdosiewicz, L.K. The effects of dietary fatty acids on the proliferation of normal human urothelial cells in vitro. *British Journal of Cancer* 74:728–34, 1996.

Soyland, E., J. Funk, G. Rajka, M. Sandberg, P. Thune, Ruistad L., et al. Effect of dietary supplementation with very-long chain n-3 fatty acids in patients with psoriasis. *New England Journal of Medicine* 1993;328(25):1812–1816, 1993.

Spagnoli, L.G., G. Palmieri, A. Mauriello, et al. Morphometric evidence of the trophic effect of L-carnitine on human skeletal muscle. *Nephron* 55:16–23, 1990.

Sparti, A., J. De. Effect of diet on glucose tolerance 36 hours after glycogen-depleting exercise. *European Journal of Clinical Nutrition* 46:377–85, 1992 Jun.

Spaulding, C.C., R.L. Walford, and R.B. Effros. Calorie restriction inhibits the age-related dysregulation of the cytokines TNF-alpha and IL-6 in C3B10RF1 mice. *Mechanisms of Ageing and Development* 93(1–3):87–94, 1997.

Spieth, L.E., et al. A low-glycemic index diet in the treatment of pediatric obesity. *Archives of Pediatrics and Adolescent Medicine* 154(9):947–51, 2000.

Spina, R.J., T. Ogawa, W.M. Kohrt, W.H.D. Martin, J.O. Holloszy, A.A. Ehsani. Differences in cardiovascular adaptations to endurance exercise training between older men and women. *Journal of Applied Physiology* 75:849–55, 1993 Aug.

Spindler, S.R. Calorie restriction enhances the expression of key metabolic enzymes associated with protein renewal during aging. *Annals of the New York Academy of Sciences* 928:296–304, 2001.

Spindler, S.R. Reversing the negative genomic effects of aging with short-term calorie restriction. *Scientific World Journal* 1(10):544–6, 2001.

Spriet, L.L., S.J. Peters. Influence of diet on the metabolic responses to exercise. *Proceedings of the Nutrition Society* 57:25–33, 1998 Feb.

Sprott, R.L. Diet and calorie restriction. *Experimental Gerontology* 32(1–2):205–14, 1997.

Stacpoole, P.W. Should NIDDM patients be on high-carbohydrate, low-fat diets? Affirmative [see comments]. *Hospital Practice* (Office Edition) 27 (Suppl 1):6–10; discussion 14–6, 1992 Feb.

Stallings, V.A., P.B. Pencharz. The effect of a high protein-low calorie diet on the energy expenditure of obese adolescents. *European Journal of Clinical Nutrition* 46:897–902, 1992 Dec.

Stallone, D.D., A.J. Stunkard, et al. Weight loss and body fat distribution: a feasibility study using computed tomography. *International Journal of Obesity* 15(11):775–80, 1991.

Stamler, J. The marked decline in coronary heart disease mortality rates in the United States, 1968–1981; summary of findings and possible explanations. *SBM Cardiology* 72:11–22, 1985.

Stampfer, M.J., F.B. Hu, J.E. Manson, E.B. Rimm, W.C. Willett. Primary prevention of coronary heart disease in women through diet and lifestyle. *New England Journal of Medicine* 343(1):16–22, 2000.

Stanko, R.T. ea. Plasma lipid concentrations in hyperlipidemic patients consuming a highfat diet supplemented with pyruvate for six weeks. *American Journal of Clinical Nutrition* 56:950–4, 1992.

Stanko, R.T. ea. Pyruvate supplementation of a low-cholesterol, low-fat diet: effects on plasma lipid concentrations and body composition in hyperlipidemic patients. *American Journal of Clinical Nutrition* 59:423–27, 1994.

Stanko, R.T., D.L. Tietze, J.E. Arch. Body composition, energy utilization, and nitrogen metabolism with a severely restricted diet supplemented with dihydroxyacetone and pyruvate. *American Journal of Clinical Nutrition* 55:771–6, 1992 Apr.

Stanko, R.T., D.L. Tietze, J.E. Arch. Body composition, energy utilization, and nitrogen metabolism with a 4.25-MJ/d low-energy diet supplemented with pyruvate. *American Journal of Clinical Nutrition* 56:630–5, 1992 Oct.

Starling, R.D., D.L. Costill, W.J. Fink. Relationships between muscle carnitine, age and oxidative status. *European Journal of Applied Physiology* 71:143–6, 1995.

Stein, O., et al. Calorie restriction in mice does not affect LDL reverse cholesterol transport in vivo. *Biochemical and Biophysical Research Communications* 308(1):29–34, 2003.

Stein, T.P., et al. Effect of nitrogen and calorie restriction on protein synthesis in the rat. *American Journal of Physiology* 230(5):1321–5, 1976.

Stemmermann, G.N. Patterns of disease among Japanese living in Hawaii. *Archives of Environmental Health* 20:266–73, 1970 Feb.

Stern, L., N. Iqbal, P. Seshadri, et al. The effects of low-carbohydrate versus conventional weight-loss diets in severely obese adults: one-year follow-up of a reandomized trial. *Annals of Internal Medicine* 140:778–85, 2004.

Stern, M.P., S.M. Haffner. Body fat distribution and hyperinsulinemia as risk factors for diabetes and cardiovascular disease. *Arteriosclerosis* 6:123–130, 1986.

Stern, J.S., et al. Calorie restriction in obesity: prevention of kidney disease in rodents. *Journal of Nutrition* 131(3):913S–7S, 2001.

Stevens, L.J., S.S. Zentall, M.L. Abate, T. Kuczek, J.R. Burgess. Omega-3 fatty acids in boys with behavior, learning and health problems. *Physiology and Behavior* 59(4/5):915–20, 1996.

Stevenson, R.W., D.R. Mitchell, G.K. Hendrick, R. Rainey, A.D. Cherrington, R.T. Frizzell. Lactate as substrate for glycogen resynthesis after exercise. *Journal of Applied Physiology* 62:2237–40, 1987 Jun.

Stoll, B.A. Breast cancer and the Western diet: role of fatty acids and antioxidant vitamins. *European Journal of Cancer* 34(12):1852–6, 1998.

Stoll, S., A. Rostock, R. Bartsch, E. Korn, A. Meichelböck, W.E. Mu. The potent free radical scavenger alpha-lipoic acid improves cognition in rodents. *Annals of the New York Academy of Sciences* 717:122–8, 1994 Jun 30.

St-Onge, M.P., P.J. Jones. Greater rise in fat oxidation with medium-chain triglyceride consumption relative to long-chain triglyceride is associated with lower initial body weight and greater loss of subcutaneous adipose tissue. *International Journal of Obesity and Related Metabolic Disorders* 27(12):1565–71, 2003.

Stookey, J.D. Energy density, energy intake and weight status in a large free-living sample of Chinese adults: exploring the underlying roles of fat, protein, carbohydrate, fiber and water intakes. *European Journal of Clinical Nutrition* 55(5):349–59, 2001.

Sudi, K.M., S. Gallistl, et al. The effects of changes in body mass and subcutaneous fat on the improvement in metabolic risk factors in obese children after short-term weight loss. *Metabolism* 50(11):1323–9, 2001.

Sugimoto, T., K. Nishiyama, F. Kuribayashi, K. Chihara. Serum levels of insulin-like growth factor (IGF) I, IGF-binding protein (IGFBP)-2, and IGFBP-3 in osteoporotic patients with and without spinal fractures. *Journal of Bone and Mineral Research* 12:1272–9, 1997 Aug.

Sun, D., et al. Effects of calorie restriction on polymicrobial peritonitis induced by ce-
cum ligation and puncture in young C57BL/6 mice. *Clinical and Diagnostic Laboratory Immunology* 8(5):1003–11, 2001.

Suzuki, Y.J., M. Tsuchiya, L. Packer. Lipoate prevents glucose-induced protein mod-
ifications. *Free Radical Research Communications* 17:211–7, 1992.

Taaffe, D.R., J.L. Thompson, et al. Recombinant human growth hormone, but not
insulin-like growth factor-I, enhances central fat loss in postmenopausal women
undergoing a diet and exercise program. *Hormone and Metabolic Research*
33(3):156–62, 2001.

Takada, Y., S. Aoe, M. Kumegawa. Whey protein stimulated the proliferation and differentiation of osteoblastic MC3T3-E1 cells. *Biochemical and Biophysical Research
Communications* 223:445–9, 1996 Jun 14.

Takada, Y., N. Kobayashi, K. Kato, H. Matsuyama, M. Yahiro, S. Aoe. Effects of whey
protein on calcium and bone metabolism in ovariectomized rats. *Journal of Nutritional Science and Vitaminology (Tokyo)* 43:199–210, 1997 Apr.

Takeda, S., P.G. Sim, D.F. Horrobin, T. Sanford, K.A. Chisholm, V. Simmons. Mechanism of lipid peroxidation in cancer cells in response to gamma-linolenic acid
(GLA) analyzed by GC-MS(I): Conjugated dienes with peroxyl (or hydroperoxyl)
groups and cell-killing effects. *Anticancer Research* 13:193–9, 1993.

Talmadge, R.J., H. Silverman. Glyconeogenic and glycogenic enzymes in chronically
active and normal skeletal muscle. *Journal of Applied Physiology* 71:182–91, 1991
Jul.

Talom, R.T., S.A. Judd, D.D. McIntosh, et al. High flaxeed (linseed) diet restores endothelial function in the mesenteric arterial bed of spontaneously hypertensive
rats. *Life Sciences* 16:1415–25, 1999.

Tanaka, H., T. Swensen. Impact of resistance training on endurance performance. A
new form of cross-training? *Sports Medicine* 25:191–200, 1998 Mar.

Tannenbaum, A. The dependence of tumor formation on the composition of the
calorie-restricted diet as well as on the degree of restriction. 1945. *Nutrition*
12(9):653–4, 1996.

Tapp, D.C., et al. Protein restriction or calorie restriction? A critical assessment of the
influence of selective calorie restriction on the progression of experimental renal
disease. *Seminars in Nephrology* 9(4):343–53, 1989.

Tataranni, P.A., D.E. Larson, S. Snitker, J.B. Young, J.P. Flatt, E. Ravussin. Effects of
glucocorticoids on energy metabolism and food intake in humans. *American Journal of Physiology* 271:E317–25, 1996 Aug.

Taylor, A., et al. Dietary calorie restriction in the Emory mouse: effects on lifespan, eye
lens cataract prevalence and progression, levels of ascorbate, glutathione, glucose,
and glycohemoglobin, tail collagen breaktime, DNA and RNA oxidation, skin in-
tegrity, fecundity, and cancer. *Mechanisms of Ageing and Development* 79(1):33–57,
1995.

Tepper, B.J., M.I. Friedman. Altered acceptability of and preference for sugar solu-
tions by diabetic rats is normalized by high-fat diet. *Appetite* 16:25–38, 1991
Feb.

Terpstra, A.H., A.C. Beynen, et al. The decrease in body fat in mice fed conjugated
linoleic acid is due to increases in energy expenditure and energy loss in the exc-
reta. *Journal of Nutrition* 132(5):940–5, 2002.

Terry, P., P. Lichtenstein, M. Feychting, A. Ahlbom, A. Wolk. Fatty fish consumption
and risk of prostate cancer. *Lancet* 357(9270):1764–6, 2001.

Tew, B.Y., X. Xu, H.I. Wang, P.A. Murphy, S. Hendrich. A diet high in wheat fiber decreases the bioavailability of soybean isoflavones in a single meal fed to women.
Journal of Nutrition 126:871–7, 1996.

The American Kidney Fund: American Kidney Fund Warns About Impact of High-
Protein Diets on Kidney Health: 25 April 2002.

The International Society for the Study of Fatty Acids and Lipids (ISSFAL). Recommendations for the essential fatty acid requirement for infant formulas (policy statement). Available at: http://www.issfal.org.uk/. Accessed January 17, 2001.

Thomas, E.L., A.E. Brynes, et al. Preferential loss of visceral fat following aerobic exercise, measured by magnetic resonance imaging. *Lipids* 35(7):767–76, 2000.

Thomson, W.A. Infant formulas and the use of vegetable protein. *Journal of the American Oil Chemists' Society* 56(3):386–8, 1979.

Tiggemann, M. Dietary restraint as a predictor of reported weight loss and affect. *Psychological Reports* 75:1679–82, 1994 Dec.

Tiikkainen, M., R. Bergholm, et al. Effects of identical weight loss on body composition and features of insulin resistance in obese women with high and low liver fat content. *Diabetes* 52(3):701–7, 2003.

Tiikkainen, M., R. Bergholm, et al. Effects of equal weight loss with orlistat and placebo on body fat and serum fatty acid composition and insulin resistance in obese women. *American Journal of Clinical Nutrition* 79(1):22–30, 2004.

Tillman, J.B., et al. Dietary calorie restriction in mice induces carbamyl phosphate synthetase I gene transcription tissue specifically. *Journal of Biological Chemistry* 271(7):3500–6, 1996.

Tisdale, M.J. Inhibition of lipolysis and muscle protein degradation by EPA in cancer cachexia. *Nutrition* 12:S31–3, 1996.

Toornvliet, A.C., H. Pijl, M. Frölich, R.G. Westerndorp, A.E. Meinders. Insulin and leptin concentrations in obese humans during long-term weight loss. *Netherlands Journal of Medicine* 51:96–102. 1997 Sep.

Torigoe, K., O. Numata, et al. Effect of weight loss on body fat distribution in obese children. *Acta Paediatrica Japonica* 39(1):28–33, 1997.

Toubro, S., A. Astrup. Randomised comparison of diets for maintaining obese subjects' weight after major weight loss: ad lib, low fat, high carbohydrate diet v fixed energy intake. *British Medical Journal* 314(7073):29–34, 1997.

Toussaint, O., et al. Approach of evolutionary theories of ageing, stress, senescence-like phenotypes, calorie restriction and hormesis from the view point of far-from-equilibrium thermodynamics. *Mechanisms of Ageing and Development* 123(8):937–46, 2002.

Trichopoulou, A., T. Costacou, C. Bamia, D. Trichopoulos. Adherence to a Mediterranean Diet and Survival in a Greek Population. *New England Journal of Medicine* 348:2599–2608, 2003.

Trichopoulou, A., K. Katsouyanni, S. Stuver, et al. Consumption of olive oil and specific food groups in relation to breast cancer risk in Greece [see comments]. *Journal of the National Cancer Institute* 87:110–6, 1995 Jan 18.

Trout, D., K.M. Behall. Prediction of glycemic index among high-sugar, low-starch foods. *International Journal of Food Sciences and Nutrition* 50(2):135–44, 1999.

Truswell, A.S., N. Choudhury. Monounsaturated oils do not all have the same effect on plasma cholesterol. *European Journal of Clinical Nutrition* 52:312–5, 1998 May.

Truswell, A.S. Food carbohydrates and plasma lipids—an update. *American Journal of Clinical Nutrition* 59:710S–8S, 1994 Mar.

Tsihlias, E.B., et al. Comparison of high- and low-glycemic-index breakfast cereals with monounsaturated fat in the long-term dietary management of type 2 diabetes. *American Journal of Clinical Nutrition* 72(2):439–49, 2000.

Tsujikawa T., J. Satoh, K. Uda, T. Ihara, T. Okamoto, Y. Araki, et al. Clinical importance of n-3 fatty acid-rich diet and nutritional education for the maintenance of remission in Crohn's disease. *Journal of Gastroenterology* 35(2):99–104, 2000.

Tuominen, J.A., P. Ebeling, H. Vuorinen-Markkola, VA. Koivisto. Post-marathon paradox in IDDM: unchanged insulin sensitivity in spite of glycogen depletion. *Diabetic Medicine* 14:301–8, 1997 Apr.

Tuominen, J.A., J.E. Peltonen, V.A. Koivisto. Blood flow, lipid oxidation, and muscle glycogen synthesis after glycogen depletion by strenuous exercise. *Medicine & Science in Sports & Exercise* 29:874–81, 1997 Jul.

Turcato, E., M. Zamboni, et al Interrelationships between weight loss, body fat distribution and sex hormones in pre- and postmenopausal obese women. *Journal of Internal Medicine* 241(5):363–72, 1997.

Tworoger, S.S., J. Chubak, et al. The effect of CYP19 and COMT polymorphisms on exercise-induced fat loss in postmenopausal women. *Obesity Research* 12(6):972–81, 2004.

Tyler, D.O., J.D. Allan, F.R. Alcozer. Weight loss methods used by African American and Euro-American women. *Research in Nursing and Health* 20:413–23, 1997 Oct.

Tzonou, A., C.C. Hsieh, A. Polychronopoulou, G. Kaprinis, N. Toupadaki. Diet and ovarian cancer: a case-control study in Greece. *International Journal of Cancer* 55:411–4, 1993.

Ullmann, D., W.E. Connor, L.F. Hatcher, S.L. Connor, D.P. Flavell. Will a high-carbohydrate, low-fat diet lower plasma lipids and lipoproteins without producing hypertriglyceridemia? *Arteriosclerosis, Thrombosis and Vascular Biology* 11:1059–67, 1991 Jul–Aug.

Urhausen, A., W. Kindermann. Blood ammonia and lactate concentrations during endurance exercise of differing intensities. *European Journal of Applied Physiology* 65:209–14, 1992.

Uribe, M., et al. Beneficial effect of vegetable protein diet supplemented with psyllium plantago in patients with hepatic encephalopathy and diabetes mellitus. *Gastroenterology* 88(4):901–7, 1985.

US Department of Agriculture, US Department of Health and Human Services. Nutrition and your health.

van Aggel-Leijssen, D.P., W.H. Saris, et al. Short-term effects of weight loss with or without low-intensity exercise training on fat metabolism in obese men. *American Journal of Clinical Nutrition* 73(3):523–31, 2001.

Van Aswegen, C.H., D.J. Du Plessis. Can linoleic acid and gamma-linolenic acid be important in cancer treatment? *Medical Hypotheses* 43:415–7, 1994.

Van de Stadt, K.D. Prostaglandins and leukotrienes in inflammation and allergy. *Netherlands Journal of Medicine* 25:22–9, 1982.

van der Kooy, K., R. Leenen, et al. Changes in fat-free mass in obese subjects after weight loss: a comparison of body composition measures. *International Journal of Obesity and Related Metabolic Disorders* 16(9):675–83, 1992.

van der Merwe, C.F., J. Booyens, H.E. Joubert, C.A. van der Merwe. The effect of gamma-linolenic acid, an in vitro cytostatic substance contained in evening primrose oil, on primary liver cancer. A double-blind placebo controlled trial. *Prostaglandins Leukotrienes and Essential Fatty Acids* 40:199–202, 1990.

Van Dokkum, W., et al. The effects of a high-animal- and a high-vegetable-protein diet on mineral balance and bowel function of young men. *British Journal of Nutrition* 56(2):341–8, 1986.

van Marthens, E. Alterations in the rate of fetal and placental development as a consequence of early maternal protein/calorie restriction. *Biology of the Neonate* 31(5–6):324–32, 1977.

Varnier, M., G.P. Leese J. Thompson, M.J. Rennie. Stimulatory effect of glutamine on glycogen accumulation in human skeletal muscle. *American Journal of Physiology* 269:E309–15, 1995 Aug.

Vazquez, J.A., U. Kazi, N. Madani. Protein metabolism during weight reduction with very-low-energy diets: evaluation of the independent effects of protein and carbohydrate on protein sparing. *American Journal of Clinical Nutrition* 62:93–103, 1995 Jul.

Verdich, C., S. Toubro, et al. Leptin levels are associated with fat oxidation and dietary-induced weight loss in obesity. *Obesity Research* 9(8):452–61, 2001.

Vergauwen, L., E.A. Richter, P. Hespel. Adenosine exerts a glycogen-sparing action in contracting rat skeletal muscle. *American Journal of Physiology* 272:E762–8, 1997 May.

Vicario, I.M., D. Malkova, E.K. Lund, I.T. Johnson. Olive oil supplementation in healthy adults: effects in cell membrane fatty acid composition and platelet function. *Annals of Nutrition and Metabolism* 42:160–9, 1998.

Vigilante, K.C. and M.M. Flynn. From Atkins to Zone: the truth about high-fat, high-protein diets for weight loss. *Medical Health Rhode Island* 83(11):337–8, 2000.

Villar-Palasí, C., J.J. Guinovart. The role of glucose 6-phosphate in the control of glycogen synthase. *FASEB Journal* 11:544–58, 1997 Jun.

Visioli, F., G. Bellomo, C. Galli. Free radical-scavenging properties of olive oil polyphenols. *Biochemical and Biophysical Research Communications* 247:60–4, 1998 Jun 9.

Visioli, F., G. Bellomo, G. Montedoro, C. Galli. Low density lipoprotein oxidation is inhibited in vitro by olive oil constituents. *Atherosclerosis* 117:25–32, 1995 Sep.

Vognild, E., E.O. Elvevoll, J. Brox, et al. Effects of dietary marine oils and olive oil on fatty acid composition, platelet membrane fluidity, platelet responses, and serum lipids in healthy humans. *Lipids* 33:427–36, 1998 Apr.

von Schacky, C., P. Angere, W. Kothny, K. Theisen, H. Mudra. The effect of dietary omega-3 fatty acids on coronary atherosclerosis: a randomized, double-blind, placebo-controlled trial. *Annals of Internal Medicine* 130:554–62, 1999.

Voskuil, D.W., E.J.M. Feskens, M.B. Katan, D. Kromhout. Intake and sources of alpha-linolenic acid in Dutch elderly men. *European Journal of Clinical Nutrition* 50:784–7, 1996.

Vukovich, M.D., R.L. Sharp, L.D. Kesl, D.L. Schaulis, D.S. King. Effects of a low-dose amino acid supplement on adaptations to cycling training in untrained individuals. *International Journal of Sport Nutrition* 7:298–309, 1997 Dec.

Wabitsch, M., H. Hauner, et al. The relationship between body fat distribution and weight loss in obese adolescent girls. *International Journal of Obesity and Related Metabolic Disorders* 16(11):905–11, 1992.

Wadden, T.A., R.V. Considine, G.D. Foster, D.A. Anderson, D.B. Sarwer, J.S. Caro. Short- and long-term changes in serum leptin dieting obese women: effects of caloric restriction and weight loss. *Journal of Clinical Endocrinology and Metabolism* 83:214–8, 1998 Jan.

Wainfan, E., L.A. Poirier. Methyl groups in carcinogenesis: effects on DNA methylation and gene expression. *Cancer Research* 52:2071s–7s, 1992.

Walford, R.L., S.R. Spindler. The response to calorie restriction in mammals shows features also common to hibernation: a cross-adaptation hypothesis. *Journal of Gerontology Series A: Biological Sciences and Medical Sciences* 52(4):B179–83, 1997.

Walford, R.L., et al. Calorie restriction in biosphere 2: alterations in physiologic, hematologic, hormonal, and biochemical parameters in humans restricted for a 2-year period. *Journals of Gerontology Series A: Biological Sciences and Medical Sciences* 57(6):B211–24, 2002.

Walford, R.L., et al. Physiologic changes in humans subjected to severe, selective calorie restriction for two years in biosphere 2: health, aging, and toxicological perspectives. *Journal of Toxicology Science* 52(2 Suppl):61–5, 1999.

Wang, T.T., N. Sathyamoorthy, J.M. Phang. Molecular effects of genistein on estrogen receptor mediated pathways. *Carcinogenesis* 17:271–5, 1996.

Wang, J., B. Laferrere, et al. Regional subcutaneous-fat loss induced by caloric restriction in obese women. *Obesity Research* 10(9):885–90, 2002.

Warren, J.M., C.J. Henry, and V. Simonite. Low glycemic index breakfasts and reduced food intake in preadolescent children. *Pediatrics* 112(5):e414.

Warwick, Z.S. Schiffman, S.S. J.J. Anderson. Relationship of dietary fat content to food preferences in young rats. *Physiology and Behavior* 48:581–6, 1990 Nov.

Watters, M.R. Organic neurotoxins in seafoods. *Clinical Neurology and Neurosurgery* 97:119–24, 1995 May.

Webb, P. and T. Abrams Loss of fat stores and reduction in sedentary energy expenditure from undereating. *Hum Nutr Clin Nutr* 37(4):271–82, 1983.

Weber, P. Management of osteoporosis: is there a role for vitamin K? *International Journal for Vitamin and Nutrition Research* 67:350–6, 1997.

Weber, P.C. The modification of the arachidonic acid cascade by n-3 fatty acids. *Advanced Prostaglandin Thromboxane Leukotriene Research* 20:232–40, 1990.

Weck, M., S. Fischer, et al. Loss of fat, water, and protein during very low calorie diets and complete starvation. *Klinische Wochenschrift* 65(23):1142–50, 1987.

Weder, A.B., et al. The antihypertensive effect of calorie restriction in obese adolescents: dissociation of effects on erythrocyte countertransport and cotransport. *Journal of Hypertension* 2(5):507–14, 1984.

Wee, S.L., et al. Influence of high and low glycemic index meals on endurance running capacity. *Medicine & Science of Sports & Exercise* 31(3):393–9, 1999.

Weed, J.L., et al. Activity measures in rhesus monkeys on long-term calorie restriction. *Physiology and Behavior* 62(1):97–103, 1997.

Weigle, D.S., D.E. Cummings, et al. Roles of leptin and ghrelin in the loss of body weight caused by a low fat, high carbohydrate diet. *Journal of Clinical Endocrinology & Metabolism* 88(4):1577–86, 2003.

Weinsier, R.L., G.R. Hunter, et al. Body fat distribution in white and black women: different patterns of intraabdominal and subcutaneous abdominal adipose tissue utilization with weight loss. *American Journal of Clinical Nutrition* 74(5):631–6, 2001.

Weintraub, M.S., Y. Rosen, R. Otto, S. Eisenberg, J.L. Breslow. Physical exercise conditioning in the absence of weight loss reduces fasting and postprandial triglyceride-rich lipoprotein levels. *Circulation* 79:1007–14, 1989 May.

Weissmann, G. Pathways of arachidonate oxidation to prostaglandins and leukotrienes. *Seminars in Arthritis and Rheumitism* 13:123–9, 1983 Aug.

Wenzel, S.E. Arachidonic acid metabolities: mediators of inflammation in asthma. *Pharmacotherapy* 17:3S–12S, 1997 Jan–Feb.

West, D.W., M.L. Slattery, L.M. Robison, T.K. French, A.W. Mahoney. Adult dietary intake and prostate cancer risk in Utah: a case-control study with special emphasis on aggressive tumors. *Cancer Causes and Control* 2:85–94, 1991.

Westman, E.C., W.S. Yancy, J.S. Edman, K.F. Tomlin, C.E. Perkins. Effect of 6-month adherence to a very low carbohydrate diet program. *American Journal of Medicine* 113:30–6, 2002.

Westphal, S., et al. Postprandial chylomicrons and VLDLs in severe hypertriacylglycerolemia are lowered more effectively than are chylomicron remnants after treatment with n-3 fatty acids. *American Journal of Clinical Nutrition* 71(4):914–20, 2000.

Wetter, T.J., et al. Effect of calorie restriction on in vivo glucose metabolism by individual tissues in rats. Am J Physiol *American Journal of Physiology* 276(4 Pt 1):E728–38, 1999.

Weyman-Daum, M., et al. Glycemic response in children with insulin-dependent diabetes mellitus after high- or low-glycemic-index breakfast. *American Journal of Clinical Nutrition* 46(5):798–803, 1987.

Wigmore, S.J., J.A. Ross, J.S. Falconer, et al. The effect of polyunsaturated fatty acids on the progress of cachexia in patients with pancreatic cancer. *Nutrition* 12:S27–30, 1996.

Willett, W.C. Is dietary fat a major determinant of body fat? *American Journal of Clinical Nutrition* 67(suppl):556S–62S, 1998.

Willett, W.C. Reduced-carbohydrate diets: No role in weight management? *Annals of Internal Medicine* 140:836–7, 2004.

Williams, K.I., G.A. Higgs, Eicosanoids and inflammation. *Journal of Pathology* 156:101–10, 1988 Oct.

Williams, P.T. Health effects resulting from exercise versus those from body fat loss. *Medicine & Science in Sports & Exercise* 33(6 Suppl): S611–21; discussion S640–1, 2001.

Williams, P.T., et al. Effects of low-fat diet, calorie restriction, and running on lipoprotein subfraction concentrations in moderately overweight men. *Metabolism* 43(5):655–63, 1994.

Williamson, J.R., P.I. Hoffmann, W.M. Kohrt, R.I. Spina, A.R. Coggan, O. Holloszy.

Endurance exercise training decreases capillary basement membrane width in older nondiabetic and diabetic adults. *Journal of Applied Physiology* 80:747–53, 1996 Mar.

Winblad, B., J. Hardy, L Ba, L.G. Nilsson. Memory function and brain biochemistry in normal aging and in senile dementia. *Annals of the New York Academy of Sciences* 444:255–68, 1985.

Wing, R.R., J.A. Vazquez, C.M. Ryan, Cognitive effects of ketogenic weight-reducing diets. *International Journal of Obesity and Related Metabolic Disorders* 19:811–6, 1995 Nov.

Winter, B.K., G. Fiskum, and L.L. Gallo. Effects of L-carnitine on serum triglyceride and cytokine levels in rat models of cachexia and septic shock. *British Journal of Cancer* 72(5):1173–9, 1995.

Wittert, G.A., H. Turnbull, et al. Leptin prevents obesity induced by a high-fat diet after diet-induced weight loss in the marsupial S. crassicaudata. *Am J Physiol Regul Integr Comp Physiol* 286(4):R734–9, 2004.

Wolever, T.M., et al. Beneficial effect of low-glycemic index diet in overweight NIDDM subjects. *Diabetes Care* 15(4):562–4, 1992.

Wolever, T.M., et al. Second-meal effect: low-glycemic-index foods eaten at dinner improve subsequent breakfast glycemic response. *American Journal of Clinical Nutrition* 48(4):1041–7, 1988.

Wolz, P., J. Krieglstein. Neuroprotective effects of alpha-lipoic acid and its enantiomers demonstrated in rodent models of focal cerebral ischemia. *Neuropharmacology* 35:369–75, 1996 Mar.

Wolzak, A., L.G. Elias, and R. Bressani. Protein quality of vegetable proteins as determined by traditional biological methods and rapid chemical assays. *Journal of Agricultural and Food Chemistry* 29(5):1063–8, 1981.

Wong, C.W., A.H. Liu, G.O. Regester, G.L. Francis, D.L. Watson. Influence of whey and purified whey proteins on neutrophil functions in sheep. *Journal of Dairy Research* 64:281–8, 1997 May.

Wong, C.W., D.L. Watson, Immunomodulatory effects of dietary whey proteins in mice. *Journal of Dairy Research* 62:359–68, 1995 May.

Wood, P.D., R.B. Terry, W.L. Haskell. Metabolism of substrates: diet, lipoprotein metabolism, and exercise. *Federal Proceedings* 44:358–63, 1985 Feb.

Woollett, L.A., D.M. Kearney, Spady DK. Diet modification alters plasma HDL cholesterol concentrations but not the transport of HDL cholesteryl esters to the liver in the hamster. *Journal of Lipid Research* 38:2289–302, 1997.

Wright, P.D., Rich., A.J. Ketosis and nitrogen excretion in undernourished surgical patients. *Acta Chirurgica Scandinavia* (Suppl) 507:41–8, 1981.

Wroble, R.R, D.P. Moxley. Weight loss patterns and success rates in high school wrestlers. *Medicine & Science in Sports & Exercise* 30:625–8, 1998 Apr.

Wu, J., X. Wang, et al. Combined intervention of soy isoflavone and moderate exercise prevents body fat elevation and bone loss in ovariectomized mice. *Metabolism* 53(7):942–8, 2004.

Wurtman, R.J. Nutrients that modify brain function. *Scientific American* 246:50–9, 1982 Apr.

Wuster, C., W.E. Blum, S. Schlemilch, M.B. Ranke, R. Ziegler. Decreased serum levels of insulin-like growth factors and IGF binding protein 3 in osteoporosis. *Journal of Internal Medicine* 234:249–55, 1993 Sep.

Wyatt, H.R., et al. Long term weight loss and very low-carbohydrate diets in the National Weight Control Registry. *Obesity Research* 8 (Suppl 1):87S., 2000.

Wyatt, H.R., et al. Long-term weight loss and breakfast in subjects in the National Weight Control Registry. *Obesity Research* 10(2):78–82, 2002.

Wymelbeke, W.H.A., J. Louis-Sylvestre, et al. Influence of medium-chain and long-chain triacylglycerols on the control of food intake in men. *American Journal of Clinical Nutrition* 68:226–34, 1998.

Wynn, V., R.R. Abraham, et al. Method for estimating rate of fat loss during treatment of obesity by calorie restriction. *Lancet* 1(8427):482–6, 1985.

Xu, X., K.S. Harris, H.J. Wang, P.A. Murphy, S. Hendrich. Bioavailability of soybean isoflavones depends upon gut microflora in women. *Journal of Nutrition*, 125:2307–15, 1995.

Xu, N., et al. Uptake of radiolabeled and colloidal gold-labeled chyle chylomicrons and chylomicron remnants by rat platelets in vitro. *Arteriosclerosis, Thrombosis and Vascular Biology* 15(7):972–81, 1995.

Xu, S., et al. Calorie restriction can increase thymocyte apoptosis through Bcl-2 and Fas pathway. *Chinese Medical Sciences Journal* 15(4):226, 2000.

Schutz, Y., J.P. Flatt, and E. JequierAm. Failure of dietary fat intake to promote fat oxidation: a factor favoring the development of obesity. *Journal of Clinical Nutrition* 50:307–14, 1989 Aug.

Yam, D., A. Eliraz, E.M. Berry. Diet and disease—the Israeli paradox: possible dangers of a high omega-6 polyunsaturated fatty acid diet. *Journal of the Israeli Medical Society* 32(11):1134–43, 1996.

Yamada, T., et al. Comparison of effects of vegetable protein diet and animal protein diet on the initiation of anemia during vigorous physical training (sports anemia) in dogs and rats. *Journal of Nutritional Science and Vitaminology (Tokyo)* 33(2):129–49, 1987.

Yan, Z., M.K. Spencer, A. Katz. Effect of low glycogen on glycogen synthase in human muscle during and after exercise. *Acta Physiologica Scandinavia* 145:345–52, 1992 Aug.

Yanagibori, R., Y. Suzuki, K. Kawakubo, Y. Makita, A. Gunji. Carbohydrate and lipid metabolism after 20 days of bed rest. *Acta Physiologica Scandinavia* (Suppl) 616:51–7, 1994.

Yancy, W.S., M.K. Olsen, J.R. Guyton, et al. A low-carbohydrate, ketogenic diet cersus a low-fat diet to treat obesity and hyerplipidemia. *Annals of Internal Medicine* 140:769–77, 2004.

Yang, M.-U. Composition of weight loss during short-term weight reduction. *Journal of Clinical Investigation* 58:722–30, 1976.

Yang, M.U., T.B. van Itallie. Composition of weight loss during short-term weight reduction. *Journal of Clinical Investigation* 55:722–30, 1976 Sep.

Yaqoob, P., J.A. Knapper, D.H. Webb, C.M. Williams, E.A. Newsholme, P.C. Calder. Effect of olive oil on immune function in middle-aged men. *American Journal of Clinical Nutrition* 67:129–35, 1998 Jan.

Yarrows, S.A. Weight loss through dehydration in amateur wrestling. *Journal of the American Dietetic Association* 88:491–3, 1988 Apr.

Yavelow, J., T.H. Finlay, A.R. Kennedy, W. Troll. Bowman-Birk soybean protease inhibitor as an anticarcinogen. *Cancer Research*, 43:2454s–9s, 1983.

Yehuda, S., S. Rabinovitz, R.I. Carasso, D.I. Mostofsky. Fatty acids and brain peptides. *Peptides* 19:407–19, 1998.

Yip, I., V.L. Go, et al. Insulin-leptin-visceral fat relation during weight loss. *Pancreas* 23(2):197–203, 2001.

York, E. Fiber/fat/carbohydrates in weight loss. *American Journal of Public Health* 77 (4):514–5, 1987.

Yoshida, T., N. Sakane, T. Umekawa, M. Kondo. Relationship between basal metabolic rate, thermogenic response to caffeine, and body weight loss following combined low calorie and exercise treatment in obese women. *International Journal of Obesity and Related Metabolic Disorders* 18:345–50, 1994 May.

Yoshida, K., et al. Calorie restriction reduces the incidence of myeloid leukemia induced by a single whole-body radiation in C3H/He mice. *Proceedings of the National Academy of Sciences USA* 94(6):2615–9, 1997.

Yoshida, K., et al. Radiation-induced myeloid leukemia in mice under calorie restriction. *Leukemia* 11 (Suppl 3) 410–2, 1997.

Yoshida, K., Y. Hirabayashi, and T. Inoue. Calorie restriction reduces the incidence of radiation-induced myeloid leukemia. *IARC Scientific Publications* 156:553–5, 2002.

Young, S.N. Behavioral effects of dietary neurotransmitter precursors:basic and clinical aspects. *Neuroscience and Biobehavioral Reviews* 20:313–23, 1996 Summer.

Young, V.R. Soy protein in relation to human protein and amino acid nutrition. *Journal of the American Dietetic Association* 91:828–35, 1991.

Young, P.C. et al. A pilot study to determine the feasibility of the low glycemic index diet as a treatment for overweight children in primary care practice. *Ambulatory Pediatrics* 4(1):28–33, 2004.

Zambón, D., J. Sabate, S. Munoz, et al. Substituting walnuts for monounsaturated fat improves the serum lipid profile of hypercholesterolemic men and women. *Annals of Internal Medicine* 132:538–46, 2000.

Zamboni, M., F. Armellini, et al. Effect of weight loss on regional body fat distribution in premenopausal women. *American Journal of Clinical Nutrition* 58(1):29–34, 1993.

Zamboni, M., R. Facchinetti, et al. Effects of visceral fat and weight loss on lipoprotein(a) concentration in subjects with obesity. *Obesity Research* 5(4):332–7, 1997.

Zemel, M.B., W. Thompson, et al. Calcium and dairy acceleration of weight and fat loss during energy restriction in obese adults. *Obesity Research* 12(4):582–90, 2004.

Zhu, P., et al. Effect of dietary calorie and fat restriction on mammary tumor growth and hepatic as well as tumor glutathione in rats. *Cancer Letters* 57(2):145–52, 1991.

Zou, B., M. Suwa, et al. Decreased serum leptin and muscle oxidative enzyme activity with a dietary loss of intra-abdominal fat in rats. *Journal of Nutritional Biochemistry* 15(1):24–9, 2004.

Zureik, M., P. Ducimetière, J.M. Warnet, G. Orssaud. Fatty acid proportions in cholesterol esters and risk of premature death from cancer in middle aged French men. *British Medical Journal* 311:1251–4, 1995.

ACKNOWLEDGEMENTS

I am grateful to the following people who helped during the writing of this book: Jo Lynn Valoff for her research assistance and suggestions; Tracy Bernstein for her editing and stewardship; Kristin Massey for helping to create the delicious *Eat to Win* Power Meals recipes; and my parents, for everything else.

ABOUT THE AUTHOR

Robert Haas, MS, graduated cum laude from Florida State University with a master's degree in nutrition and food science. He is a world-renowned sports nutritionist and is a feature writer and columnist for various health and fitness publications, including *Fitness Rx for Women* and *Fitness Rx for Men*.